1990 YEAR BOOK OF ORTHOPEDICS®

The 1990 Year Book® Series

Year Book of Anesthesia®: Drs. Miller, Kirby, Ostheimer, Roizen, and Stoelting

Year Book of Cardiology®: Drs. Schlant, Collins, Engle, Frye, Kaplan, and O'Rourke

Year Book of Critical Care Medicine®: Drs. Rogers and Parrillo

Year Book of Dentistry®: Drs. Meskin, Ackerman, Kennedy, Leinfelder, Matukas, and Rovin

Year Book of Dermatology®: Drs. Sober and Fitzpatrick

Year Book of Diagnostic Radiology®: Drs. Bragg, Hendee, Keats, Kirkpatrick, Miller, Osborn, and Thompson

Year Book of Digestive Diseases®: Drs. Greenberger and Moody

Year Book of Drug Therapy®: Drs. Hollister and Lasagna

Year Book of Emergency Medicine®: Dr. Wagner

Year Book of Endocrinology®: Drs. Bagdade, Braverman, Halter, Horton, Kannan, Korenman, Molitch, Morley, Odell, Rogol, Ryan, and Sherwin

Year Book of Family Practice®: Drs. Rakel, Avant, Driscoll, Prichard, and Smith

Year Book of Geriatrics and Gerontology®: Drs. Beck, Abrass, Burton, Cummings, Makinodan, and Small

Year Book of Hand Surgery®: Drs. Dobyns, Chase, and Amadio

Year Book of Hematology®: Drs. Spivak, Bell, Ness, Quesenberry, and Wiernik

Year Book of Infectious Diseases®: Drs. Wolff, Barza, Keusch, Klempner, and Snydman

Year Book of Infertility: Drs. Mishell, Paulsen, and Lobo

Year Book of Medicine®: Drs. Rogers, Des Prez, Cline, Braunwald, Greenberger, Wilson, Epstein, and Malawista

Year Book of Neonatal and Perinatal Medicine: Drs. Klaus and Fanaroff

Year Book of Neurology and Neurosurgery®: Drs. Currier and Crowell

Year Book of Nuclear Medicine®: Drs. Hoffer, Gore, Gottschalk, Sostman, Zaret, and Zubal

Year Book of Obstetrics and Gynecology®: Drs. Mishell, Kirschbaum, and Morrow

Year Book of Occupational and Environmental Medicine: Drs. Emmett, Brooks, Harris, and Schenker

Year Book of Oncology: Drs. Young, Longo, Ozols, Simone, Steele, and Weichselbaum

Year Book of Ophthalmology®: Drs. Laibson, Adams, Augsburger, Benson, Cohen, Eagle, Flanagan, Nelson, Reinecke, Sergott, and Wilson

Year Book of Orthopedics®: Drs. Sledge, Poss, Cofield, Frymoyer, Griffin, Hansen, Johnson, Springfield, and Weiland

Year Book of Otolaryngology–Head and Neck Surgery®: Drs. Bailey and Paparella

Year Book of Pathology and Clinical Pathology®: Drs. Brinkhous, Dalldorf, Grisham, Langdell, and McLendon

Year Book of Pediatrics®: Drs. Oski and Stockman

Year Book of Plastic, Reconstructive, and Aesthetic Surgery: Drs. Miller, Bennett, Haynes, Hoehn, McKinney, and Whitaker

Year Book of Podiatric Medicine and Surgery®: Dr. Jay

Year Book of Psychiatry and Applied Mental Health®: Drs. Talbott, Frances, Frances, Freedman, Meltzer, Schowalter, and Yudofsky

Year Book of Pulmonary Disease®: Drs. Green, Loughlin, Michael, Mulshine, Peters, Terry, Tockman, and Wise

Year Book of Speech, Language, and Hearing: Drs. Bernthal, Hall, and Tomblin

Year Book of Sports Medicine®: Drs. Shephard, Eichner, Sutton, and Torg, Col. Anderson, and Mr. George

Year Book of Surgery®: Drs. Schwartz, Jonasson, Peacock, Shires, Spencer, and Thompson

Year Book of Urology®: Drs. Gillenwater and Howards

Year Book of Vascular Surgery®: Drs. Bergan and Yao

Editor
Clement B. Sledge, M.D.
Chairman, Department of Orthopaedic Surgery, Brigham and Women's Hospital, Professor of Orthopaedic Surgery, Harvard Medical School, Boston

Co-Editor
Robert Poss, M.D.
Associate Professor of Orthopaedic Surgery, Harvard Medical School; Orthopaedic Surgeon, Brigham and Women's Hospital, Boston

Associate Editors
Robert H. Cofield, M.D.
Professor of Orthopedic Surgery, Mayo Medical School; Consultant, Department of Orthopedics, Mayo Clinic, Rochester

John W. Frymoyer, M.D.
Professor of Orthopedic Surgery, University of Vermont; Director, McClure Musculoskeletal Research Center, Burlington

Paul P. Griffin, M.D.
Professor of Orthopedic Surgery, Medical University of South Carolina, Charleston

Sigvard T. Hansen, Jr., M.D.
Orthopedist-in-Chief, Department of Orthopedics, Harborview Medical Center; Professor of Orthopaedics, University of Washington School of Medicine, Seattle

Kenneth A. Johnson, M.D.
Professor of Orthopedic Surgery, Mayo Clinic Scottsdale; Past President, American Orthopaedic Foot and Ankle Society

Dempsey S. Springfield, M.D.
Associate Professor of Orthopaedic Surgery, Harvard Medical School; Visiting Orthopaedic Surgeon, Massachusetts General Hospital, Boston

Andrew J. Weiland, M.D.
Surgeon in Chief, Hospital for Special Surgery, New York; Professor of Surgery (Orthopedics and Plastic), Cornell University Medical College

Assistant Editor to Dr. Johnson
David A. Friscia, M.D.
Fellow in Foot and Ankle Surgery, Mayo Clinic Scottsdale

The Year Book of ORTHOPEDICS®

1990

Editor
Clement B. Sledge, M.D.

Co-Editor
Robert Poss, M.D.

Associate Editors
Robert H. Cofield, M.D.
John W. Frymoyer, M.D.
Paul P. Griffin, M.D.
Sigvard T. Hansen, Jr., M.D.
Kenneth A. Johnson, M.D.
Dempsey S. Springfield, M.D.
Andrew J. Weiland, M.D.

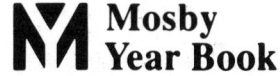
Mosby
Year Book

St. Louis   Baltimore   Boston   Chicago   London   Philadelphia   Sydney   Toronto

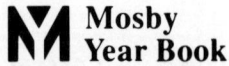
Mosby
Year Book
Dedicated to Publishing Excellence

Editor-in-Chief, Year Book Publishing: Nancy Gorham
Sponsoring Editor: Nancy G. Puckett
Manager, Medical Information Services: Edith M. Podrazik
Senior Medical Information Specialist: Terri Strorigl
Assistant Director, Manuscript Services: Frances M. Perveiler
Assistant Managing Editor, Year Book Editing Services: Wayne Larsen
Production Coordinator: Max F. Perez
Proofroom Supervisor: Barbara M. Kelly

Copyright © November 1990 by Mosby–Year Book Medical Publishers, Inc.
A Year Book Medical Publishers imprint of Mosby-Year Book, Inc.

Mosby–Year Book, Inc.
11830 Westline Industrial Drive
St. Louis, MO 63146

All rights reserved. No part of this publication may be reproduced, stored in a retrieval system, or transmitted, in any form or by any means, electronic, mechanical, photocopying, recording, or otherwise, without prior written permission from the publisher.
Printed in the United States of America.

Permission to photocopy or reproduce solely for internal or personal use is permitted for libraries or other users registered with the Copyright Clearance Center, provided that the base fee of $4.00 per chapter plus $.10 per page is paid directly to the Copyright Clearance Center, 21 Congress Street, Salem, MA 01970. This consent does not extend to other kinds of copying, such as copying for general distribution, for advertising or promotional purposes, for creating new collected works, or for resale.

Editorial Office:
Mosby–Year Book, Inc.
200 North LaSalle St.
Chicago, IL 60601

International Standard Serial Number: 0276-1092
International Standard Book Number: 0-8151-1894-5

Table of Contents

The material in this volume represents literature reviewed through January 1990.

JOURNALS REPRESENTED ix
PUBLISHER'S PREFACE xi
INTRODUCTION xiii

1. **Pediatrics,** *edited by* PAUL P. GRIFFIN, M.D.. 1

    Introduction 1
    PEDIATRIC HIP 1
    SPINE 15
    FOOT 24
    LIMB LENGTHENING 36
    INFECTION 40
    TRAUMA 42

2. **Trauma,** *edited by* SIGVARD T. HANSEN, JR., M.D. 49

    Introduction 49
    COLLES' FRACTURES 49
    FRACTURE CARE 59
    TRAUMATOLOGY 67
    STIMULATION OF THE HEALING RESPONSE 78
    COMPLICATIONS AND THEIR MANAGEMENT 83
    AMPUTATION 89
    IMAGING 93
    MISCELLANEOUS 95

3. **Shoulder, Elbow, and Forearm,** *edited by* ROBERT H. COFIELD, M.D. . . . 97

    Introduction 98
    SHOULDER 98
        Trauma and Related Conditions 98
        Rotator Cuff and Related Syndromes 113
        Prosthetic Arthroplasty and Arthrodesis 124
    ELBOW AND FOREARM 128
        Elbow Trauma 128
        Prosthetic Arthroplasty and Other Reconstructive Procedures. . . 132
        Forearm Trauma 138

4. **Adult Reconstruction,** *edited by* ROBERT POSS, M.D. AND CLEMENT B.
   SLEDGE, M.D.. 141

    Introduction 141
    GENERAL 142
    TOTAL HIP RECONSTRUCTION 163
    LIGAMENTS AND MENISCAL INJURIES 184
    KNEE PAIN 189

CARTILAGE DAMAGE 190
MAGNETIC RESONANCE IMAGING. 196
VASCULAR DAMAGE TRAUMA 201
COMPARTMENT SYNDROME 203
OSTEOTOMY. 205
INFECTION IN TOTAL JOINT REPLACEMENT 211
TOTAL KNEE RECONSTRUCTION 219
HIP FRACTURES 232
OSTEOPOROSIS 235

5. **Hand,** *edited by* ANDREW J. WEILAND, M.D. 241

   Introduction 241

6. **The Spine,** *edited by* JOHN W. FRYMOYER, M.D.. 265

   Introduction 265
   CERVICAL FRACTURES AND FUSION TECHNIQUES 266
   SPINAL STENOSIS—CAUSES AND TREATMENT 270
   THORACIC SPINAL FRACTURES—TYPE/COMPLICATIONS. 276
   BASIC DIAGNOSIS IN LOW BACK PAIN 287
   VERTEBRAL INFECTIONS 294
   SACROILIAC JOINTS 295
   SURGICAL TECHNIQUES AND RESULTS 296

7. **The Foot and Ankle,** *edited by* KENNETH A. JOHNSON, M.D., AND ASSISTANT EDITOR DAVID A. FRISCIA, M.D. 315

   Introduction 315
   PROBLEMS OF THE FOREFOOT 315
   TRAUMA AND SEQUELAE 325
   PEDIATRIC 338
   MISCELLANEOUS 341

8. **Musculoskeletal Neoplasia,** *edited by* DEMPSEY S. SPRINGFIELD, M.D. . . . 345

   Introduction 345
   METASTATIC CARCINOMA. 346
   ASSESSMENT AND PROGNOSIS OF MUSCULOSKELETAL TUMORS 352
   MISCELLANEOUS BONE LESIONS 359

Subject Index 371
Author Index 389

Journals Represented

Mosby–Year Book subscribes to and surveys nearly 850 U.S. and foreign medical and allied health journals. From these journals, the Editors select the articles to be abstracted. Journals represented in this YEAR BOOK are listed below.

Acta Chirurgica Scandinavica
Acta Dermato-Venereologica
Acta Orthopaedica Scandinavica
Acta Radiologica
American Journal of Clinical Nutrition
American Journal of Epidemiology
American Journal of Neuroradiology
American Journal of Physical Medicine & Rehabilitation
American Journal of Roentgenology
American Journal of Sports Medicine
American Surgeon
Annales de Chirurgie de la Main
Annals of Rheumatic Diseases
Annals of the Royal College of Surgeons of England
Archives of Internal Medicine
Archives of Orthopedic and Traumatic Surgery
Archives of Physical Medicine and Rehabilitation
Arthritis and Rheumatism
Cancer
Clinical Treatment Reviews
Clinical Orthopaedics and Related Research
Developmental Medicine and Child Neurology
Diabetic Medicine
Foot and Ankle
French Journal of Orthopedic Surgery
Human Pathology
Injury
International Journal of Radiation, Oncology, Biology, and Physics
Italian Journal of Orthopedics and Traumatology
Journal of Arthroplasty
Journal of Bone and Joint Surgery (American volume)
Journal of Bone and Joint Surgery (British volume)
Journal of Clinical Microbiology
Journal of Clinical Oncology
Journal of Computer Assisted Tomography
Journal of Gerontology
Journal of Hand Surgery (American)
Journal of Hand Surgery (British)
Journal of Neurology, Neurosurgery and Psychiatry
Journal of Orthopaedic Research
Journal of Orthopedic Surgical Techniques
Journal of Orthopedic Trauma
Journal of Pediatric Orthopedics
Journal of Trauma
Journal of the National Cancer Institute
Neurology
Neurosurgery
New England Journal of Medicine

Orthopaedic Review
Orthopedics
Pain
Plastic and Reconstructive Surgery
Radiology
Radiotherapy and Oncology
Scandinavian Journal of Rheumatology
Skeletal Radiology
Southern Medical Journal
Spine

STANDARD ABBREVIATIONS

The following terms are abbreviated in this edition: acquired immunodeficiency syndrome (AIDS), the central nervous system (CNS), cerebrospinal fluid (CSF), computed tomography (CT), electrocardiography (ECG), and human immunodeficiency virus (HIV).

Publisher's Preface

We welcome Andrew J. Weiland, M.D., as an Editor of the YEAR BOOK OF ORTHOPEDICS. Doctor Weiland is Surgeon-in-Chief at the Hospital for Special Surgery, New York, and Professor of Surgery (Orthopedics and Plastic), Cornell University Medical College. He selected and commented on material related to hand surgery.

Introduction

This edition of the YEAR BOOK OF ORTHOPEDICS is the second effort of a new editorial team. The only change has been that Andrew Weiland, M.D., has replaced Richard Gelberman, M.D., as the Associate Editor for Hand Surgery.

The rapid pace of development, change, and technical innovation in orthopedic surgery continues to produce a large volume of exciting literature. The Editors have attempted to provide a good cross section of that literature, selecting papers that confirm earlier concepts or verify operative procedures with long-term follow-ups or point out exciting new concepts and procedures. In addition, we have tried to include significant examples of laboratory research when we believe that research soon will have application in clinical management.

Each chapter begins with an introduction by an Associate Editor that outlines the interesting and innovative areas of a subject. We believe these introductory comments, in addition to the comments after each included paper, are useful. We recognize, however, that they represent the bias of the editors. The usefulness of such editorial comments is determined finally by the reader; I invite any comments about the organization of the YEAR BOOK OF ORTHOPEDICS so that we can make it a more useful adjunct to your effort to stay abreast of the current literature.

Clement B. Sledge, M.D.

1 Pediatrics

Introduction

The pediatric orthopedic literature for the past year reflects the continued interest in and ambiguities of surgical treatment of clubfoot. Whose operative procedure is best, and at what age is the surgical result more likely to be better? Opinions about these problems are expressed in the abstracts to follow, but answers are far from clearly being determined.

For years we have seen post-spinal fusion progression of scoliosis in the presence of a solid fusion. This phenomenon has been explained by Dubousset. He has shown increasing rotation and change in the sagittal and coronal deformities by growth of the vertebral bodies with the posterior spine tethered by a solid fusion. In the young patient, fusion anteriorly and posteriorly possibly will be the most effective treatment if surgery cannot be delayed safely.

The treatment of spondylolisthesis is still a controversy. Should the displacement be reduced or fused in situ? One good study in our current series shows excellent results for severe spondylolisthesis by fusion in situ. It also addresses the problem of cosmesis. To date, reduction has the possibility of nerve root injury. The answers are still evasive.

Congenital hip or developmental hip dysplasia and the problems associated with diagnosis and treatment were subjects of a number of articles. Ultrasonography continues to progress as an important tool for diagnosis and follow-up of infants and young children. Avascular necrosis is still the most serious complication in management. It is iatrogenic, but how to prevent it with certainty is not clear. Its occurrence affects development of the acetabulum as well as the capital epiphysis. Some of the sequelae to this problem and treatment are reported. Several abstracted articles deal with the overall management of hip dysplasia.

Paul P. Griffin, M.D.

Pediatric Hip

Ultrasound for Hip Assessment in the Newborn
Terjesen T, Bredland T, Berg V (Trondheim Univ Hosp, Trondheim, Norway)
J Bone Joint Surg [Br] 71-B:767–773, November 1989   1–1

Clinical screening of neonates for congenital hip dislocation is not completely reliable. Ultrasound is useful in the evaluation of hips in infants, but its place in screening neonates remains controversial. Graf's method of angle measurements by ultrasound is unreliable in infants aged less than 3 months because the reference points are often difficult to define. A technique based on the measurement of distances rather than angles for interpretation of neonatal pelvic ultrasound scans was described.

The hips of 1,000 consecutively seen newborns were examined clinically on the first day of life and with ultrasound scanning on the third day of life. There were 470 girls and 530 boys. Ultrasound assessment was based on measurements of the coverage of the femoral head by the bony acetabular roof. Measured were the distance from the acetabular floor to the lateral bony rim of the acetabular roof and the distance from the same point on the acetabular fossa to the lateral joint capsule. Both distances were measured along a line perpendicular to the long axis of

Bony Rim Percentage (BRP) at Birth, 2 Months, and 4 to 5 Months in Each Group, Including Only Affected Hips

Group	Characteristics	Number of patients	Number of hips	BRP Birth Mean	s.d.	2 months Mean	s.d.	4 to 5 months Mean	s.d.
I	Positive Ortolani, instability by ultrasound	7	8	35.9	9.2	55.0	4.8	57.7	6.8
II	False positive Ortolani, normal by ultrasound	9	11	56.9	5.3	59.9	6.3	60.5	6.0
III	Normal clinical findings, suspected pathology by ultrasound	29	33	43.9	3.6	52.9	6.6	57.1	6.4
IV	Family CDH	12	24	54.7	4.6	56.6	8.0	61.7	8.5
V	Breech position	12	24	56.2	5.5	60.8	5.3	62.6	3.8

(Courtesy of Terjesen T, Bredland T, Berg V: J Bone Joint Surg [Br] 71-B:767–773, November 1989.)

the transducer. The percentage of the femoral head covered by the osseous acetabular roof was called the bony rim percentage (BRP).

Infants with unstable hips or suggestive findings on clinical or ultrasound examination and all newborns in high-risk groups were followed up and reexamined. The infants were classified into 5 groups. Group I infants had unstable hips both clinically and by ultrasound examination, group II infants had a falsely positive Ortolani test with normal ultrasound, group III infants had normal clinical findings but suggestive findings on ultrasound evaluation, group IV infants had family history of congenital hip dislocation, and group V infants were delivered breech-first.

The mean BRP was 55.3% for girls and 57.2% for boys. The difference was statistically significant. Seven infants (0.7%), all girls, had clinical instability confirmed with ultrasound. The mean BRP was 35.9%, and all hips had head coverage below the lower normal limit (table). At reexamination 4–5 months later, all hips had become normal, and the mean BRP had increased to 53%. At a mean late follow-up of 27 months, none of the infants had signs of late dislocation.

Ultrasound evaluation of the hips of newborns using the BRP method for interpretation is effective for detecting congenital dislocation of the hip and for resolving inconclusive clinical findings; it is as reliable as radiography in the follow-up of infants with manifest or suspected hip abnormalities and those in the high-risk groups.

▶ Ultrasound is becoming more available in hospitals and is excellent for detecting widening of the joint space, a shallow acetabulum, and subluxation of the hip. Instability can be detected with it even when clinical and radiologic evaluations are normal; the degree of instability or widening demonstrated with sonography that does or does not need treatment remains to be determined.—P.P. Griffin, M.D.

Reliability of Radiological Measurements in the Assessment of the Child's Hip
Broughton NS, Brougham DI, Cole WG, Menelaus MB (Royal Children's Hosp, Melbourne)
J Bone Joint Surg [Br] 71-B:6–8, January 1989

Pelvic radiography has an important role in the diagnosis of congenital dislocation of the hip (CDH) in children. Several different measurements have been suggested to facilitate interpretation of radiographs of the hip and define normal ranges for the acetabular index at different ages. However, few studies have assessed the accuracy of these radiologic measurements. To quantify differences in the radiologic assessment of CDH, hip radiographs for children aged 4 months to 15 years were studied.

Of the 474 evaluated radiographs, 179 had been obtained before and after treatment for CDH, 79 were of a hip contralateral to a hip with CDH, and 216 were of apparently normal hip joints seen on radiographs taken during micturating cystourethrography. The acetabular index, Smith's c/b and h/b ratios (Fig 1–1), the amount of femoral head uncovering, the head-teardrop distance, and the neck-shaft angle were measured in all radiographs. The ACM angle, the M–Z distance, and the center-edge angle were measured in 170 hips of children aged more than 5 years. One observer assessed 126 radiographs twice, with the 2 sessions separated by at least 2 weeks. Two observers each assessed 100 hip radiographs independently, and 1 observer assessed 60 hips that had been radiographed twice on the same day.

A wide spread was found between values recorded by the same observer on different occasions. For example, intraobserver differences for the acetabular index ranged from −10 degrees to +9 degrees. The 95% prediction interval was ±6 degrees (table). Similar differences were found between interobserver measurements, and between measurements of the same hip on 2 radiographs taken on the same day and interpreted by the same observer. The acetabular index was the most helpful measurement for evaluating children aged up to 8 years. The center-edge angle was

Measurements Undertaken and Variation Between Observations

	Range of observations	Differences – 95% prediction intervals Intra-observer	Inter-observer
Acetabular index (degrees)	4 to 47	± 6.1	± 5.5
Centre-edge angle (degrees)	0 to 42	± 9.3	± 9.1
Head–teardrop distance (mm)	5 to 21	± 2.8	± 2.7
Femoral uncovering (degrees)	−3 to 16	± 3.5	± 3.8
ACM angle (degrees)	40 to 58	± 4.7	± 4.5
M–Z distance (mm)	0 to 17	± 3.3	± 3.1
Neck–shaft angle (degrees)	121 to 188	± 10.4	± 12.6
Smith's c/b ratio	0.57 to 1.05	± 0.04	± 0.06
Smith's h/b ratio	0.00 to 0.22	± 0.05	± 0.05

(Courtesy of Broughton NS, Brougham DI, Cole WG, et al: *J Bone Joint Surg [Br]* 71-B:6–8, January 1989.)

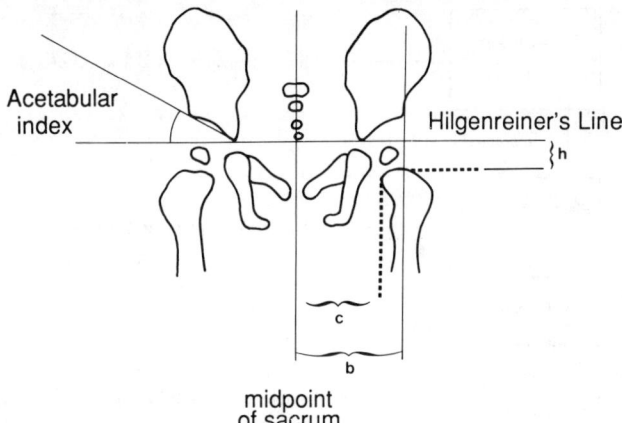

Fig 1–1.—Diagram to show the distances used to calculate Smith's c/b and h/b ratios. (Courtesy of Broughton NS, Brougham DI, Cole WG, et al: *J Bone Joint Surg [Br]* 71-B:6–8, January 1989.)

helpful for children aged more than 5 years, and Smith's c/b ratio and neck-shaft angle were helpful measurements for all ages. However, single readings of all measurements were unreliable.

▶ The authors have shown that the reproducibility of the various measurements about the hip for evaluating hip development is difficult. The most reproducible and reliable measurement appears to be the C-B ratio of Smith, which shows progressive subluxation as the ossification irregularities do not affect it. This plus the acetabular index (AI) are the 2 most reliable parameters to show the persistence of hip dysplasia even though the AI is influenced significantly by pelvic rotation.—P.P. Griffin, M.D.

Prospective Study of Congenital Dislocation of the Hip
Tredwell SJ, Davis LA (BC Children's Hosp; Univ of British Columbia, Vancouver)
J Pediatr Orthop 9:386–390, July–August 1989   1–3

A retrospective study of congenital dislocation of the hip in a large population of newborns showed that immediate flexion–abduction splinting for screened subluxable and dislocatable hips had a beneficial effect on the natural history of the disease. Data from subsequent retrospective studies supported that conclusion. A prospective study was done to test the previous conclusions and examine the incidence of hip dysplasia in an unselected infant population.

A 5-year screening program for hip dysplasia comprising 5,900 consecutive newborns yielded 62 infants with dislocated, dislocatable, or subluxable hips. All newborns with positive findings had a flexion–abduction cascade initiated within the first week of life (Fig 1–2). A soft abduction splint was used for the first 7–10 days of life. Hips that were

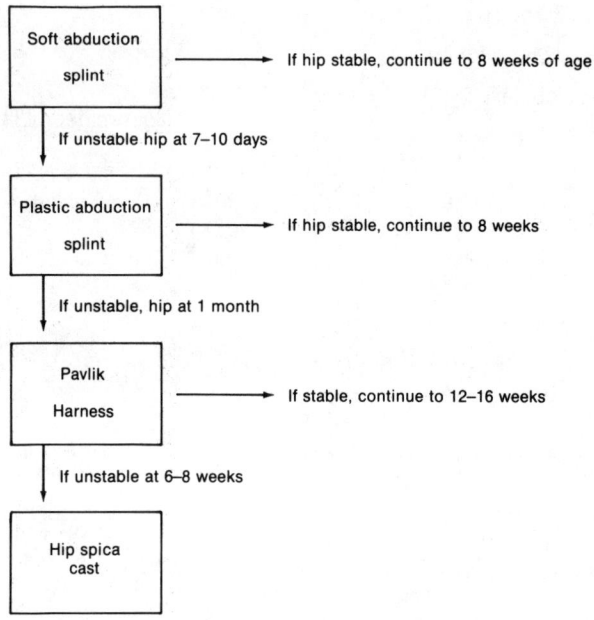

Fig 1–2.—Flexion–abduction cascade. (Courtesy of Tredwell SJ, Davis LA: *J Pediatr Orthop* 9:386–390, July–August 1989.)

clinically stable thereafter were maintained in the soft abduction splint until the infant was aged 8 weeks. Hips that were still clinically unstable after soft abduction splinting were placed in a plastic abduction brace, and those that were still unstable after 4–6 weeks of plastic abduction bracing were placed in a Pavlik harness. A hip spica was used if splinting or bracing did not stabilize the hip. All patients with an acetabular index (AI) greater than 30 degrees were put back into splints until their AI was below 30 degrees. Routine clinical examinations were performed at 4-month intervals. Radiographic follow-up examinations were performed when the infants were aged 4 months. Fifty-two infants completed all protocols of the study.

Thirty-two of the 52 evaluable patients had clinical hip stability after the use of a soft abduction splint only. Of the 20 patients who needed further treatment with a plastic abduction brace, 17 became clinically stable and 3 progressed to a Pavlik harness. Two of these 3 infants attained hip stability, and 1 had to be placed in a hip spica. Radiographic follow-up examinations at age 4 months showed that 2 of the 32 infants believed to have been stable after the use of a soft abduction splint required further treatment. One patient with an AI of 35 degrees at age 4 months was placed in a plastic abduction brace full-time for 2 months and part-time for the next 4 months. The child had AIs of 29 degrees at age 12 months and 25 degrees at age 18 months. The other child who had an AI of 35 degrees at 8 months needed a hip spica from age 11 to 14 months. At 2 years of age, the child's AI was 25 degrees.

Thus, immediate flexion–abduction splinting for screened subluxable and dislocatable hips in 52 children followed through the first year of life had a 100% success rate with no iatrogenic complications.

▶ This excellent study supports early treatment of hip instability in the newborn. Barlow found that hips stabilized within 5 days without treatment. Soft splints are not likely to be effective in hips that would not spontaneously become stable, but their use is not likely to cause avascular necrosis, which can occur with the Pavlik harness and the plastic abductor orthosis. Therefore if one follows the regimen described, successful treatment of the unstable hip recognized at birth should be expected. Of the hips that are stable at 5 to 10 days, some will have pelvic obliquity caused by contralateral abduction contracture and will have persistent acetabular dysplasia of the hip opposite the contracture (1).—P.P. Griffin, M.D.

Reference

1. Green NE, Griffin PP: *J Bone Joint Surg [Am]* 64-A:1273, 1982.

Avascular Necrosis in Congenital Hip Dysplasia: The Effect of Treatment
Robinson HJ Jr, Shannon MA (Univ of Minnesota, Minneapolis)
J Pediatr Orthop 9:293–303, May–June 1989   1–4

Despite major advances in the treatment of congenital dislocation of the hip, avascular necrosis (AVN) remains a significant complication of both closed and open reduction. The records of all patients who had treatment for congenital dislocations of the hip between 1948 and 1967 and in whom AVN developed were reviewed to assess the outcomes of treatment for AVN and to identify the most beneficial treatment.

The retrospective review yielded 39 available patients with 50 involved hips. Twenty-one patients came in for follow-up examinations. Radiographs were reviewed for acetabular index, center edge angle, Mose sphericity, and Severin classification. The mean age at initial treatment of the 39 patients was 18 months. All patients underwent closed reduction with casting in the flexed and abducted position. Avascular necrosis was diagnosed within 1 year of closed reduction, but by the time AVN was confirmed, 16 of the 50 hips already had redislocated, 14 hips had only limited coverage, and 20 hips still were well contained.

Eighteen patients with 20 involved hips received only conservative nonoperative treatment consisting of abduction, bracing, and physical therapy. A review of those 18 patients showed that the greater the initial extent of necrosis, the worse the function and radiographic outcome at final follow-up (Fig 1–3). Patients with the best outcomes had final center edge angles of greater than 15 degrees, Harris hip scores of greater than 90 degrees, Mose ratings of good, and Severin IA or B classifications.

Twenty-five patients eventually underwent some form of operation in

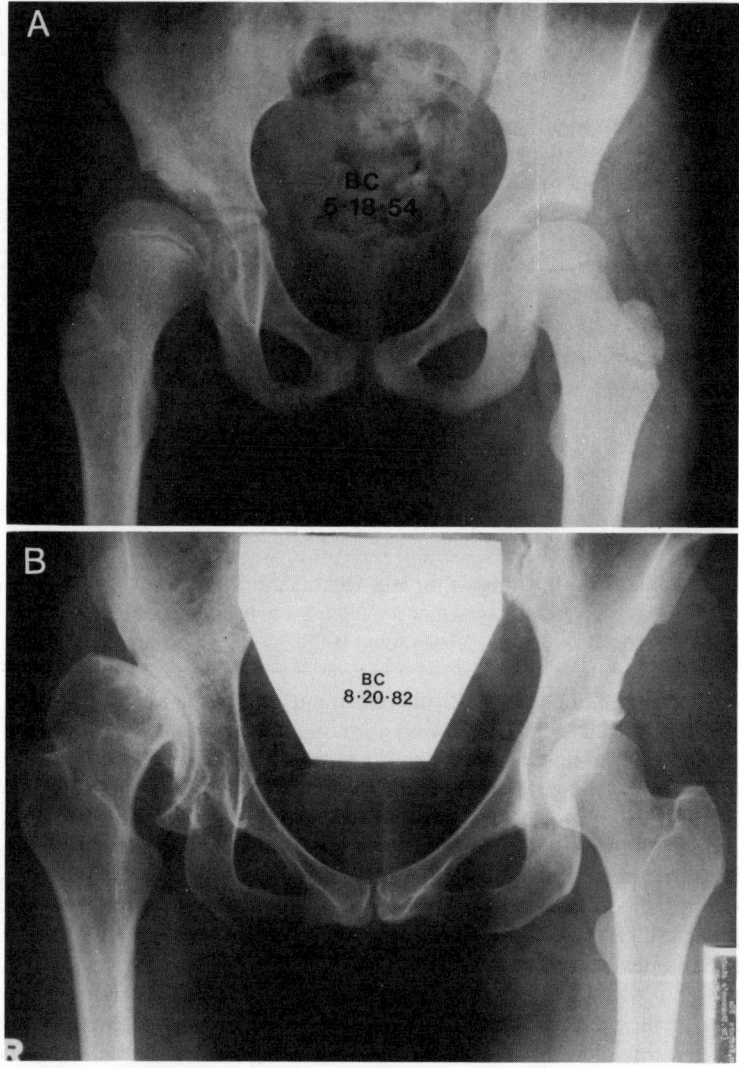

Fig 1–3.—**A,** follow-up roentgenogram 5 years after closed reduction of the right hip shows completely restored epiphysis but coxa magna and a shallow acetabulum; **B,** 28 years later, significant acetabular dysplasia and osteoarthritis are observed. (Courtesy of Robinson HJ Jr, Shannon MA: *J Pediatr Orthop* 9:293–303, May–June 1989.)

30 involved hips, including open reduction, varus derotational osteotomy, innominate osteotomy, and shelf procedures, but operations were only minimally successful. Seven hips had conventional cemented total replacement. However, at a mean follow-up of only 4 years, 3 prostheses already were showing evidence of progressive radiolucent lines, and mechanical failure was anticipated.

Nonoperative maintenance of a reduced femoral head remains the best option in AVN. If reduction cannot be maintained, an early pelvic or femoral osteotomy appears to have the best prognosis. Many patients end up with salvage procedures, including hip fusion because even conventional cemented total hip replacement holds little promise for a favorable long-term outcome.

▶ This article shows the devastating effect of AVN in congenital dislocation of the hip. Hips that remained reduced did better than those that subluxated or redislocated. Surgical treatment was shown not to be effective in changing the outcome. I believe that if the femoral head can recover and if the physis is not completely destroyed, maintenance of coverage of the femoral head will prevent progressive subluxation. The coxa magna that follows partial AVN is associated with a poorly developed acetabulum. An innominate osteotomy in the hip that has coxa magna and a low center edge angle will improve the long-term result. Little else can be done to alter the outcome of AVN, and at all cost the risk for producing AVN should be reduced by observing all guidelines that possibly could prevent it.—P.P. Griffin, M.D.

Treatment of Failed Open Reduction for Congenital Dislocation of the Hip
McCluskey WP, Bassett GS, Mora-Garcia G, MacEwen GD (Alfred I duPont Inst, Wilmington, Del)
J Pediatr Orthop 9:633–639, November–December 1989   1–5

Congenital dislocation of the hip can be treated with closed reduction in infants, but older children who are walking are likely to need open reduction. The problem of redislocation after open reduction has received little attention. In this study of 23 patients (25 hips), all of whom had had previous attempts at open reduction, the causes of redislocation, the incidence of avascular necrosis, and the results of treatment were investigated.

Congenital dislocation of the hip in these patients was diagnosed at a mean age of 13 months. Open reduction first was performed at a mean age of 1 year 8 months; final successful reduction was achieved at a mean age of 2 years 10 months. Before the final open reduction, 19 osteotomies had been performed in 14 hips and open reduction attempted twice in 8 hips and 3 times in 1 hip. Sixteen patients had had difficulties with the postoperative case immobilization. Fifteen hips were not concentrically reduced at the time of initial open reduction, and 2 had postoperative infections.

The hips that were stiff were treated before surgery with a physical therapy program and traction to regain motion. After satisfactory motion was obtained, an anterior surgical approach was used to reduce the hip. At the time of surgery, the reduction was confirmed both clinically and arthrographically. At the final evaluation, Severin scores were determined for 23 hips. Three that were classified as Severin grade I and 9 classified as grade II had center-edge angles normal for age. Seven grade III hips had mild dysplasia, 1 grade IV hip was subluxated, and 3 grade VII hips had significant arthritic changes.

Eleven hips (44%) had evidence of avascular necrosis. Four had a lateral physeal growth disturbance, 4 had a central physeal growth arrest, and 3 had complete femoral head necrosis. Previous failed procedures are likely to affect long-term outcome in these children. Many will need additional reconstructive procedures as young adults for premature osteoarthritis.

▶ Open reduction for a dislocated hip is a demanding procedure. To achieve a satisfactory reduction requires release of the capsule and isthmus, the iliopsoas tendon, and the transverse acetabular ligament. Stability of the reduction has to be assured at the operating table. Repeated open reduction is difficult, and failure to achieve a good result was shown by the 44% rate of avascular necrosis and only 12% of 23 hips with normal center edge angles after repeated open reductions.—P.P. Griffin, M.D.

Congenital Dislocation of the Hip: Acetabular Deficiency in Adolescence (Absence of the Lateral Acetabular Epiphysis) After Limbectomy in Infancy
O'Hara JN (Royal Orthopaedic Hosp, Birmingham, England)
J Pediatr Orthop 9:640–648, November–December 1989   1–6

Excision of the limbus in infants with congenital dislocation of the hip is associated with degenerative changes in adolescence and early adulthood. To determine the effects of limbectomy, records of 61 patients treated for receiving treatment for congenital dislocation of the hip were reviewed.

In 31 cases, anterolateral arthrotomy and limbectomy had been performed. Many patients underwent additional procedures during childhood. Normal development of the lateral acetabular epiphysis usually could be seen at about the age of 11 years. The second side appeared up to a year later, possibly a result of differences in radiographic technique. Nevertheless, variations from one side to another and from patient to patient were apparent.

At age 11 years, the lateral acetabular epiphysis appears to be an anterolateral structure. At age 14 years, the epiphysis is larger and the cartilaginous gap is partly obscured by bone. All 31 patients who underwent limbectomy failed to have a lateral acetabular epiphysis on the treated side; all 30 patients in whom the limbus was preserved developed normally.

The germinal cells that form the lateral acetabular epiphysis are excised at limbectomy. The result is deterioration in acetabular cover, appearing in previously sound hips in adolescence. Excision of the limbus can be avoided; its retention contributes to postrelocation stability of the hip and is essential to normal acetabular development.

▶ This study should teach us not to excise the limbus. I never could find a reason to excise the "limbus" and had always believed the excision would impair the growth of the acetabulum and lead to subluxation of the head. I hope all of us take heed.—P.P. Griffin, M.D.

The Place of Acetabuloplasty in the Treatment of Residual Acetabular Dysplasia Before the Age of Four Years: A Study of 14 Cases With a Follow-Up of More Than Five Years
Jacquemier A, Ferreira E, Tallet J-M, Bollini G, Bouyala JM (Hôpital de la Timone, Marseille, France)
Fr J Orthop Surg 3:155–161, June 1989   1–7

Problems with the use of innominate osteotomy of the Salter type for persistent acetabular dysplasia have led to the use of simple acetabuloplasty in hips with a normal amount of anteversion. Downward displacement of the acetabular roof is achieved with a supra-acetabular osteotomy, and the Y-cartilage is used as a hinge to tilt the acetabulum.

Fourteen acetabuloplasties were performed in 10 children with acetabular dysplasia. Eight procedures were for dysplasia secondary to congenital dislocation, and 6 were for primary dysplasia. All 10 patients were aged 16 to 37 months at operation. Follow-up was a minimum of 5 years.

The clinical results were good in all but 1 case. Determination of Wiberg's C and CE angles on anteroposterior radiographs showed satisfactory acetabular development in all but 3 hips. In these cases there was a preexisting lesion of the acetabular growth plates, defective centering of the hip, or a deformity of the femoral head after postreduction osteochondritis.

Surgical correction of acetabular dysplasia persisting after the age of 18 months is warranted. The acetabular orientation in the horizontal plane should be assessed with computed tomographic scanning. If the orientation is not defective, acetabuloplasty is safe and allows for acetabular growth. Innominate osteotomy may be needed if anteversion is increased.

▶ This procedure may have more versatility in the direction of coverage than others have. Care not to cross the triradiate cartilage must be taken to prevent early physeal closure. I have used this procedure in cerebral palsy patients and found it to be a satisfactory way to stabilize the hip.

The authors' studies of version of the acetabulum is interesting; with increasing availability of CT-3D reconstruction we may be able to be more selective not only of the procedure but also in identifying a patient who will continue to have spontaneous improvement. The increased acetabular angle on an anteroposterior radiograph is not evidence alone that a hip needs surgical treatment.—P.P. Griffin, M.D.

Femoral Capital Osteonecrosis: MR Finding of Diffuse Marrow Abnormalities Without Focal Lesions
Turner DA, Templeton AC, Selzer PM, Rosenberg AG, Petasnick JP (Rush-Presbyterian-St Luke's Med Ctr; Rush Med College, Chicago; Meriter Hosp, Madison, Wis)
Radiology 171:135-140, April 1989   1-8

Osteonecrosis of the head of the femur usually is characterized by focal abnormalities at the femoral head on magnetic resonance (MR) imaging. In the past 4 years 5 patients with 6 painful hips later shown to have femoral capital osteonecrosis lacked these focal signs initially, but had diffuse signal abnormalities instead.

These patients were aged 24 to 71 years and had pain in the affected hip for 1 week to 4 months. Prior scintigraphy had shown intense radionuclide uptake in the head of the femur, and radiographs had yielded normal results or had shown subtle osteopenia.

Magnetic resonance images obtained with short repetition and echo times showed low signal intensity, with isointensity or diffuse hyperintensity on long echo and repetition time images. The marrow above the acetabulum showed edema in 2 cases. Focal abnormalities were not evident until 6 or 8 weeks or 4 months later in 5 cases, by which time the diffuse signals had disappeared.

Diffuse hypointensity on short echo time MR images and isointensity or diffuse hyperintensity on long repetition and echo time images should raise the possibility of femoral capital osteonecrosis. This nonspecific pattern probably indicates bone marrow edema and may be an early sign of osteonecrosis.

▶ These 2 studies are interesting in that the 5 adults for whom MR imaging showed a diffuse edema pattern later had diagnoses of osteonecrosis, but the 3 children with hip pain and a diffuse edema pattern later had resolution of both their clinical symptoms and the MR imaging abnormalities. Children may have a greater capacity for recovery from marrow ischemia, but regardless of reason we should be slow to diagnose osteonecrosis in a child with an MR imaging study that shows a pattern of interosseous edema.—P.P. Griffin, M.D.

Hip Pain in Three Children Accompanied by Transient Abnormal Findings on MR Images
Pay NT, Singer WS, Bartal E (St Francis Regional Med Ctr, Wichita, Kan; Univ of Kansas, Wichita)
Radiology 171:147-149, April 1989   1-9

Legg-Calvé-Perthes disease has been detected early with magnetic resonance (MR) imaging. In 3 cases clinical and MR imaging pointed to this condition, but eventual resolution of the images and improvement in the patients' symptoms led to a final diagnosis of transient bone marrow edema.

Girl, 10 years, reported persistent mild hip pain for several months. Findings on radiography, bone scintigraphy, and hip aspiration were negative. The T_1-weighted images showed an inhomogeneous, poorly marginated area of hypointensity involving the epiphysis. After 2 weeks of traction, the girl's symptoms were relieved. A follow-up T_1-weighted image revealed complete resolution of the abnormal signal pattern in the epiphysis.

The other 2 cases followed a similar course. In 1 child, however, follow-up images still showed a focal hypointense area in the metaphysis, perhaps an area of fibrosis or an old infarct. Transient abnormal findings on MR images and hip pain in children may suggest edema rather than avascular necrosis. In such cases conservative management is indicated.

Relationship Between Femoral Anteversion and Osteoarthritis of the Hip
Kitaoka HB, Weiner DS, Cook AJ, Hoyt WA Jr, Askew MJ (Akron City Hosp; Northeastern Ohio Univs, Akron; Children's Hosp Med Center of Akron, Ohio)
J Pediatr Orthop 9:396–404, July–August 1989   1–10

The relationship between mechanical trauma and the development of osteoarthritis has been well studied. Femoral anteversion is defined as anterior inclination of the femoral neck axis relative to the transcondylar plane. It has been proposed that excessive femoral anteversion causes osteoarthritis of the hip. Prophylactic derotational operations are being performed in children with increased femoral anteversion, to prevent the development of osteoarthritis in adulthood. A study was done to determine the relationship between femoral anteversion and osteoarthritis of the hip.

Eight men and 8 women with a mean age of 68 years underwent total hip arthroplasty because of severe disabling primary osteoarthritis, and 18 volunteers with a mean age of 63 years had no history of hip disease. Most controls underwent anteroposterior radiography of the hip to confirm the absence of arthritis in the hip. Ten of the 16 patients had unilateral osteoarthritis; the other 6 patients had bilateral disease.

Femoral anteversion angles were measured with a modified CT technique. Defining the femoral neck axis is the most difficult and most critical aspect of all radiographic techniques used to determine anteversion. For this study, a composite of multiple tomograms was constructed to represent the femoral neck axis more accurately. Based on data obtained in 12 trial measurements, the modified CT technique demonstrated a mean error of -0.8 degree with a standard deviation of 2.2 degrees (Table 1).

Femoral anteversion in patients with osteoarthritis ranged from -12 degrees to 20 degrees (Table 2), whereas femoral anteversion in the controls ranged from -18 degrees to 24 degrees. The difference between patients and controls was not significant statistically. In patients with osteoarthritis, anteversion ranged from -12 degrees to 20 degrees in the 22 involved hips and from -5 degrees to 18 degrees in the 10 uninvolved hips. This difference also was not significant statistically.

TABLE 1.—Accuracy of Modified CT Techniques

Trial	Set angle (S, degrees)	Measured femoral anteversion (degrees) C	ΔC	Error (S − ΔC) (degrees)*
1	0	13	—	—
2	0	18	0	0
3	0	20	2	−2
4	8	30	12	−4
5	15	29	11	4
6	22	40	22	0
7	−4	14	−4	0
8	−4	9	−9	1
9	−13	7	−11	−2
10	−20	3	−15	−5
11	−26	−7	−25	−1
12	−35	−17	−35	0

*Mean ± SD in 12 trials −0.8 ± 2.2.
(Courtesy of Kitaoka HB, Weiner DS, Cook AJ, et al: J Pediatr Orthop 9:396–404, July–August 1989.)

TABLE 2.—Femoral Anteversion in Osteoarthritic Subjects

Subject	Involved hip	Sex	Femoral anteversion (degrees)* Left hip	Right hip
1	Bilateral	M	1	1
2	Bilateral	F	3	10
3	Left	M	15	3
4	Bilateral	F	20	20
5	Left	M	3	18
6	Left	M	−2	−5
7	Bilateral	M	6	9
8	Left	M	2	−5
9	Left	M	19	18
10	Left	F	−8	−4
11	Bilateral	F	−10	−12
12	Right	F	5	0
13	Left	F	10	0
14	Right	M	−3	4
15	Right	F	10	3
16	Bilateral	F	10	8

Note: Sixteen research subjects and 32 hips were studied.
*Mean ±SD in 22 involved, osteoarthritic hips 5.1 ± 8.7; in 10 uninvolved hips 2.7 ± 8.9, and in all 32 hips 4.3 ± 8.8.
(Courtesy of Kitaoka HB, Weiner DS, Cook AJ, et al: J Pediatr Orthop 9:396–404, July–August 1989.)

Performing prophylactic derotation femoral osteotomy in children with excessive femoral anteversion is not warranted because factors other than femoral anteversion are also involved in the etiology of primary osteoarthritis of the hip.

▶ Although the numbers are small, the consistency is meaningful. No one yet has been able to show a significant correlation of anteversion and the development of osteoarthritis.—P.P. Griffin, M.D.

Spine

Comparison of Cotrel-Dubousset and Harrington Rod Instrumentations in Idiopathic Scoliosis
Fitch RD, Turi M, Bowman BE, Hardaker WT (Duke Univ)
J Pediatr Orthop 10:44–47, January 1990   1–11

Harrington rod instrumentation (HRI) is the standard against which newer systems of treatment for idiopathic scoliosis must be measured. Researchers compared Cotrel-Dubousset instrumentation (CDI) with HRI in 62 patients who had surgical treatment for idiopathic scoliosis. Group I included 32 patients having CDI, bony fusion, and no postoperative immobilization. Group II included 30 patients having HRI, Bobechko hooks, fusion, and 4-month postoperative bracing. To evaluate the ability of the 2 systems to correct associated sagittal plane deformities, each group was divided into those with preoperative thoracic hypokyphosis and those with normal kyphosis. A single examiner reviewed preoperative, immediately postoperative, and follow-up radiographs of the thoracolumbar spine.

The 2 groups were similar with regard to curve magnitude, age, and

TABLE 1.—Results of Spinal Instrumentation for
Idiopathic Scoliosis in the Frontal Plane

Variable	CDI	HRI
Preoperative curves		
Mean	54.5°	52.7°
Range	38–78°	32–76°
Postoperative curves		
Mean	17.2°	25.6°
Range	0–37°	5–63°
Immediate correction		
Mean	68.2%	52.8%
Range	26–100%	7–87%
Loss of correction		
Mean	1.8°	8.1°
Range	0–8°	0–21°

Abbreviations: CDI, Cotrel-Dubousset instrumentation; HRI, Harrington rod instrumentation.
(Courtesy of Fitch RD, Turi M, Bowman BE, et al: J Pediatr Orthop 10:44–47, January 1990.)

TABLE 2.—Complications

Procedure/complication	n
CDI	
Prominent rod requiring trimming	2
Ileus	2
HRI	
Fracture of laminae	2
Cutout of Bobechko hooks	1
Slippage of rod within upper hooks	1
Lateral femoral cutaneous neuropathy	1
Urinary tract infection	2
Ileus	1

Note: Abbreviations as in Table 1.
(Courtesy of Fitch RD, Turi M, Bowman BE, et al: *J Pediatr Orthop* 10:44–47, January 1990.)

type. The CDI treatment provided significantly improved immediate frontal plane correction (Table 1). This treatment was also more effective in improving thoracic kyphosis, especially in patients with preoperative hypokyphosis. Operative procedures were similar in duration, blood loss, and low complication rates (Table 2).

Cotrel-Dubousset treatment compared favorably with HRI in outcome. Any loss of correction was not significant, even without the use of postoperative bracing, and operative time, blood loss, and complication rate were not increased.

▶ The CD system produced a greater improvement in both the lateral curve and the hypokyphosis than the Harrington; although the differences were not large, they may well be significant. However, for patients whose lose of kyphosis is not excessive, I believe the curve can be corrected satisfactorily and maintained with less risk by a Harrington distraction rod plus a Luque rod with Wisconsin (Drummond) wire fixation.— P.P. Griffin, M.D.

The Crankshaft Phenomenon
Dubousset J, Herring JA, Shufflebarger H (St Vincent de Paul Hosp, Paris; Texas Scottish Rite Hosp, Dallas; Miami Children's Hosp)
J Pediatr Orthop 9:541–550, September–October 1989   1–12

It previously was assumed that posterior fusion of the spine in young patients with congenital scoliosis would arrest all remaining spinal growth. However, increasing deformity has followed posterior surgical fusion in these patients. Progression occurred with growth and was not the result of pseudarthrosis or hardware failure. This progression is called the crankshaft phenomenon, as the entire spine and trunk gradually rotate and deform as the scoliosis progresses. The case reports of young children operated on for idiopathic or paralytic scoliosis were reviewed to determine whether progression of a posteriorly fused scoliosis is inevitable in children who have considerable remaining growth.

Between 1966 and 1984, spinal fusion was performed in 14 children with idiopathic scoliosis and in 26 children with paralytic scoliosis. Thirty-nine patients had posterior fusion alone, and 1 patient had both anterior and posterior fusion. The mean age at the time of fusion was 9 years 6 months. All patients were Risser zero at the time of operation.

Thirty-nine of the 40 evaluated patients had progressive postfusion angulation and rotation of the spine. The mean Cobb angle progressed from 37 degrees at 1 year after fusion to 52 degrees after a mean follow-up of 5 years 6 months. The mean Perdriolle angle increased from 29.5 degrees at 1 year to 45 degrees at final follow-up. The more immature patients who had the most remaining growth at the time of fusion showed the greatest progression. The single patient who showed no progression had undergone anterior and posterior arthrodesis for a lordoscoliosis. The scoliosis in this patient was 15 degrees at 1 year after fusion, and 17 degrees at follow-up. The Perdriolle was not measurable.

The remaining asymmetric growth in young children will cause curve progression after a posterior spinal fusion. The amount of curve progression is proportional to the number of unfused growth centers and the number of years of remaining growth. Using computerized 3-dimensional reconstruction of the spine and its deformity showed how an asymmetric growth arrest produces spinal deformity. In the presence of a solid posterior fusion, the remaining anterior spinal growth will produce angulation and rotation in the direction opposite the growth tether. The findings therefore refute the previously held assumption that posterior spinal fusion would arrest all remaining spinal growth.

▶ This interesting concept of a crankshaft phenomenon does explain both curve progression and increasing rotation after a solid posterior fusion that we have seen occur after posterior spinal fusion in a young child. Asymmetric fusion of a physis in an extremity is expected to cause deformity so why not in the spine! With the structure of the vertebral column resembling a cylinder it is reasonable that asymmetric growth after asymmetric fusion would cause the vertebral column to bend, translate, and rotate. This is what these authors have found. For a young child we have to consider both posterior and anterior fusion as the preferred treatment.—P.P. Griffin, M.D.

Scoliosis in Spinal Muscular Atrophy: Natural History and Management
Merlini L, Granata C, Bonfiglioli S, Marini ML, Cervellati S, Savini R (Istituto Ortopedico Rizzoli, Bologna, Italy)
Dev Med Child Neurol 31:501–508, August 1989

Infantile and juvenile spinal muscular atrophy (SMA) is an autosomal recessive disorder that causes degeneration of anterior-horn cells in the spinal cord, leading to symmetric muscle weakness and paralysis. Spinal muscular atrophy is classified as severe, intermediate, or mild disease. Severe SMA is almost always fatal within the first year of life. Children with intermediate SMA may survive into adolescence or adulthood, but they always have vertebral deformities. Mild SMA also may cause progressive spinal deterioration. Scoliosis is the most serious problem in patients with intermediate SMA or in those with mild SMA who have stopped walking.

During a 12-year period, 109 patients received treatment for SMA. Spinal muscular atrophy was severe in 18 cases, intermediate in 52, and mild in 39. All 18 children with severe SMA died between the ages of 1.5 and 22 months. Five children with intermediate SMA died between the ages of 5 and 13 years. At the last follow-up examination, the 47 surviving patients with intermediate SMA were aged 3 to 35 years, and the 39 patients with mild SMA were aged 3 to 47 years. Unaided sitting was the highest functional level attained by the intermediate SMA patients. Sixteen patients with mild SMA lost the ability to walk when they were aged 4 to 15 years.

A brace was used by patients with more than 50 degrees of kyphosis in the sitting position or with a scoliotic curve of more than 20 degrees. Twenty-four patients with intermediate SMA showed an average 8 degrees increase per year in curve severity, even though they were wearing the brace as prescribed. In patients with mild SMA, curve severity was directly proportional to muscle weakness in the lower limbs. Patients who had stopped walking had nearly 3 degrees progression in curve severity per year despite daily use of the brace (Fig 1–4). On the other hand, the deformity in those who were still able to walk and who were not using a brace was always less than 60 degrees, and the deformity did not progress greatly with age (Fig 1–5).

Seven patients had a total of 12 operations; 4 had late complications.

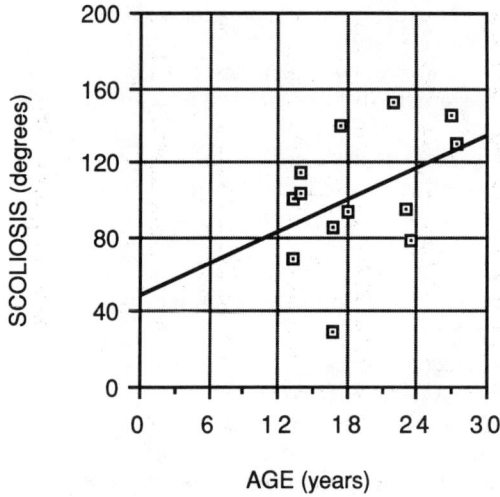

Fig 1–4.—Scoliosis in 13 patients with mild SMA, aged 13 to 27 years, unable to walk for an average of 10 years. Regression analysis between scoliosis and age (y = 49.03 + 2.84x) shows that scoliosis increased on the average by 3 degrees each year. At 18 years, scoliosis averaged 100 degrees, compared with 140 degrees in patients with intermediate SMA. (Courtesy of Merlini L, Granata C, Bonfiglioli S, et al: *Dev Med Child Neurol* 31:501–508, August 1989.)

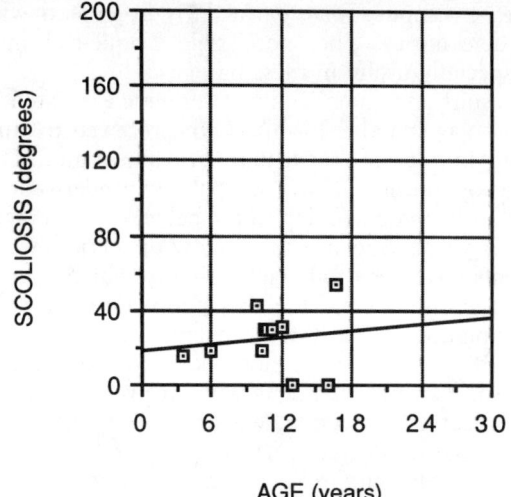

Fig 1-5.—Scoliosis in 10 patients with mild SMA, aged 6 to 17 years, and still able to walk. All scoliotic curves were less than 60 degrees (average, 30 degrees) and increased only slightly (0.6 degree each year) with age (y = 17.8 + 0.6x). (Courtesy of Merlini L, Granata C, Bonfiglioli S, et al: *Dev Med Child Neurol* 31:501–508, August 1989.)

Two patients needed reinsertion of their sacral rods when they were displaced after surgery, 1 had a new cervicothoracic curve when the rod became too short because of skeletal growth, and 1 had pseudoarthrosis at the lumbosacral level that required refusion. All patients had improved balance and comfort in the sitting position that resulted in improved function in the upper limbs.

Scoliosis in SMA is still largely an unresolved problem as nonoperative treatment does not control or arrest scoliosis. New surgical procedures to correct and stabilize the spine at an earlier age therefore should be developed.

▶ This article clearly shows the association of progressive scoliosis with ambulatory status and severity of the muscle weakness. Bracing had little influence on curve progression; in selected patients early fusion seems appropriate.—P.P. Griffin, M.D.

Spinal Fusion Augmented by Luque-Rod Segmental Instrumentation for Neuromuscular Scoliosis
Broom MJ, Banta JV, Renshaw TS (Newington Children's Hosp, Newington, Conn; Orlando Regional Med Ctr, Orlando, Fla)
J Bone Joint Surg [Am] 71A:32–44, January 1989   1–14

Luque-rod segmental instrumentation with posterior spinal fusion in the treatment of scoliosis provides more rigid fixation than does traditional Harrington-rod system. Rod instrumentation is associated with a high incidence of complications, particularly in patients with neuromuscular spinal deformities. The more rigid Luque-rod instrumentation seems to be especially useful in these patients.

Long-term results and complication rates were evaluated in 74 patients with neuromuscular spinal deformities who received treatment with the relatively new Luque-rod segmental instrumentation. Four patients needed 2-stage operations. Thirty-six patients underwent spinal fusion only, and 38 had fusion extending to the pelvis. The average age at operation was 14.7 years. The average follow-up period was 42 months. Thirteen patients have been followed for more than 5 years.

Spinal fusion did not change the ability to walk in any of the patients. The mean preoperative curve was 73 degrees, and the mean postoperative curve was 38 degrees. At the most recent follow-up, the average loss of correction was 4 degrees. Patients who received 4.8 mm rods had lost a mean of 4.5 degrees correction, whereas those who received 6.4 mm rods had an average 1.5 degrees correction loss (table). In addition to the scoliosis, kyphotic deformity in 7 patients was more than 60 degrees. Kyphosis in these patients that averaged 91 degrees preoperatively improved to a mean of 55 degrees postoperatively. Pelvic obliquity seen in 47 patients improved from a mean of 17.3 degrees to 10.9 degrees. At follow-up, 29 patients had asymptomatic migration and 5 patients had rotation of a rod, but none had a consequent delay in fusion. One severely retarded 14-year-old boy died of cardiopulmonary arrest 18 hours after surgery. No major perioperative neurologic complications occurred. Other complications included 3 deep wound infections, 2 pressure sores, 6 sets of broken Luque rods, and 1 instance of distal rod rotation and migration. A tendency for cephalad progression of deformity was noted when the fusion ended cephalad at or below the fourth thoracic vertebra: 7 patients needed cephalad extension of the fusion because of increasing deformity. Fourteen patients needed reoperation for repair of pseudoarthrosis, incision and drainage of wound infection, or hardware problems.

Luque-rod segmental instrumentation with posterior spinal fusion is effective in the treatment of patients with scoliosis secondary to a variety of neuromuscular disorders.

Results According to Major Diagnostic Categories

Diagnosis	No. of Patients	Preop.	Max.-Bend. Radiograph	Postop.	Final	Correction (Per cent)
All patients	74	73	41	38	42	48
Cerebral palsy	30	75	46	41	45	45
Myelomeningocele	8	75	29	35	43	53
Duchenne muscular dystrophy	7	62	23	28	33	55
Spinal muscular atrophy	6	94	62	51	56	46
Severe mental retardation	7	76	51	47	52	38

(Courtesy of Broom MJ, Banta JV, Renshaw TS: J Bone Joint Surg [Am] 71A:32–44, January 1989.)

▶ The segmental fixation with Luque rods is shown to be effective in the treatment of scoliosis in neuromuscular patients. Patients with neuromuscular scoliosis must have fused of the T2 to T3 to prevent cephalad progression of the curve. The unit Luque rod is more effective in controlling pelvic oblique than the 2 separate rods. Migration of the rod on the high side will allow the pelvic obliquity to recur, as was seen in some of these patients.—P.P. Griffin, M.D.

The Management of Rotatory Atlanto-Axial Subluxation in Children
Phillips WA, Hensinger RN (Univ of Michigan, Ann Arbor)
J Bone Joint Surg [Am] 71A:664–668, June 1989

Rotatory atlantoaxial subluxation is an uncommon condition of unknown etiology that occurs primarily in children. Affected children have torticollis and decreased motion of the neck, with or without pain. Most atlantoaxial subluxations are easily reduced with traction. However, irreducible subluxations have been reported in children who were given late diagnoses. Factors that influence the success of traction in reducing rotatory atlantoaxial subluxation, and the utility of dynamic computed tomography (CT) in its diagnosis were studied. During a 12-year period in 23 children with an average age of 7 years 6 months.

Nine children had sustained minor trauma, but in only 2 were the falls severe enough to have been predisposing factors to torticollis. Nine children had had upper respiratory infections just before the onset of torticollis. One child had juvenile rheumatoid arthritis. No predisposing inflammatory or traumatic factors could be identified in the remaining 4 children. Of the 23 children, 11 were seen within a week after onset of torticollis, 5 between 1 week and 1 month after onset, and 7 were seen more than 1 month after symptom onset.

Using the radiographic Fielding-Hawkins classification, 8 children had type 1 and 14 had type 2 subluxations. The radiographs for 1 child were unavailable. None of the children had type 3 subluxations. Five children underwent dynamic CT examination of the neck to document the presence of subluxation. A positive CT scan showed no motion, or limited asymmetric motion between the first and second cervical vertebrae (Fig 1–6). All children had cervical halter traction, and halo traction if halter traction was not effective. The end point of therapy was active, equal lateral rotation to each side.

The subluxation reduced spontaneously with bed rest in 3 of the 11 children who were seen within a week after onset of symptoms. A short period of traction reduced the subluxation in the other 8 children and in the 5 children seen within a month after onset of symptoms. Of the 7 children who were seen more than a month after symptom onset, 1 needed posterior atlantoaxial arthrodesis. Reduction initially was achieved in the other 6 children, but 4 children had recurrences, and 2 eventually needed arthrodesis of the first and second cervical vertebrae. Dynamic CT examination clearly documented the subluxation. Acquired torticollis in children should arouse suspicion of rotatory atlantoaxial

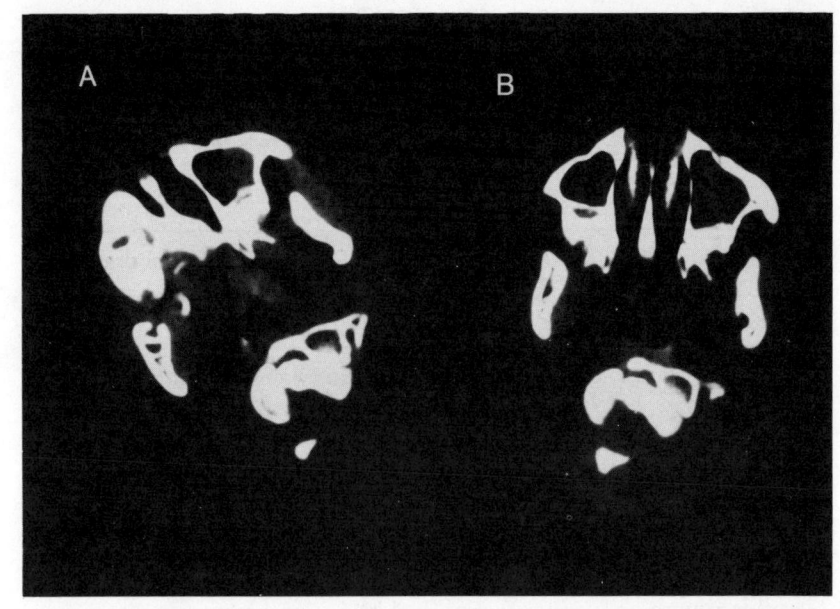

Fig 1-6.—Dynamic CT scans of the upper cervical spine in a patient who had rotatory atlantoaxial subluxation. **A,** the head is rotated approximately 45 degrees to 1 side, with the contralateral lateral mass of the first cervical vertebra moving forward on the cephalad articulating facet of the second cervical vertebra. **B,** the head cannot be rotated past the midline, and the relationship of the first and second cervical vertebrae is unchanged. (Courtesy of Phillips WA, Hensinger RN: *J Bone Joint Surg [Am]* 71-A:664-668, June 1989.)

subluxation, particularly in the presence of a recent history of minor infection or trauma.

▶ All too frequently symptoms of acute torticollis are treated lightly. Not all children with acute torticollis have rotatory subluxation. In those who have trauma or torticollis that persists for a week, a CT scan or appropriate radiograph to evaluate C1-C2 for subluxation should be done. Procrastination of treatment may lead to an irreversible rotatory subluxation that may need an arthrodesis of C1-C2. I have not been successful in reducing the subluxation that has been present for 1 month or more.—P.P. Griffin, M.D.

Spinal Arthrodesis for Severe Spondylolisthesis in Children and Adults: A Long-Term Follow-Up Study
Freeman BL III, Donati NL (Univ of Tennessee, Memphis)
J Bone Joint Surg [Am] 71-A:594-598, April 1989   1-16

Surgery is the usually accepted treatment for patients with severe spondylolisthesis, but controversy exists over whether arthrodesis should be performed with or without reduction. Long-term results were compared for 14 children and adolescents, 2 of whom had open reduction as well as spinal arthrodesis.

All patients had a slip of 50% or greater (Myerding grade III or IV). The 12 who had a posterior spinal arthrodesis in situ ranged in age from 7 to 22 years at the time of surgery and were followed up for 3 to 26 years. Preoperative symptoms included tight hamstrings, pain, no ankle

Patient Data

Case	Age at Operation (Yrs.)	Age at Follow-up (Yrs.)	Grade of Slip	Per Cent of Slip	Slip Angle (Degrees)	Postop. Pain	Cosmetic Result
1	7	23	III	65	35	None	Satis.
2	9	20	IV	100	70	None	Unaware of deform.
3	16	36	IV	85	45	Mild	Dissatis.
4	14	19	IV	90	35	None	Satis.
5	17	29	IV	90	55	None	Satis.
6	22	25	IV	95	40	None	Unaware of deform.
7	13	17	III	75	50	None	Satis.
8	13	19	III	55	20	None	Unaware of deform.
9	13	16	III	55	15	None	Unaware of deform.
10	13	18	III	55	25	Mild	Unaware of deform.
11	17	31	III	60	40	Mild	Dissatis.
12	16	32	IV	100	60	None	Unaware of deform.
13	13	39	IV	60	35	None	Unaware of deform.
14	13	39	III	55	35	Mild	Satis.

(Courtesy of Freeman BL III, Donati NL: *J Bone Joint Surg [Am]* 71-A:594–598, April 1989.)

jerk, increased lordosis, flat buttocks, and a prominent sacrum with a step-off. All had an isthmic spondylolisthesis.

Eight of these patients reported no pain at the most recent follow-up. Four had occasional mild pain with strenuous activity but were not limited in their activities. Six patients said they were not aware of any deformity. None had the characteristic waddling gait associated with the disorder. All had a solid fusion with no progression of the slip.

The 2 patients having open reduction and internal fixation lost correction when the rods were removed. Both needed additional operative procedures, and 1 was left with a mild nerve root deficit. Both were aware of their deformities, but they were satisfied with their appearance, free of back pain, and not limited in their activity (table).

Predictably good results are obtained by in situ posterior arthrodesis with no attempt at reduction. Most children and adolescents with severe spondylolisthesis can benefit from this method of treatment. Reduction can be successful, but is not reliable and may result in serious complications.

▶ A solid fusion in spondylolisthesis almost uniformly produces good results as shown in this study. A trend is to consider reduction as favorable for improving results. Reduction does improve the appearance, but is not significantly better in relieving pain or hamstring tightness with a successful solid fusion. The trade-off for this cosmetic improvement is the risk of nerve root damage.— P.P. Griffin, M.D.

Foot

Correction of Idiopathic Clubfoot: A Comparison of Results of Early Versus Delayed Posteromedial Release
DePuy J, Drennan JC (Yale Univ; Newington Children's Hosp, Newington, Conn)
J Pediatr Orthop 9:44–48, January–February 1989

One-stage posteromedial release is effective for idiopathic talipes equinovarus, but the timing of the procedure is controversial. To study the effect of timing on the results, data for 15 feet operated on at age 4.4 months, 15 operated on at age 9.1 months, and 14 operated on at age 16.1 months were reviewed. Preoperative deformity and serial casting were similar in all 30 patients (44 feet). All had a complete 1-stage posteromedial release with 2-pin fixation and similar postoperative management.

Results were best in patients who had the earliest surgery. Failure to achieve an angle of more than 20 degrees on a Kite anteroposterior view was evident in 13% of the early group, 40% of the middle group, and 64% of the late group. The early group also had significantly better hindfoot-to-forefoot alignment on radiographs than the middle and late groups. The relationship between average postoperative talo-first metatarsal angle to timing of surgery was −1.86 degrees for the early group,

+3.4 degrees for the middle group, and +6.46 degrees for the late group. Only 7% in the early group had tarsal distortions, compared with 28% in the middle group and 35% in the late group.

Early, middle, and late posteromedial releases produce satisfactory results. Early correction, however, yields better alignment of the forefoot, correction of hindfoot varus, and tarsal configuration. Experience with more patients who are observed for a longer time after surgery is needed to confirm these preliminary results.

▶ The results in the later age group were not dramatically different but did support early surgery (3–4 months). Numbers in each group were small, and the difference in angle between groups was small. Longer follow-up and larger numbers may give the same or different results.—P.P. Griffin, M.D.

Comparative Review of Surgical Treatment of the Idiopathic Clubfoot by Three Different Procedures at Columbus Children's Hospital
Magone JB, Torch MA, Clark RN, Kean JR (Columbus Children's Hosp, Columbus, Ohio; Ohio State Univ)
J Pediatr Orthop 9:49–58, January–February 1989   1–18

The initial treatment of clubfoot consists of manipulation and serial casting. Surgical soft tissue release is indicated when the clubfoot shows resistance to closed treatment. However, what constitutes the best surgical procedure is not agreed upon. Three surgical procedures, the Turco, the Carroll, procedure, and the McKay, are presently used to treat clubfoot at a large pediatric care center. The early results of treatment of 76 cases of clubfoot in 54 children were evaluated clinically and radiographically after 1 of the 3 procedures of soft tissue clubfoot release.

Of 37 boys and 17 girls, 22 had bilateral clubfoot. Twenty-five patients underwent the Carroll procedure on 35 clubbed feet, 13 had the McKay procedure in 17 clubbed feet, and 16 had the Turco procedure in 24 clubbed feet. All 54 patients underwent orthopedic and neurologic follow-up examinations. In addition, all patients had their feet traced. A new rating system that weighs dynamic functional results more heavily than other factors was used to compare results. Radiographic evaluation included measuring the talocalcaneal angle and talo-first metatarsal angle on anteroposterior and lateral radiographs of the foot (table).

The average postoperative follow-ups were 25 months for the Carroll procedure, 16 months for the McKay procedure, and 64 months for the Turco procedure. Sixteen feet had follow-ups of less than 1 year. For the Carroll procedure, postoperative functional results were rated excellent in 11% of the feet, good in 37%, fair in 29%, and poor in 23%. For the McKay procedure, outcomes were rated excellent in 12.5% of the feet, good in 50%, fair in 12.5%, and poor in 25%. For the Turco procedure, results were rated excellent in 12.5% of the feet, good in 33.3%, fair in

Radiographic Evaluation Summary

	Group I	Group II	Group III	Normal feet
	\multicolumn{4}{c}{Degrees measured}	
Anteroposterior talocalcaneal angle				
Mean	32	46	37	33
SD	11	9	10	6
Anteroposterior talo-first metatarsal angle				
Mean	+1	−8	−8	−10
SD	12	7	7	7
Lateral talocalcaneal angle				
Mean	26	35	24	37
SD	6	12	10	7
Lateral talo-first metatarsal angle				
Mean	14	15	14	10
SD	10	11	8	8
Lateral calcaneal-first metatarsal angle				
Mean	142	145	146	149
SD	9	10	10	9
Total ankle motion				
Mean	21	16	24	51
SD	8	7	17	12

(Courtesy of Magone JB, Torch MA, Clark RN, et al: *J Pediatr Orthop* 9:49–58, January–February 1989.)

16.7%, and poor in 37.5%. Radiographically evident complications included overcorrection and undercorrection at the talonavicular articulation; avascular necrosis of the talus, navicular, and calcaneus; and talar dome flattening.

Because the results are only preliminary, it is too early to identify the most effective of the 3 procedures. However, on the basis of available data, the following technical suggestions pertaining to all 3 procedures are offered: use of a more physiologic orientation of the bimalleolar axis, anatomical alignment at the talonavicular joint, and postoperative use of a hinged ankle cast brace to increase final ankle range of motion.

▶ These 3 procedures have more similarities than differences. A significant number of feet have poor results after treatment with any of these procedures. This is to be expected when all the experts doing "their" operations to the best of their ability still have a significant number of poor results. Until the unknown that is responsible for these poor results is identified, we will make little progress in improving the results of treatment.— P.P. Griffin, M.D.

Arterial Abnormalities in Talipes Equinovarus as Assessed by Angiography and the Doppler Technique

Sodre H, Bruschini S, Mestriner LA, Miranda F Jr, Levinsohn EM, Packard DS Jr, Crider RJ Jr, Schwartz R, Hootnick DR (Escola Paulista de Medicina, São Paulo, Brazil; State Univ of New York, Syracuse; New York Univ)
J Pediatr Orthop 10:101–104, January 1990   1–19

Arteriographic studies performed in limbs with talipes equinovarus showed that 89% had reduced or absent anterior tibial arteries and medial plantar arteries, compared with only 2% to 7% in an otherwise normal general population. In patients studied no relationship was found between the severity of the clinical condition and the degree of arterial deficiency. Abnormalities consisted primarily of hypoplasia or premature termination of the anterior tibial artery, found in 93% of limbs (Fig 1–7). The medial plantar artery was absent from 93%

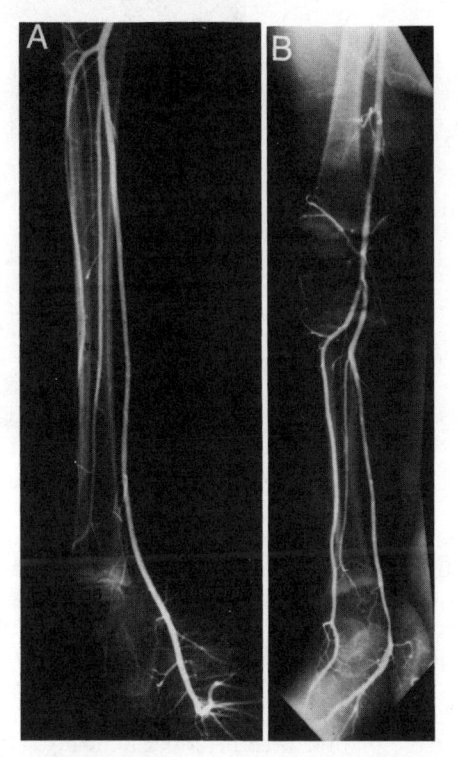

Fig 1–7.—**A**, lateral radiograph of the leg and foot of a patient with talipes equinovarus demonstrating that a single large vessel, the posterior tibial artery, supplies the foot. The anterior tibial artery *(TA)* terminates at the midleg level. The peroneal artery descends to the level of the ankle before terminating. (Courtesy of Sodre H, Filho JL, Napoli MMM, et al: *Rev Bras Ortop* 22:43–48, 1987.) **B**, lateral arteriogram of a normal limb for comparison. The anterior and posterior tibial arteries are of equal caliber. (Courtesy of Sodre H, Bruschini S, Mestriner LA, et al: *J Pediatr Orthop* 10:101–104, January 1990.)

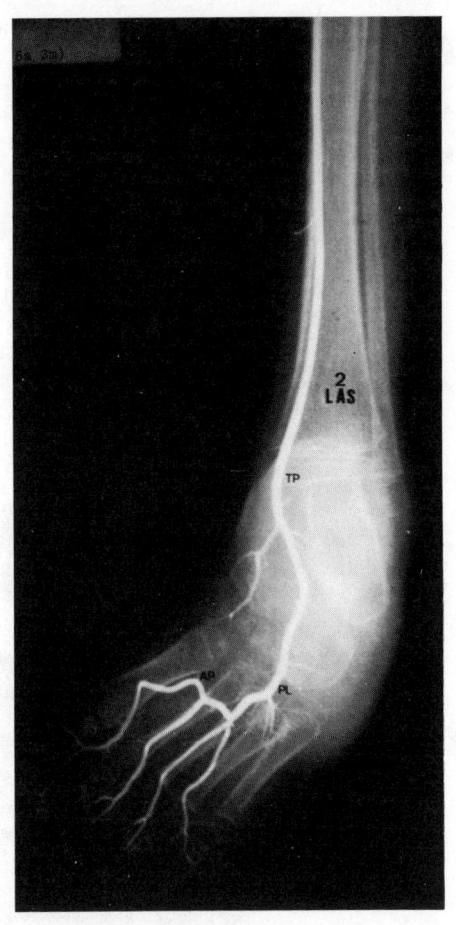

Fig 1-8.—Anteroposterior radiograph of a foot and ankle with talipes equinovarus demonstrating the arteriographic filling of a single vessel, the posterior tibial artery *(TP)*, entering the foot on its posteromedial aspect. A reduced medial plantar artery is present. The major artery in the foot is the lateral plantar *(PL)*, which provides all the common digital branches. (Courtesy of Sodre H, Filho JL, Napoli MMM, et al: *Rev Bras Ortop* 22:43–48, 1987. From Sodre H, Bruschini S, Mestriner LA, et al: *J Pediatr Orthop* 10:101–104, January 1990.)

of limbs (Fig 1–8). All posterior tibial and peroneal arteries were normal.

Arteriographic findings of arterial deficiencies conflict with data obtained by the doppler technique. To delineate the relationship between results obtained by iodinated contrast angiography and by continuous-wave Doppler examination, researchers studied 9 limbs in 5 patients using both techniques. Angiography was performed before surgical intervention and Doppler studies were performed postoperatively. None of the 9 limbs had complete filling of the anterior tibial artery, the medial plantar artery, or the plantar arch arteriographically. However, all limbs had pulses with the Doppler technique at all anatomical locations examined (table).

Continuous-wave Doppler studies are less useful for identifying major arteries than is dissection or angiography. From these findings, it is apparent that arterial dysgenesis may play a role in the etiology of clubfoot. Because the posterior tibial artery usually provides the only arterial sup-

Results of Doppler Examination

Patient no.	Age (yr,mo)	Arteriographic data Side	Anterior tibial[†]	Plantar arch	Age (yr,mo)	Anterior tibial	Doppler data[*] Dorsalis pedis	Posterior tibialis	Brachial right arm
1	8,10	R [‡] L	Normal Proximal	Deficient Deficient	12,6	100 100	100 100	100 100	90
7	0,9	R L	Middle Middle	Deficient Deficient	3,1	60 60	60 60	100 100	70
12	1,1	R L	Middle Middle	Deficient Deficient	3.6	80 70	80 70	80 80	80
13	0,11	R L	Distal hypoplasia throughout	Deficient Complete	3.3	70 70	70 70	90 90	70
16	5,0	R L	Distal Distal	Deficient Deficient	8.3	60 40	25 70	80 80	80

[*]Pressure (mm Hg) at which the sound disappeared.
[†]Point of termination of the anterior tibial artery in proximal, middle, and distal third of the leg.
[‡]Only normal limb in this set of limbs. All other limbs had a clubfoot deformity.
(Courtesy of Sodre H, Bruschini S, Mestriner LA, et al: *J Pediatr Orthop* 10:101–104, January 1990.)

ply to the foot, this vessel must be preserved at surgery and during later ankle dorsiflexion.

▶ This study compared arteriography with continuous-wave Doppler in identifying arterial anomalies or deficiencies in clubfoot. The preoperative studies were done by angiography, and the postoperative studies were done by Doppler. This comparison would seem to be invalid, but the authors reported on arteriographic studies in 3 patients preoperatively and postoperatively in which no changes were observed; consequently, the authors believed that Doppler fails to show deficiencies in arterial structure and flow. It is important to recognize that in clubfoot the posterior tibial artery may be the only adequate artery to the clubfoot.—P.P. Griffin, M.D.

Development of the Child's Arch
Gould N, Moreland M, Alvarez R, Trevino S, Fenwick J (Univ of Vermont, Burlington)
Foot Ankle 9:241–245, April 1989   1–20

The neutral foot is one that is neither flat nor highly arched. Pediatric patients aged from 11 months up to 5 years were studied to determine whether the development of a neutral foot would be enhanced footwear that supports arches. Studies were made in 125 beginning walkers aged 11–14 months; weight-bearing; anteroposterior, lateral, and Harris view x-ray films; pedotopography; and clinical examination of the lower extremities were used for assessment. Fifty children (group 1) were randomized to receive straight-last shoes; 25 (group 2) to receive straight-last shoes plus longitudinal arch cookies; 25 (group 3) to receive orthopedic shoes with long counters, solid shanks, Thomas heels, and 0.312-cm inside heel wedges; and 25 (group 4) to receive the same shoes as group 3 plus a supplemental thin longitudinal arch support. Shoes were to be the main footwear until children reached the age of 5 years. Children were evaluated at age 2 and 3 years, and at the end of the study.

In the first year all children had pes planus—flatfoot. There were no cases of cavus foot. At 2 years of age, all children had longitudinal arch improvement. Arch-support footwear—shoes 2, 3, and 4—appeared to aid in more rapid development of the arch than did shoe 1. At 3 years of age, all feet showed improved arch development regardless of the type of footwear worn, but arch development occurred sooner with shoes 2, 3, and 4, particularly with shoe 2.

At 5 years of age, 60% of children wearing shoe 1 had normal arches, 40% had pes planus, 79% had hyperpronation, and 88% had genu valgum; 75% of children wearing shoe 2 had normal arches, 25% had pes planus, 75% had hyperpronation, and 95% had genu valgum; 71% of children wearing shoe 3 had normal arches, 29% had pes planus, 85% had hyperpronation, and 93% had genu valgum; 60% of children wearing shoe 4 had normal arches, 40% had pes planus, 80% had hyperpronation, and 90% had genu valgum.

Arches developed regardless of the footwear worn, but development was more rapid until the age of 3 years with arch-support footwear. Rapidity of arch development continued up to 5 years of age in children who wore longitudinal arch cookies. Hyperpronation and genu valgum are apparently normal in 5-year-old children.

▶ The numbers in the study are too small in that 52 patients were evaluated at 5 years. The controls wore straight last shoes and had responses the same as those of patients who wore "orthopedic" shoes with arch support. This study does not provide evidence to support treating flat feet in children. (Compare this study with that of Wenger et al. [1]).—P.P. Griffin, M.D.

Reference

1. Wenger et al: *J Bone Joint Surg [Am]* 71-A:800, 1989.

Corrective Shoes and Inserts as Treatment for Flexible Flatfoot in Infants and Children
Wenger DR, Mauldin D, Speck G, Morgan D, Lieber RL (Texas Scottish Rite Hosp, Dallas; Univ of California, San Diego)
J Bone Joint Surg [Am] 71-A:800–810, July 1989
1–21

Opinions on the need to treat flexible flatfoot vary widely, but results with corrective shoes or inserts have not previously been tested scientifically. The effect of such treatment was studied prospectively in infants and children, aged 1 to 6 years old, with flatfeet meeting radiographic criteria. The patients were randomly assigned to group I, controls; group II, those given corrective orthopedic shoes; group III, those given a Helfet heel-cup; and group IV, those with a custom-molded plastic insert. Results were assessed blindly with photographs and radiographs at the end of at least 3 year's treatment.

In the 98 children completing the study, no significant difference was found between control and treated groups in angle between talus and sole of the foot, angle between talus and first metatarsal, or in talocalcaneal angle. All groups, including controls, had significant improvement. The greatest change in radiographic angle was found in patients with the largest initial angle, irrespective of treatment.

Children with typical flexible flatfoot do not need treatment with corrective shoes or inserts. Parents can be assured that the condition is a normal variation and that it will improve with time.

▶ The management of painless flexible flatfeet is controversial. Although the numbers of patients are not large, the statistics appear valid. I have always believed the conclusion made in this study. It is the best-controlled study ever published, to my knowledge. Orthopedists now have a scientific study to quote that supports nontreatment of the typical flexible flatfoot. However, children with pathologic musculoskeletal disorders may benefit from treatment of pes planus—not to correct the deformity, as it will not—but only to relieve fatigue and to improve function.—P.P. Griffin, M.D.

Subtalar Joint Coalition in Children: New Observations
Lee MS, Harcke HT, Kumar SJ, Bassett GS (Alfred I duPont Inst, Wilmington, Del)
Radiology 172:635–639, September 1989

Subtalar coalition is a cause of peroneal spastic flatfoot. Its diagnosis in preadolescents is difficult because skeletal maturation has not progressed to the point at which osseous bridging can be demonstrated with radiography. New observations on the nature of subtalar coalition in children were evaluated (Fig 1–9).

Two groups of children with clinical and radiographic findings suggesting tarsal coalition were studied. The first group of 11 children had sur-

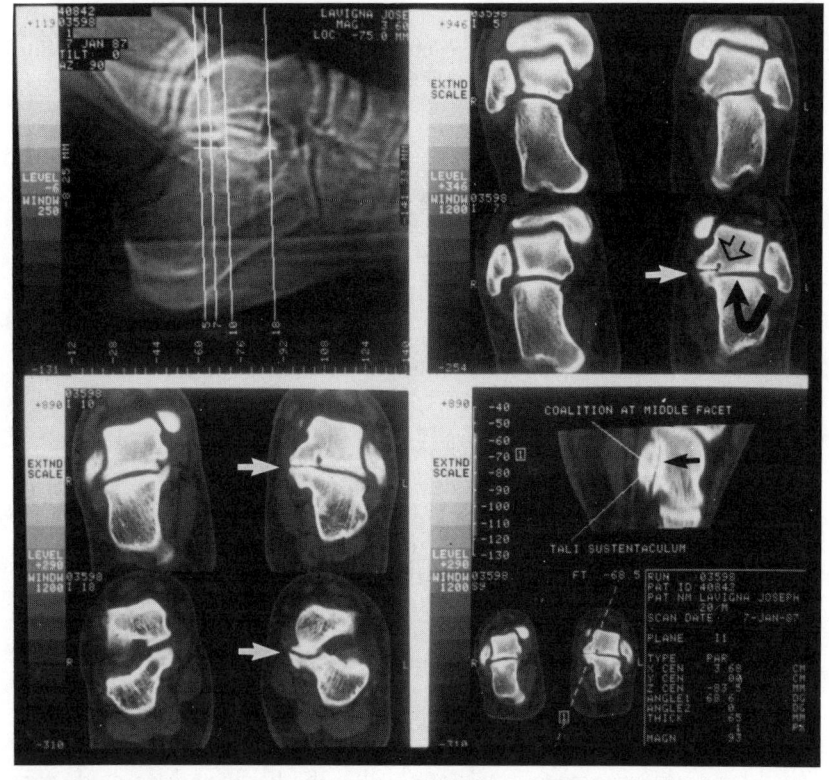

Fig 1–9.—Images of a 12-year-old boy. Surgically confirmed middle-facet coalition *(white arrow)*, fibro-osseous type, seen on coronal CT sections. Note associated narrowing of the tarsal canal *(open arrow)* and posterior facet *(curved arrow)*. Note off-axis CT reconstruction image displaying fibro-osseous coalition on the middle facet joint *(straight black arrow)*. (Courtesy of Lee MS, Harcke HT, Kumar SJ, et al: *Radiology* 172:635–639, September 1989.)

gery that helped confirm a subtalar joint pathologic condition. The second group, consisting of 14 children with radiologic findings similar to those of the first group, had treatment without surgery. Four additional children with a radiographically obvious bone coalition also were studied. The ages of patients ranged from 8 to 17 years. In patients with surgical treatment, release of the fibrocartilaginous bridge restored hindfoot motion. In 4 of the 18 patients not having surgery, the subtalar coalition was osseous. Radiographic studies were definitive in these cases. None of the patients had falsely negative radiographic findings. Coalition posterior to the sustentaculum tali was the most common site of occurrence.

Diagnosing nonosseous coalition requires careful evaluation with CT. Physicians must pay close attention to subtle changes in the hindfoot, especially posterior to the sustentaculum tali, which is a common site of nonosseous subtalar coalition.

▶ The histologic material found in the subtalar coalition varies in its content of fibrous cartilage and bone. Complete osseous coalitions are demonstrated easily. Coalitions that are not completely ossified are more difficult to diagnose. In the nonosseous subtalar coalition the sustentaculum talus is hypoplastic and misshapen, and the articular surface is irregular. In the foot with painful, limited subtalar motion and normal results of radiographs, a nonosseous coalition of the subtalar joint in the middle facet, but more commonly, posterior to the middle facet, must be considered as a possibility.—P.P. Griffin, M.D.

Subtalar Arthrodesis in Children
Gallien R, Morin F, Marquis F (Quebec City)
J Pediatr Orthop 9:59–63, January–February 1989

The Grice-Green extra-articular arthrodesis of the subtalar joint for the correction of paralytic flatfeet in children with cerebral palsy did not yield good results. The Batchelor procedure, a modification of the Grice-Green subtalar arthrodesis, was not better. Subtalar arthrodesis by grafting cancellous bone and the use of metallic internal fixation also has been used. A retrospective study was done to compare the advantages of extra-articular with those of intra-articular subtalar arthrodesis in the treatment of children with valgus deformities.

The study population consisted of 7 patients with cerebral palsy, 10 patients with myelomeningocele, and 13 patients with agenesis of the corpus callosum associated with progressive polyneuropathy. The average age at operation was 6 years, and ranged from 4 to 10 years. The 30 patients underwent 3 different procedures in 51 affected feet, and 21 patients had bilateral procedures. A modified Grice-Green procedure was done on 14 feet, simultaneous Grice-Green and Batchelor procedures were done on 21 feet, and intra-articular subtalar fusion with a fibular bone graft was done on 16 feet.

After postoperative follow-up of 8 months to 11 years, results were rated excellent in 51% of the operated feet, satisfactory in 22%, and un-

TABLE 1.—Results With Subtalar Arthrodesis According to Pathology and Procedure

	FEET	SUCCESSFUL= EXCELLENT + SATISFACTORY	UNSATIS- FACTORY
ALL PATIENTS (30)	51	73%	27%
CEREBRAL PALSY	11	81%	19%
MYELOMENINGOCELE	14	61%	39%
AGENESIS CORPUS CALLOSUM	26	84%	16%
MODIFIED GRICE-GREEN	14	61%	39%
GRICE-GREEN BATCHELOR	21	84%	16%
INTRA-ARTICULAR FUSION	16	72%	28%

(Courtesy of Gallien R, Morin F, Marquis F: *J Pediatr Orthop* 9:59–63, January–February 1989.)

TABLE 2.—Subtalar Arthrodesis: Unsatisfactory Results According to Pathology and Procedure

	VARUS	VALGUS	NON UNION
MATERIAL (FEET)	7 (13%)	6 (11%)	10 (19%)
MYELOMENINGOCELE	1 (7%)	4 (28%)	4 (28%)
AGENESIS CORPUS CALLOSUM	4 (15%)	2 (8%)	6 (23%)
CEREBRAL PALSY	2 (18%)	0	0
MODIFIED GRICE-GREEN	0	4 (28%)	6 (33%)
GRICE-GREEN BATCHELOR	3 (14%)	1 (4%)	1 (4%)
INTRA-ARTICULAR FUSION	4 (25%)	1 (6%)	3 (18%)

(Courtesy of Gallien R, Morin F, Marquis F: *J Pediatr Orthop* 9:59–63, January–February 1989.)

satisfactory in 27% (Table 1). The modified Grice-Green procedure was successful in 61% of the feet and unsatisfactory in 39%. The combined Grice-Green-Batchelor procedure was successful in 84% of the feet and unsatisfactory in 16%. Intra-articular subtalar fusion yielded successful results in 72% of the feet and unsatisfactory results in 28%. Only 1 patient had wound dehiscence. No infections occurred.

Of the 3 procedures, the modified Grice-Green operation was the least successful, resulting in 4 instances of valgus and 6 nonunions (Table 2). The combined Grice-Green-Batchelor procedure gave the best results, as 96% of the cases had bony union. There were only 3 instances of varus deformity. One patient had both nonunion and valgus. Intra-articular subtalar arthrodesis led to varus in 4 patients, valgus in 2, and nonunion in 3. One patient had displacement of the fibular graft that needed reoperation.

Subtalar arthrodesis is considered a stabilizing, rather than a corrective, procedure. A flexible or passively corrected hindfoot is the most important prerequisite for a successful outcome. The bone or metallic block is used merely to maintain the corrected position. The Batchelor procedure, using a dowel bone block between the talus and calcaneum, combined with the Grice-Green procedure, using a bone block in the sinus tarsi, led to the best results.

▶ The Grice-Green procedure is a demanding one if undercorrection and overcorrection are to be avoided. In some feet the configuration of the calcaneus and talus may make it impossible to place the graft in a stable position with the hindfoot in a neutral abduction and adduction. By first immobilizing the subtalar joint with a Steinmann pin or a screw through the neck of the talus across the posterior facet and into the calcaneus with the hindfoot in neutral varus-valgus, the graft more easily can be inserted firmly across the sinus tarsi without overcorrection of the foot.—P.P. Griffin, M.D.

The Grice Extra-Articular Subtalar Arthrodesis in the Treatment of Spastic Hindfoot Valgus Deformity
Drvaric DM, Schmitt EW, Nakano JM (Emory Univ; Hall Orthopaedic Clinic, Grand Junction, Colo)
Dev Med Child Neurol 31:665–669, October 1989   1–24

Many reports have been made on the Grice extra-articular arthrodesis since it was originally described. However, most have centered on patients with valgus hindfoot secondary to poliomyelitis. The treatment of spastic hindfoot valgus with the Grice procedure, performed between 1965 and 1980, was evaluated in 102 feet in 60 patients.

Eighty-eight feet had heel-cord lengthening before subtalar arthrodesis, which usually was done 3 weeks or more before the arthrodesis. After the Grice procedure was performed, the feet were immobilized in a long-leg cast with knee extended, hindfoot in neutral or minimal valgus, and ankle dorsiflexed at 10–15 degrees. Postoperative immobilization consisted of either 6 weeks in a long-leg cast followed by 4–6 weeks in a short-leg cast, or 10–12 weeks in a non-weight-bearing long-leg cast. A result was judged to be satisfactory if the hindfoot was in a neutral position or with less than 5 degrees valgus on clinical examination and if an anteroposterior radiograph of the foot showed a talocalcaneal angle of 25–35 degrees. A result was satisfactory only if no clinical recurrence of deformity or varus occurred. If adequate correction was maintained, lack of radiographic evidence of bony union was not classified as unsatisfactory. Results in 96 feet in 54 patients were satisfactory. Four feet had nonunion of the graft, 3 of which occurred at the graft-calcaneus junction. All 4 of these patients maintained their alignment and did not need revision.

The extra-articular subtalar arthrodesis as described by Grice yields a high rate of satisfactory results in patients with hindfoot valgus secondary to spasticity. Performed correctly, the Grice technique effectively maintains proper alignment of the hindfoot, and the need for triple arthrodesis can be postponed indefinitely.

▶ The Grice-Green extra-articular subtalar arthrodesis is an operation that appears to be simple, but in reality is extremely demanding. Inserting a graft of the proper length and in the proper direction supports the talocalcaneus orientation to neutral or slight valgus. When done well it is a satisfactory procedure. The addition of internal fixation with a screw or a Steinmann pin placed across the talus and os calcis with the foot in the corrected position has improved the results from this procedure in cerebral palsy, in my experience.—P.P. Griffin, M.D.

Limb Lengthening

Femoral Lengthening in Children and Adolescents: A Comparative Study of a Series of 82 Cases
Pouliquen JC, Gorodischer S, Verneret C, Richard L (Hôpital Raymond Poincaré, Garches, France)
Fr J Orthop Surg 3:162–173, June 1989   1–25

Various methods have been advocated for femoral lengthening, but all have had associated complications. Results of 6 methods used in a succession of 82 cases in 71 children followed-up at least 1 year since 1972 were compared.

Immediate lengthening, used in 14 cases, was associated with a 35% rate of complications (table). Also carrying a significant number of serious complications were oblique division and gradual lengthening by the method of Judet, used in 20 cases; gradual lengthening with transverse osteotomy and routine bone grafting, used in 11 instances; the Wagner technique, undertaken in 13 cases; and the Ilizarov method, used in 4 instances. The best results were achieved with callus distraction (callotasis), performed by the method of de Bastiani and colleagues, which produced only 1 serious complication and only 10 instances of superficial pin track infection. The difference in the incidence of complications did not appear to be related to differences in age of the patient or cause of the lesion or to the need for repeated lengthenings.

The callotasis technique provides rapid union without many complications. Good results are attributable to deferment of lengthening for 10 to 15 days while the callus organizes, and then gradual lengthening of the callus based on its radiologic appearance.

▶ This article is another that supports the new biology of lengthening by a rate of distraction compatible with the callus "growing" longer. It also shows the

Infective and Bony Complications

Techniques	Periods	Complic. Vas.	Nerv.	Inf. Sup.	Deep	Non-union	Fract.	Duration of treat.	% of bone and inf. compl.
Immediate 14 cases	1975-84	0	1 (rec.)	0	1	0	4	4M	35 %
Oblique div. Judet 20 cases	1973-85	0	0	5	1†	1	4	5.2m*	30 %
Trans. div. + graft 11 cases	1974-84	0	0	4	0	1	2	6.2m*	27 %
Wagner 13 cases	1979-85	0	0	2	1	0	3	6.6m	31 %
Ilizarov 4 cases	1986-87	0	0	3	0	0	1	5.1m	25 %
Callotasis Verona techn. 20 cases	1986-87	0	0	10	0	0	1	4.9m	5 %
All techniques	1973-87	0	1 (rec.)	24	3	2	15		C.U : 20.5 % Inf : 3.6 %
82 cases				3.6 %		2.5 %	18 %		Tot : 24.1 %

Abbreviations: rec, recovery; *C.U.,* Complications of union; *Inf.,* Infection.
*Duration assessed on radiographs because of routine protection by a caliper.
†Septic arthritis complicating treatment of a fracture.
(Courtesy of Pouliquen JC, Gorodischer S, Verneret C, et al: *Fr J Orthop Surg* 3:162–173, June 1989.)

seriousness of choosing lengthening as a way of correcting limb length discrepancies. The incidence of serious complications was 24%. Lengthening still should be reserved for the patient's who would not be candidates for epiphysiodesis or limb shortening. I am afraid doctor ego too frequently is dictating the use of lengthening as a procedure of choice.—P.P. Griffin, M.D.

The Modified Wagner Method for Surgical Lengthening of the Limbs
Mastragostino S, Bagliani GP, Boero S, Formica C, Origo C (Istituto Scientifico Giannina Gaslini; Ospedale Regionale San Martino, Genova, Italy)
Ital J Orthop Traumatol 15:133–144, June 1989   1–26

The traditional Wagner method for limb lengthening in the correction of disharmonic dysmetria and hypometria has certain limitations and disadvantages, including the need for open osteotomy and multistage procedures. A modification of the traditional Wagner technique involves performing a corticotomy instead of the traditional osteotomy. The advantages of this modification are that it takes less time to perform, the risk of deep infections is decreased, and the continuity of the entire medullary canal is preserved, allowing more bone regeneration. The experience with the modified Wagner external fixation system at this institution since 1982 is evaluated.

During a 5-year period, 15 patients with hypometria, aged 12–20 years, and 25 patients with dysmetria, aged 11–24 years, underwent bone-lengthening procedures in 51 limbs, using the modified Wagner method. Achondroplasia and hypochondroplasia were the most common causes of hypometria, whereas congenital and traumatic etiologies were the most common causes of dysmetria. The extent of dysmetria ranged from 3 to 25 cm, with an average of 7.5 cm.

Limb length equalization was attained in 13 of the 25 patients with dysmetria, correction was incomplete in 7 patients, and 5 patients had overlengthening. Overlengthening in these 5 patients was performed as a precaution against recurrence. The growth cartilage was still open in all 5 patients. The consolidation time is defined as the period between the end of the lengthening procedure and the removal of instrumentation. Time to consolidation after femoral lengthening to correct dysmetria averaged 10 months and to correct hypometria averaged 11 months. In this series, only 1 patient with congenital dysmetria and 1 patient with hypometria underwent tibial lengthening. The average consolidation time after tibial lengthening in these 2 patients was 6 months. None of the patients had deep infection, and only 1 patient had delayed consolidation.

When used correctly, the Wagner external fixator associated with a modified operation in which open osteotomy is replaced with corticotomy achieves excellent results in patients who need femoral lengthening. The Ilizarov external fixation system is more effective in patients who need tibial lengthening.

▶ The corticotomy instead of the osteotomy and lengthening of 3 times a day of 1 mm per day resulted in sufficient callus to make the osteosyntheses plate unnecessary. Complications and problems associated with lengthening by other techniques occurred in these patients. Lengthening of an extremity is not a simple procedure, and in spite of the current wave of enthusiasm we must be selective in recommending lengthening and in the external fixator we choose. The most significant fact learned from Ilizarov is the importance of the rate of elongation of the callus.— P.P. Griffin, M.D.

Correction of Complicated Extremity Deformities by External Fixation
Grill F (Speising Hosp, Vienna)
Clin Orthop 241:166–176, April 1989   1–27

Orthofix and Ilizarov systems are external fixation devices that allow 3-dimensional fixation of fractures and osteotomies. Both systems can be used for compression, distraction, angular correction, full weight bearing, and bone-lengthening procedures, and indications for their use still are expanding. However, the use of external fixation in children has not been well reported.

During a 9.5-year period, external fixators were applied to 33 limb segments in 28 children, aged 3–19 years, with lower extremity deformities of different etiologies that had not improved with previous treatment. All except 6 deformities were congenital. External fixators were applied for an average of 20.7 weeks. The Wagner device was used in 6 cases of high iliac hip dislocation; the Orthofix system was used in 2 hips, 4 femurs, 12 tibias, and 2 feet; and the Ilizarov system was applied in 4 feet and 3 lower legs.

Of 22 limb deformities associated with length discrepancies in 19 patients, 2 had treatment with the Ilizarov fixator; 14 had the Orthofix fixator; and 6 had the Wagner fixator. Experience with these 3 fixation systems led to a clear preference for the Orthofix system. The Ilizarov distractor was preferred when different interventions at various points were done simultaneously.

Angular deformities in 11 limbs were corrected during or after the growth period with the Orthofix articulated dynamic axial fixator fitted with an articulated body and a T-clamp. In axial deviations of less than 20 degrees treated with callus distraction, use of a simple dynamic axial fixator without the articulated body proved sufficient. After a lengthening of about 2–3 cm, these axial deformities were corrected by closed manipulation with the unlocked fixator in situ. The average elongation gained in the treatment of axial limb deformities was 6.7 cm.

Of 4 patients with congenital or acquired pseudarthroses, only 1 patient having the Ilizarov method attained all therapeutic goals, which included bony union, correction of length discrepancy, cosmetically acceptable lower leg length, and normal foot function. Although bony union was also achieved in 3 Orthofix-treated limbs, the other treatment goals were not attained. Two patients with bilateral limb deformities, but no length discrepancies had good results with the Orthofix system. Three other patients with neglected clubfeet also were well corrected with the Ilizarov system.

The results obtained with Orthofix or Ilizarov external fixation systems in children with nontraumatic lower limb deformities show that even very severe lower-limb deformities can be treated successfully with dynamic external fixation.

▶ The use of the most satisfactory external fixator is important in terms of complications and enhancement of the goal of treatment. The versatility of the Ilizarov external fixator makes it preferable for complex and multiple deformities in the same limb. The Orthofix is effective in correcting axial deformities with or without a length discrepancy. I find that correcting the axial angulation at the time of the corticotomy followed by a 10- to 14-day delay before distraction begins is both simple and successful and equal to the results of gradual correction of the deformity.—P.P. Griffin, M.D.

Infection

The Value of Ultrasound in Acute Osteomyelitis
Dargouth M, Essadam H, Ben Hamida H, Kooli M, Gharbi HA, Hammou A, Bardi I (Hôpital Aziza Othmana; Hôpital d'Enfants, Tunis, Tunisia)
Fr J Orthop Surg 3:174–180, June 1989   1–28

In acute osteomyelitis, the organism travels through the blood stream and multiplies in the metaphysis of long bones. Although antibiotics have greatly altered the mortality associated with this disease, chronic lesions can develop when a subperiosteal abscess ruptures into the soft tissues. Forty-three cases in which ultrasound provided timely diagnosis and precise localization of the abscess were studied.

During a period of 2 years, 45 of 50 children with acute osteomyelitis had subperiosteal abscesses. Two had ruptured before hospital admission. Of the 43 patients with unruptured abscesses, 29 were boys and 14 were girls. The peak age for the condition was between 6 and 9 years. Abscesses appeared soon after the onset of clinical signs; 36 (85%) were discovered during the first week. In most cases (90%), the site was the lower limb, particularly the tibia (60%).

Ultrasound was performed daily on all aspects of the suspected limb. The limb was immobilized, and systemic antibiotic treatment was begun. In a comparison with normal bone, the abcess appeared as an enlargement of a transsonic band corresponding to the periosteum. The operation was performed as an emergency as soon as the subperiosteal abscess was diagnosed.

Rapid relief of pain followed surgery. The children were hospitalized for 3 weeks. Plaster mobilization continued for 45 to 90 days, and antibiotic treatment lasted for 45 to 120 days. Long-term follow-up available for 30 patients classified results as resolving (13), stabilizing (16), or chronic (1). Because of the high incidence of subperiosteal abscesses, ultrasound examination should be performed routinely and repeated daily for at least a week after the onset of clinical signs. Surgical treatment prevents the development of chronic lesions, allows early isolation of the organism, and ensures good penetration for the antibiotics.

▶ Ultrasound will show subperiosteal pus. I would prefer aspiration to obtain a culture and start antibiotics immediately; if no pus is obtained on aspiration but the clinical findings support the diagnosis of osteomyelitis, ultrasound may be a preferred way of secondarily evaluating the response of treatment. If pus is aspirated, surgical decompression should be done.— P.P. Griffin, M.D.

Technetium Phosphate Bone Scan in the Diagnosis of Septic Arthritis in Childhood
Sundberg SB, Savage JP, Foster BK (Adelaide Childrens Hosp, North Adelaide, Australia)
J Pediatr Orthop 9:579–585, September–October 1989

The differentiation of septic from nonseptic arthritis is often difficult. The reliability of technetium phosphate bone scanning in distinguishing these arthropathies and in differentiating pathologic disorders of adjacent bone from primary disorders of the joint was studied by reviewing technetium scans of 106 patients aged 2 weeks to 17 years who were suspected of having septic arthritis.

Blind interpretation of scans by strict grading of joint uptake correctly identified only 13% of cases of proved septic arthritis. Interpretation of scans made after review of pertinent clinical information was incorrect in 30% of cases. Septic arthritis was incorrectly identified in 32% of cases, with no evidence of joint sepsis.

Findings of increased activity around the joint on the blood pool and delayed phases of the scan and reduced activity of the head of the femur were not significantly different in children with and without infectious arthritis, and there was no specific correlation between findings on scanning and the occurrence or absence of septic arthropathy.

The value of technetium phosphate bone scanning in investigating suspected septic arthritis is limited, except for differentiating this disorder from osteomyelitis or for evaluating suspected multifocal involvement. Findings on scans are not specific and may be misleading. The diagnosis of joint sepsis should not be based on findings on technetium phosphate bone scans alone.

▶ The specificity of a technetium phosphate scan is low. It is not diagnostic of disease, but simply allows discovery of areas of increased blood flow and osteoblastic activity. It can demonstrate increased uptake in the bone adjacent to a swollen joint when there is osteomyelitis. This is its only value in evaluating a painful joint effusion and seldom should be used.— P.P. Griffin, M.D.

Trauma

Acetabular Fractures in Children and Adolescents
Heeg M, Klasen HJ, Visser JD (Univ Hosp, Groningen, The Netherlands)
J Bone Joint Surg [Br] 71-B:418–421, May 1989

Acetabular fractures in children and adults are rare. Although well described in adults, such fractures in children have received little attention. The long-term results after treatment of traumatic acetabular fractures in 27 children aged less than 17 were evaluated retrospectively.

Two children died immediately, and 2 could not be traced. Twenty-three patients with an average age of 13 years at the time of injury were available for evaluation. All patients had injury severity scores of 18 or more; 10 patients had associated limb fractures. Eighteen patients had conservative treatment, 4 patients underwent open reduction and internal fixation, and 1 had an arthrotomy to remove loose osteochondral fragments. Conservative treatment included bed rest and skeletal traction for an average of 4.2 weeks, followed by progressive weight-bearing. The average interval between fracture and full weight-bearing was 10.1 weeks. Postoperative treatment consisted of bed rest in suspended traction for 6 weeks, followed by progressive weight-bearing for 6 weeks, and full weight bearing after 3 months. Follow-up examination performed an average of 8 years after the accidents included clinical and radiographic evaluation.

Congruency at reduction was achieved in 20 of the 23 patients, all of whom had excellent or good functional results, but was not achieved in the other 3 patients (Table 1). Of these 3 patients, 1 had sustained a type 5 triradiate cartilage fracture with gross disruption, 1 had a comminuted transverse fracture with posterior dislocation of the hip, and 1 had a posterior column fracture that could not be reduced surgically. Good or excellent radiographic results were seen in 16 patients, in all of whom congruency had been attained (Table 2). Two patients with subluxation of the hip caused by a type 5 triradiate cartilage fracture and 1 patient with severe heterotopic calcification had poor radiographic outcomes. The remaining 4 patients had fair radiographic results. Eight patients had early

TABLE 1.—Functional Results in Relation to Congruency After Reduction

	Number	Congruent	Not Congruent
Excellent	19	19	–
Good	2	1	1
Fair			
Poor	2	–	2

(Courtesy of Heeg M, Klasen HJ, Visser JD: *J Bone Joint Surg* [Br] 71-B:418–421, May 1989.)

TABLE 2.—Radiographic Results at Least 3
Years After Injury, in Relation to Congruency

	Number	Congruent	Not Congruent
Excellent	11	11	–
Good	5	5	–
Fair	4	3	1
Poor	3	1	2

(Courtesy of Heeg M, Klasen HJ, Visser JD: *J Bone Joint Surg [Br]* 71-B:418–421, May 1989.)

complications, which resolved uneventfully. In 3 patients, late complications developed that required reoperation; 1 of these patients needed fusion of the involved hip.

Conservative treatment had good results in fractures with minimal initial displacement, stable posterior fracture dislocations, and Salter-Harris type 1 and type 2 triradiate cartilage fractures. Type 5 triradiate cartilage fractures and comminuted fractures did not respond as well to conservative treatment, but operative treatment did not improve outcomes.

▶ A congruent reduction and continued growth of the triradiate cartilage are necessary for good long-term results of acetabular fractures in children. When the 2 criteria are met, a good result can be expected. Most fractures can be treated conservatively. One can do nothing to prevent a Salter-Harris type V injury from early closure, which if it occurs will prevent further acetabular development and cause subluxation of the hip. Primary operative treatment is not recommended by these authors. However, if the acetabular dome is not reduced, particularly posteriorly, subluxation may occur and late arthritis is inevitable. For these reasons, I would advise operative reduction in selected cases.—P.P. Griffin, M.D.

Management of Femoral Shaft Fractures in the Adolescent
Herndon WA, Mahnken RF, Yngve DA, Sullivan JA (Univ of Oklahoma, Oklahoma City)
J Pediatr Orthop 9:29–32, January–February 1989

The management of femoral shaft fractures in adolescents is controversial. Intramedullary fixation has been advocated for femur fractures in adolescents with head injury, multiple trauma, and failure of closed methods and in the treatment of midshaft fractures in boys nearing skeletal maturity. Other authors, however, prefer closed treatment. One recent experience with the management of femur fractures in adolescents was evaluated.

Forty-four patients with 45 fractures with open physes were treated at

1 center. The patients were aged 11–16 years. In 24 fractures having nonoperative treatment, 7 malunions occurred; none of the 21 fractures treated with intramedullary nailing had malunion. Length of hospital stay was significantly shorter for the patients having surgery. The surgical group had no premature growth arrest or infections.

Closed intramedullary nailing is the preferred treatment for virtually all femoral shaft fractures in adolescents. This procedure results in a significant decrease in the incidence of malunion and in length of hospitalization. It seems to be safe, with a low incidence of complications when done by a surgeon comfortable with closed intramedullary techniques.

▶ All treatment methods have 2 major arms that affect outcome. One is inherent to the method and its limitations; the other is dependent on the expertise in using the method. Intramedullary immobilization of femoral fracture shortens hospital stay and rehabilitation time for the adolescent. In the child aged less than 11 or 12 years the residual cartilage on the superior femoral neck that contributes to the appositional growth of the neck can be injured sufficiently to cause narrowing at the base of the neck. The closed intramedullary nailing of the femur is the procedure of choice in the adolescent, but if traction is to be used, close attention to the appropriate forces for correction of alignment is necessary and usually can be successful in preventing significant nonunion.— P.P. Griffin, M.D.

Physeal Arrest About the Knee Associated With Non-Physeal Fractures in the Lower Extremity
Hresko MT, Kasser JR (Children's Hosp Med Ctr, Boston; Univ of Massachusetts, Worcester)
J Bone Joint Surg [Am] 71-A:698–703, June 1989   1–32

Children and adolescents commonly fracture long bones, but few studies have reported on concurrent epiphyseal fractures about the knee. Growth arrest subsequent to long bone fractures has been attributed to treatment, but little is known about the condition of the physis at the time of the initial injury. The case reports of 7 children, aged 11–14 years, who were seen because of a physeal arrest about the knee associated with previous nonphyseal fractures of the lower extremity were studied. The time between the original injury and physeal arrest ranged from 1 to 3 years.

Five patients had an anterior arrest of the proximal tibial physis, and 2 patients had posterolateral arrest of the distal femoral physis. At the time of the initial injury, there was no clinical evidence of a knee injury. Five of the 7 long bone fractures had been caused by a severe traumatic event, 1 had been caused by a fall on ice, and 1 fracture had been incurred through a unicameral bone cyst after a fall. Three patients had had traction as treatment. In 2 of these patients, the traction pin was not placed in the bone that eventually had the physeal arrest. In the third patient, a traction pin initially had been placed in the proximal part of the tibia in anticipation of later intramedullary fixation of the femoral fracture. However, 3 days later, the pin was moved to a distal femoral location. All 7 patients wore casts for periods ranging from 6 weeks to 3 months. A hip-spica cast was used in patients with femoral fractures, and a long cast was used for tibial fractures. The anterior arrest of the proximal tibial physis came after a femoral fracture in 4 patients and a tibial fracture plus a fibular diaphyseal fracture in 1 patient. The 2 distal femoral arrests came after a femoral fracture in 1 patient and a tibial fracture plus a fibular fracture in the other patient. A retrospective review of the radiographs taken at the time of injury revealed an avulsion fracture at the posterolateral corner of the distal femoral physis. No iatrogenic physeal injuries were identified in any of the 7 patients.

In children, trauma to the knee concomitant with femoral or tibial fractures may well be overlooked. Therefore, a thorough clinical and radiographic examination of the knee is recommended for all patients who are seen with traumatic injury to a lower extremity, even if the most apparent injury is proximal or distal to the knee.

▶ As many as 10% of femoral fractrures in children are associated with inhibition of growth. I believe this is the result of an occult compression (Salter 5) injury to the physis.— P.P. Griffin, M.D.

Nonunion of Slightly Displaced Fractures of the Lateral Humeral Condyle in Children: An Update
Flynn JC (Orlando Regional Med Ctr, Orlando, Fla)
J Pediatr Orthop 9:691–696, November–December 1989

Slightly displaced fractures of the lateral humeral condyle in children result in nonunion if treated inadequately. Controversy exists on the management of these cases of nonunion. To determine the need for intervention and the best method of treatment, 23 cases of nonunion of the lateral condyle were studied.

The patient group consisted of 1 adult aged 24 years and 22 children aged between 18 months and 12 years. Inadequate treatment was the most common cause of nonunion. Some fractures may not be detected on radiograph. The fracture may be displaced in the cast, or the cast may be removed too soon. In this series, 8 children had no treatment. Fifteen elbows were casted or reduced and casted, although 3 should have been treated with opening and pinning.

The condylar fragment was united with bone grafting and pinning in 11 cases. At follow-up, 5 patients who have reached skeletal maturity and 6 who still are growing have satisfactory function and no significant deformity in the elbow. Union was also achieved in 3 patients who underwent graft and internal fixation, even though salvage procedures were performed too late to take advantage of the growth potential of the fragment.

Successful treatment of nonunion is dependent on the position of the distal fragment, which should not be rotated or displaced too much. Treatment done when the fragment is in a poor position may result in aseptic necrosis and degenerative arthritis. Another prerequisite for successful treatment is an open growth plate of the distal fragment. Early treatment is desirable. With delay, the physis of the condylar fragment will close prematurely and the elbow may not be salvaged.

▶ Symptoms from nonunion of the lateral condyle may range from none to a severe cubitus valgus and ulna neuropathy. Treatment of nonunion should be individualized according to duration, presence of pain, which is rare, the position of the fragment, and the amount of valgus. The radius and ulna adapt to the position of the lateral fragment; when nonunion has been present more than a year, efforts to change the position of the condyle may result in loss of motion. Osteosyntheses in situ is preferable. As in this study, diagnosis and failure to evaluate progression of healing and inadequate treatment all contribute to the incidence of nonunion. For a child with a swollen elbow, radiographs of the distal humerus and the proximal radius should be made rather than an anteroposterior view of the flexed elbow, which frequently will fail to show a fracture of the lateral condyle.—P.P. Griffin, M.D.

Assessment of a Treatment Plan for Managing Acute Vascular Complications Associated With Supracondylar Fractures of the Humerus in Children
Clement DA (Queen's Med Ctr, Nottingham, England)
J Pediatr Orthop 10:97–100, January 1990   1–34

Ischemic contracture of the forearm is a rare but disabling complication of supracondylar fractures of the humerus in children. Assessing the effectiveness of treatment is difficult in a condition seen so rarely. Researchers identified the site and cause of vascular lesions in 9 children and evaluated the outcome of treatment.

In all cases the diagnosis of vascular compromise was determined on the basis of changes in skin color, tenderness, and induration of the musculature of the forearm; pain on passive extension of the fingers; and absence of a radial pulse. All patients had some degree of sensory disturbance. Ischemia did not improve after manipulation of fractures with patients under general anesthesia, and the surgeon explored the antecubital fossa. Several different procedures were used to restore flow and reestablish adequate perfusion in the distal limb.

Wound healing by primary intention was achieved without complication in all cases. Scars were noticeable. Two children had unsatisfactory functional results because of residual deformity, but both had full range of motion. All 9 patients regained full active and passive movements of the fingers, thumb, and wrist, and all had normal distal pulses. One patient had slight, nondisabling numbness in the tip of the index finger. No patients had wasting of the forearm. Grip strength in the injured limb was >85% of that in the normal limb.

Prompt treatment to restore circulation and to control or monitor compartment pressure is essential in these cases. Management by exploration of the antecubital fossa and flexor compartment fasciotomy is recommended.

▶ The diagnosis of vascular compromise of the forearm and hand was determined solely on the clinical signs of impending Volkmann's contracture. There were no disrupted arteries or intimal tears recognized. In my opinion, injury of the brachial artery at the elbow seldom results in compartment ischemia unless there is venous obstruction. In 1 patient the brachial artery was divided and ligated and the radial pulse returned in 48 hours; I have also experienced this. Although the patients in this series did well, the forearm fasciotomy was not adequate to assure complete decompression. I believe that if there is a vascular compromise of the forearm and hand on clinical grounds it is desirable to have it confirmed by pressure measurements; if the brachial artery is to be explored, the forearm should be decompressed in its entirety.—P.P. Griffin, M.D.

The Triceps-Dividing Approach to Open Reduction of Complex Distal Humeral Fractures in Adolescents: A Cybex Evaluation of Triceps Function and Motion .
Kasser JR, Richards K, Millis M (Children's Hosp, Boston)
J Pediatr Orthop 10:93–96, January 1989   1–35

Intercondylar and comminuted condylar fractures rarely occur in children, and few recommendations have been made for their treatment. Researchers evaluated such fractures after treatment with open reduction, internal fixation with early motion, and prompt removal of hardware. Triceps function and elbow motion were assessed in 9 elbows in 8 patients with distal humeral fractures treated with open reduction and internal fixation by a triceps-dividing approach. Patients' ages at the time of fracture ranged from 10 to 20 years. Follow-up ranged from 1 year to 5 years.

At the 3-year 6-month follow-up, the patients had an average flexion–extension of 136 degrees to −6 degrees. Cybex testing revealed a slight decrease in triceps peak torque, showing a deficit of 6% at 60 degrees per second, 3% at 120 degrees per second, and 3% at 180 degrees per second.

Triceps division in children apparently does not cause significant muscle dysfunction. Open reduction through division of the triceps yields good results in children with complex distal humeral fractures. With this method, olecranon osteotomy is unnecessary.

▶ The approach described is excellent for exposure of complex fractures of the distal humerus. It heals well without significant weakness and should be the preferred approach to the elbow for open reduction of multiple-part fractures.— P.P. Griffin, M.D.

2 Trauma

Introduction

Literature on trauma, wound and fracture healing, and amputation has been extensive and generally of high quality in 1989. Choosing articles to abstract became progressively more difficult, and many meritorious papers are mentioned only in references. Each year has its own topic of special focus, and 1989 was the year of the distal radius or Colles' fracture, which is the first of several topics that are discussed.

"Fracture care," the mainstay of a general orthopedic practice, comprises approximately 80% of all orthopedic injuries. These injuries are different from high-energy fractures that involve multiple-system injuries, which are designated to the subspecialty of "orthopedic traumatology." Most papers can be separated easily into one group or the other because traumatology papers now usually originate in trauma centers. Fracture care and traumatology are the second and third topics discussed.

The Ilizarov technique continues to be a topic of interest. Its indications and ramifications are discussed from different points of view in several different sections.

The rest of the sections in this chapter discuss stimulation of the healing response, complications and their management, amputation, and musculoskeletal imaging.

Sigvard T. Hansen, Jr., M.D.

Colles' Fractures

The Unstable Colles' Fracture
Jenkins NH (Univ of Wales, Cardiff)
J Hand Surg [Br] 14B:149–154, May 1989   2–1

Malunion is a common complication of the displaced Colles' fracture. To determine which radiographic features might dispose to malunion, 115 Colles' fractures were classified (Fig 2–1) and followed prospectively.

Radiographs allowing assessment of the dorsal angle of the radius, the radial shortening, and the flattening of the radial angle were obtained at presentation, after reduction, and at fracture union. Fractures were classified according to the systems of Gartland and Werley (Table 1), Lidström (Table 2), Older et al (Table 3), and Frykman (Table 4). Fractures were also classified on the basis of comminution (Table 5, Fig 2–2).

The fracture's position at union was correlated significantly with the extent of its initial displacement. Chronic instability in these fractures led

50 / Orthopedics

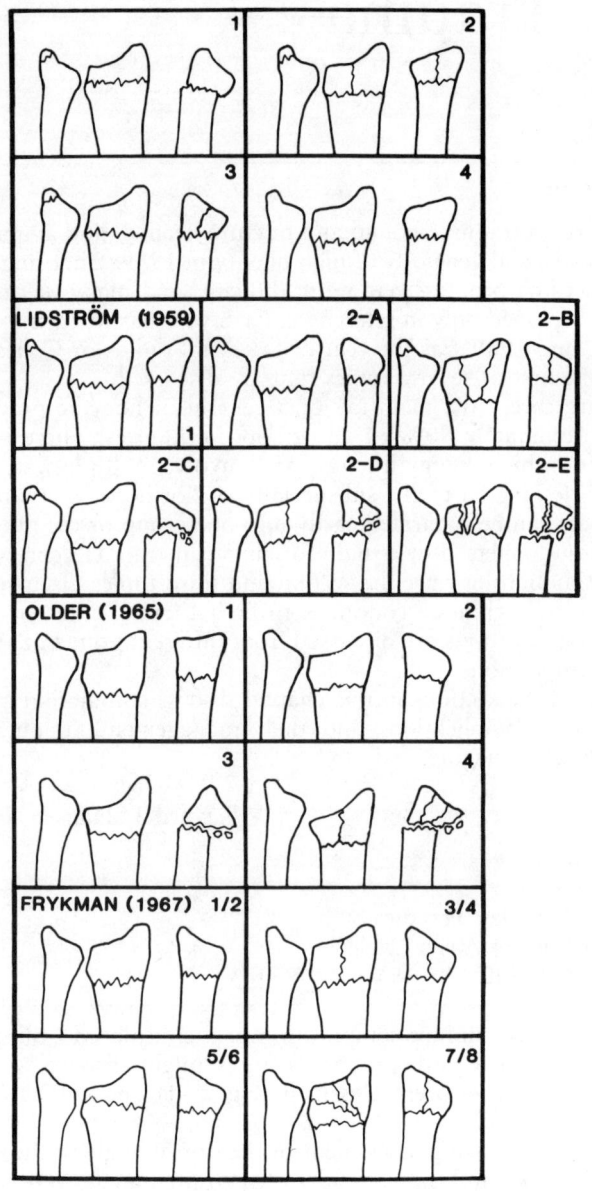

Fig 2–1.—Some classifications of Colles' fractures. (Courtesy of Jenkins NH: *J Hand Surg [Br]* 14B:149–154, May 1989.)

TABLE 1.—Classification of Gartland and Werley (1951)

Group 1	Extra-articular, displaced.
Group 2	Intra-articular, undisplaced.
Group 3	Intra-articular, displaced.
Group 4	Extra-articular, undisplaced (added for completeness by Solgaard, 1985).

Note: based on the presence, but not the extent, of displacement and radiocarpal involvement.
(Courtesy of Jenkins NH: *J Hand Surg [Br]* 14B:149–154, May 1989.)

TABLE 2.—Classification of Lidström (1959)

Group 1	Undisplaced.
Group 2a	Dorsal angulation, extra-articular.
Group 2b	Dorsal angulation, intra-articular but without gross separation of fragments.
Group 2c	Dorsal angulation plus dorsal displacement, extra-articular.
Group 2d	Dorsal angulation plus dorsal displacement, intra-articular but without gross separation of fragments.
Group 2e	Dorsal angulation plus dorsal displacement, intra-articular with separation of fragments.

Note: based on the presence, but not the extent, of displacement (dorsal angle and dorsal displacement), articular involvement, and comminution.
(Courtesy of Jenkins NH: *J Hand Surg [Br]* 14B:149–154, May 1989.)

TABLE 3.—Classification of Older et al (1965)

Group 1	"Non-displaced"—up to 5° dorsal angulation, radial articular surface at least 2 mm above ulnar head.
Group 2	"Displaced with minimal comminution"—dorsal angulation or displacement, radial articular surface no lower than 3 mm below ulnar head, minimal comminution of dorsal radius.
Group 3	"Displaced with comminution of dorsal radius"—comminution of dorsal radius: Radial articular surface below ulnar head; Minimal comminution of distal fragment.
Group 4	"Displaced with severe comminution of radial head"—marked comminution of dorsal and distal radius; Radial articular surface 2—8 mm below ulnar head.

Note: based on the extent of displacement (dorsal angle and radial shortening) and the presence of comminution.
(Courtesy of Jenkins NH: *J Hand Surg [Br]* 14B:149–154, May 1989.)

TABLE 4.—Classification of Frykman (1967)

Groups 1 and 2	Extra-articular.
Groups 3 and 4	Involve radio-carpal joint.
Groups 5 and 6	Involve distal radio-ulnar joint.
Groups 7 and 8	Involve both radio-carpal and distal radio-ulnar joints.
Groups 1, 3, 5	Have an intact ulnar styloid.
Groups 2, 4, 6 and 8	Have a fractured ulnar styloid.

Note: based on the pattern of intra-articular involvement.
(Courtesy of Jenkins NH: J Hand Surg [Br] 14B:149–154, May 1989.)

to a mean increase of 8.22 degrees dorsal angulation, a mean loss of 5.61 degrees radial angle, and 3.26 mm radial shortening.

Colles' fractures usually are radiographed about 1 week after injury and manipulated again if acute loss of position is found. Nevertheless, 95% of these fractures subsequently lost some of their position despite stability at 1 week. This late deterioration illustrates the chronic instability of the Colles' fracture. Malunion occurs regularly in most fractures in which dorsal comminution has occurred. Fractures resistant to malunion in dorsal angulation can be distinguished at radiography by an intact dorsal radial cortex. Articular involvement has no effect on the development of malunion.

▶ This excellent paper follows 115 Colles' fractures prospectively, which is a somewhat unusual approach. It reminds us of something that experienced fracture surgeons already know, that is, that most Colles' fractures gradually lose position during the 4- to 6-week healing period in casts and return to the position of dorsal angulation that was determined by the original deformity. The authors call this a "chronic instability" of Colles' fracture. They point out that comminution of the dorsal radial cortex, which occurred in 78% of their cases, predicts a gradual return to radial shortening and dorsal radial tilt. They also point out that remanipulating the fracture 1 or 2 weeks after the injury is not

TABLE 5.—A Classification Based Entirely on Comminution

Group 1	No radiographically visible comminution.
Group 2	Comminution of the dorsal radial cortex without comminution of the fracture fragment.
Group 3	Comminution of the fracture fragment without significant involvement of the dorsal cortex.
Group 4	Comminution of both the distal fragment and the dorsal cortex. As the fracture line involves the distal fracture fragment in Groups 3 and 4, intra-articular involvement is very common within these groups. Such involvement is not, however, inevitable and nor does it affect the fracture's placement within the classification.

(Courtesy of Jenkins NH: J Hand Surg [Br] 14B:149–154, May 1989.)

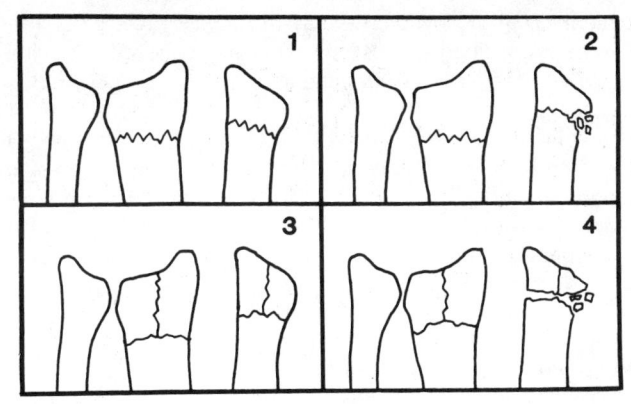

Fig 2–2.—A classification of Colles' fractures based entirely on comminution. (Courtesy of Jenkins NH: *J Hand Surg [Br]* 14B:149–154, May 1989.)

particularly helpful. This paper sets the tone for more specific discussions of the problem that follow.— S.T. Hansen, Jr., M.D.

Algodystrophy Following Colles' Fracture

Atkins RM, Duckworth T, Kanis JA (Royal Hallamshire Hosp, Sheffield, England)
J Hand Surg [Br] 14B:161–164, May 1989   2–2

Estimates of the incidence of algodystrophy after Colles' fracture have ranged from 2% to 29%. Because the syndrome is ill defined and its cause unknown, some studies may have missed transient forms of the disorder. In 109 unselected patients with Colles' fracture evidence of any of the 10 features commonly associated with algodystrophy was sought.

The mean age of the patients was 66 years, and 93 were women. Symptoms of the disorder, which is characterized by residual abnormalities at sites distant from the fracture itself, include pain and tenderness, vasomotor and sudomotor instability, swelling and dystrophy, and impairment of joint mobility. At 9-week follow-up, most (82) had no evidence of algodystrophy. Twenty-seven patients had more than 1 feature of the syndrome. If they were considered to have algodystrophy, its prevalence at 9 weeks after fracture was 24.8%.

Of the 72 patients without signs of algodystrophy who were available for study at 6 months, none had symptoms of the disorder. Twelve of 19 affected patients seen at 6 months still had evidence of instability, swelling, or stiffness. Algodystrophy appears to be fairly common after Colles' fracture, although it is a transient disorder in most patients.

▶ "Algodystrophy," a new term for me, is known more commonly as reflex sympathetic dystrophy syndrome or Sudeck's atrophy. We are beginning to recognize the many manifestations and variations of this dystrophy. This paper notes 10 features that commonly are associated with this problem, but points out that patients with this syndrome may manifest as few as 2. These symptoms can involve the fingers, wrist, or shoulder of the affected limb. By the 9-week follow-up, only 25% of the patients manifested any symptoms of this syndrome, and the syndrome developed in no new patients later. Nearly one third of those affected had resolution of all symptoms by 6 months. The paper offers no recommendations about how to treat this disorder, but simply brings to our attention that our usual method of treating Colles' fractures has a significant early incidence of algodystrophy. This disorder needs considerably more study and eventually should be correlated with treatment.—S.T. Hansen, Jr., M.D.

Carpal Malalignment in Colles' Fractures
Bickerstaff DR, Bell MJ (Royal Hallamshire Hosp, Sheffield, England)
J Hand Surg [Br] 14B:155–160, May 1989   2–3

The Colles' fracture is associated with significant morbidity. One study of more than 2,000 patients found that the average permanent loss of function was 24%. Although previous research has attributed disability after Colles' fracture to variations in the distal radius, changes in carpal alignment contributed to poor functional result.

Thirty-two patients (mean age, 63 years) were evaluated 1 year after they had sustained a Colles' fracture. All cases had been treated with standard methods. Function and carpal alignment was assessed both clinically and radiographically. X-ray films of the fractured wrists were compared with those of the normal wrists. Radiologic parameters were correlated with a functional score.

Except for the scapholunate gap, the difference between the injured and uninjured wrists was highly significant. The degree of carpal alignment as measured by the radial tilt and the radiolunate, lunate-capitate, and scapholunate angles was the most significant indicator of a poor result. Radiographic features before treatment were not predictive of the final outcome.

Carpal instability appears to be a response of the carpus to the altered mechanics caused by malunion with dorsal radial tilt. As this tilt increases, the carpus adopts the dorsal instability pattern to realign the hand upon the forearm. This abnormal position then may become fixed.

▶ An interesting new analysis of late disability that appears after a Colles' fracture is offered. The authors first referenced a significant body of literature, which confirms a high rate of disability from this injury. Then they carefully compared the injured and uninjured wrists of 32 patients for changes in dorsal radial tilt, which was previously identified as a major cause of carpal instability in Colles'-type fractures. They determined that carpal malalignment is probably a secondary complication of distal radial malalignment and is not caused by the original injury. By avoiding dorsal instability during management of the original fracture, we should be able to prevent later carpal malalignment and any related disability.—S.T. Hansen, Jr., M.D.

Plaster Cast Versus External Fixation for Unstable Intraarticular Colles' Fractures
Kongsholm J, Olerud C (Solleftea Hosp, Solleftea, Sweden; Univ Hosp, Uppsala, Sweden)
Clin Orthop 241:57–65, April 1989   2–4

Traditional closed reduction and plaster splinting were compared with primary external fixation for the stabilization of comminuted intra-articular Colles' fractures. A total of 75 consecutive patients with Frykman type VIII fractures of the distal forearm treated with primary external fixation were compared with 32 control patients who sustained similar injuries and were treated by closed reduction and cast immobilization. The mean age of the study group was 58.3 years, and the mean age of the control group was 63.8 years.

The study patients underwent anesthesia or brachial block, and the external fixators were applied in the operating room. Just distal to its midpoint, 2 pins were driven into the radial diaphysis, and 2 pins were introduced from the radial side into the diaphysis of the second metacarpal. Both sites were exposed operatively before pin insertion to avoid tendon and nerve injuries and to assure good pin placement. The fixators were removed after 5 weeks. The control group received local anesthesia, and the fracture was reduced and splinted. After 10 days, patients with displaced fractures were offered rereduction. Splintage was maintained for 5 weeks. The patients stabilized with an external fixator had maintained their reduced positions, but a significant loss of reduction had occurred in the traditionally treated group at the 10-day examination. One third of

Results at Follow-Up Examination

Variable*	External fixation	Casts
Functional outcome		
Excellent	44	1
Good	17	7
Fair	6	11
Poor	1	6
Loss of range of motion		
Pronation/supination	6.0°	16.2°
Extension/flexion	9.2°	21.0°
Grip strength		
Healed in acceptable position	90%	65%
	88%	12%
Union of ulnar styloid	66%	38%

*Differences between the operative group and the conservatively treated group are highly significant ($P < .001$) for the first 4 variables, and significant ($P < .05$) for the final variable (union of ulnar styloid).
(Courtesy of Kongsholm J, Olerud C: Clin Orthop 241:57–65, April 1989.)

the control group was rereduced, and the overall results were worse than those at 10 days. Follow-up evaluation revealed that 15 of 31 fractures had redisplaced enough at 10 days to merit rereduction; 88% of the control group and 12% of the fractures treated with external fixation healed in a displaced position (table).

Most of the patients having external fixation had good or excellent functional outcomes. Injury-related complications included 4 shoulder-hand syndromes, 6 radial nerve irritations, and 4 pin infections. Significantly better anatomical and functional results were achieved with primary external fixation than with closed reduction and casting.

▶ Having set the stage by demonstrating the poor prognosis of distal radial fractures with the previous 3 papers, we now look at the first of several papers that describes treatment. External fixation has long been a recommended alternative to casting for distal radius fractures. Although this study is not prospective, it reiterates a point that was made in previous years: that open placement of pins in the radius and in the second metacarpal is necessary to avoid impaled nerves and other complications. All the major advantages of adequate external fixation are mentioned. External fixation is shown to be more effective than casting for maintaining satisfactory alignment because the radial length and volar angle tend to return slowly to the original fracture position when treated with casting.

The authors do not mention 2 areas of concern with external fixation that are mentioned in other studies of external fixation: a significant problem with late collapse and stiffness. They do mention the standard complications associated with external fixation, including nerve injury and pin tract infection. All the fractures in this study were classified as Frykman type VIII fractures of the distal forearm (comminuted intra-articular fractures). It is interesting that the authors removed the external fixator at 5 weeks but did not notice any collapse. This relatively short immobilization perhaps was the reason that they saw no more stiffness than was noted. They have subsequently extended the indications for using external fixation to include distal radius fractures that do not involve the intra-articular surface.—S.T. Hansen, Jr., M.D.

Treatment of Unstable Colles' Fractures by External Fixation
Riis J, Fruensgaard S (Horsens Hosp, Horsens, Denmark)
J Hand Surg [Br] 14B:145-148, May 1989   2-5

Simple fractures of the distal part of the radius usually present no problem, but badly comminuted or intra-articular fractures often have poor outcomes. Various methods of treatment have been proposed, with varying degrees of success. The outcome was evaluated in 26 patients who underwent external fixation with the Hoffmann apparatus.

The average age was 55 years, and 15 patients were women. Follow-up, for an average of 29 months, was possible in 19 patients. Most of the fractures resulted from falls on the outstretched hand and were classified as types VII and VIII. External fixation was chosen when a fracture could not be reduced to an acceptable position, or when a primarily reduced fracture later caused an unacceptable loss of radial length or angulation. Exercise was started as soon as possible, and the external fixator was removed an average of 41 days after surgery.

Anatomical results were judged to be excellent or good in 85% of the patients, indicating that the external fixator was effective in immobilizing the fracture. The remaining results were fair (10%) or poor (5%). Many patients had diminished extension and flexion and limited wrist motion. Three of 14 complications were classified as major. No deep infections occurred.

In this patient group the best results were obtained when the external fixation device was applied within a few days of the injury. Although the method studied here is effective for fractures of types VII and VIII, it is not recommended as routine treatment.

▶ The second paper on external fixation is also from Scandinavia, this time from Denmark. The authors report a 6-year follow-up of 26 patients with unstable comminuted fractures of the distal radius, but include both comminuted metaphyseal fractures and intra-articular fractures in this study. They applied external fixation only to those fractures that they could not reduce or hold in an acceptable position and did not perform open pin placement. They immobilized the patients' wrists for an average of 6 weeks and reported 85% good or excellent results, although they found a significant incidence of stiffness in the wrists. Because of their method of selecting patients, a longer interval usually elapsed between fracture and application of the fixation. The most important point the authors noted was that when less time elapsed between injury and placement of the external fixation device, a better functional result was obtained. This may explain the apparently better results that were reported in the previous paper, in which selected patients were put into a fixator immediately.—S.T. Hansen, Jr., M.D.

Ligamentotaxis and Bone Grafting for Comminuted Fractures of the Distal Radius
Leung KS, Shen WY, Leung PC, Kinnimonth AWG, Chang JCW, Chan GPY (Prince of Wales Hosp, Hong Kong)
J Bone Joint Surg [Br] 71-B:838–842, November 1989   2–6

Conventional treatment of comminuted fractures of the distal radius is unsatisfactory. In a prospective study, a combination of ligamentotaxis and primary cancellous bone grafting was employed as a uniform method of treatment for 72 patients with comminuted fractures of the distal radius. Average follow-up was 11 months (range, 7–40 months).

Technique.—After application of a half-frame Hoffmann external fixator, the fracture is reduced by distraction and manipulation under fluoroscopic control. With a short longitudinal incision at the dorsum of the wrist, the fracture site is exposed and packed with cancellous bone chips. The pins and external fixator are removed at 3 weeks. A carefully monitored program of rehabilitation is begun, and full wrist mobilization is allowed at 6 weeks.

Reduction was maintained during healing, with nearly normal angles of volar tilt and only a very small loss of radial articular angle (mean, 2.2 degrees). More than 80% of patients regained good ranges of movement of wrists and forearms, with strong and pain-free wrist function. All patients obtained normal active hand movements. There were no serious pin-track infections or donor site complications.

The combination of distraction, external fixation, and bone grafting is a simple and excellent method of treating comminuted fractures of the distal radius. The method is recommended for all comminuted fractures of the distal radius except those in elderly patients and those in patients in whom a perfect closed reduction can be obtained.

▶ The third paper concerning external fixation is from Hong Kong. Yet again, the authors applied external fixation because they observed that comminuted Colles' fractures treated conservatively in casts resulted in chronic dysfunction. They stressed the principle of ligamentotaxis, or reducing the metaphyseal and articular fragments by applying tension on the capsule and the ligaments. They kept the external fixator in place for only 3 weeks and found that the reduction could then be maintained during an aggressive rehabilitation program.

A slightly higher rate of return to full range of motion and pain-free wrist function than that in the 2 previous papers was reported. The major difference in the treatment method was grafting of the metaphyseal defect produced by the distraction, which of course accounts for the earlier union. Also, during the rehabilitation phase, the authors used a brace that limited extension but allowed flexion so that the fixator could be removed earlier to begin early motion without displacing the fracture. This treatment program incorporates all the recommendations for using external fixators and reports the lowest incidence of complications because fixation is applied only for a short period. It is the most aggressive treatment program that currently is recommended in the literature, and appears to be giving the best results.—S.T. Hansen, Jr., M.D.

▶ This series of papers seems to indicate that we should be considerably more aggressive in treating Colles' fractures that cannot be reduced in an anatomical and stable manner in all but elderly or osteoporotic patients. This rule certainly fits with my own prejudice. Precise pin-placement technique, an open approach to avoid nerves, and a bone graft to shorten the period of external fixation and ensure solid union seem to be the future course of treating Colles' fractures.—S.T. Hansen, Jr., M.D.

Several other papers on this topic also make worthwhile reading:

References

1. Meléndez EM, et al: *J Hand Surg [Am]* 14-A:807, 1989.
2. Solgaard S: *Acta Orthop Scand* 60:387, 1989.
3. Howard PW, et al: *J Bone Joint Surg [Br]* 71-B:68, 1989.
4. Bennett GL, et al: *Orthop Rev* 18:210, 1989.

Fracture Care

Trimalleolar Fractures: Late Results After Fixation of the Posterior Fragment
Heim UFA (Kreuzspital, Chur, Switzerland)
Orthopedics 12:1053–1059, August 1989   2–7

For 20 years, internal fixation and functional posttreatment of displaced malleolar fractures generally have been accepted. Additional injury involving the posterolateral tibial fragment may influence the position and stability of the fibula itself. Open reduction with internal fixation is recommended. From 1969 to 1982, 60 trimalleolar fractures were operated on with fixation of the posterior fragment. A late follow-up (average, 8 years) including radiographs was possible in 45 patients.

The patients were evaluated by radiographic records and clinical examination. The average patient age at the time of the injury was 50 years. About half of the fragments had been judged large and half as small or probably small. No early complications occurred. At periods ranging from 2 years 4 months to 5 years 10 months, 4 patients showed severe arthrosis, which was a result of technical errors; correctly stabilized posterior fragments do not lead to arthrosis. Later follow-up revealed that 35 patients regained full function, had no pain, and were in radiologic stage 0 or 1. Age had no effect on the development of arthrosis. The screw technique from the dorsal approach gave better results than the indirect technique especially when small fragments and depressions were present. Dislocation of the talus and depressed areas in the articular surface were associated with a worse prognosis.

▶ Recent literature on ankle fractures indicates that a trimalleolar fracture has a significantly worse prognosis than a simple bimalleolar ankle fracture, even when the posterior fragment is small. This paper reports a 12-year documentation of trimalleolar fractures with an average 8-year follow-up. Most of the fractures were managed with operative fixation of the posterior fragment. Heim not only indicates that anatomical stable fixation improves results, but also illustrates both direct and indirect stabilization techniques. He concludes that an anatomically stabilized posterior fragment will decrease significantly or preclude arthrosis, which frequently occurs when anatomical stabilization is not done. My experience indicates that this is a valid conclusion.

Another reference that strongly backs Heim's conclusions is by Jaskulka (1).—S.T. Hansen, Jr., M.D.

Reference

1. Jaskulka RA, et al: *J Trauma* 29:1565, 1989.

Unrecognized Injuries of the Lateral Ligaments Associated With Lateral Malleolar Fractures of the Ankle
Whitelaw GP, Sawka MW, Wetzler M, Segal D, Miller J (Boston City Hosp)
J Bone Joint Surg [Am] 71-A:1396–1399, October 1989   2–8

Four patients who had lateral malleolar fractures between May 1985 and November 1987 were found to have damaged lateral ligaments when the ankles were stressed to test for stability at internal fixation of the fractures. The torn ligaments were repaired with absorbable suture after completion of internal fixation.

Three patients were followed for 9, 12, and 15 months, and none had test results positive for instability of the ankle. At most recent follow-up all 3 had returned to their previous employment and level of activity.

Possible disruption of the lateral ligaments should be suspected in a patient with a fracture of the ankle, particularly when the injury is caused by high-energy trauma. During open reduction of the fracture, the ankle should be examined for stability with both the anterior drawer and talar tilt tests or stress radiographs. The ligaments should be repaired because the procedure markedly increases the chances for a stable ankle and involves only minimal prolongation of anesthesia.

▶ New information is presented in this interesting and possibly controversial discussion of lateral liagment injuries associated with lateral malleolar fracture of the ankle. Most of us usually don't expect to find a ligament injury along with a lateral malleolar fracture. Even if we do, our usual experience with lateral ligament injuries is that they heal rather well with casting and don't require operative fixation even though a significant number of patients need later lateral ligament reconstruction. My experience is that lateral ligament injuries with late sequelae generally result from grade III ankle sprains; I don't remember seeing one in association with a lateral malleolar fracture. However, the observations described here seem to be valid, and it is certainly worth looking for them in all high-energy ankle fractures with major displacement.—S.T. Hansen, Jr., M.D.

Tibial Shaft Fractures Treated With Functional Braces: Experience With 780 Fractures
Sarmiento A, Gersten LM, Sobol PA, Shankwiler JA, Vangsness CT (Univ of Southern California)
J Bone Joint Surg [Br] 71-B:602–609, August 1989   2–9

Functional bracing is an effective approach to selected tibial shaft fractures. The results of functional bracing in 780 patients with tibial shaft fractures were followed to union. Patients' average age was 30 years. Nearly one third of the fractures were comminuted. Fractures with excessive initial shortening and those with increasing angular deformity in the initial cast were excluded.

Closed fractures healed after an average of 17.4 weeks, and open fractures healed after 21.7 weeks. Ninety percent of injuries healed with 10 mm or less of shortening. Twelve patients had more than 10 degrees of varus at the time of healing, and 6 had more than 10 degrees of anterior angulation. The incidence of nonunion was 2.5%. Bracing was discontinued in 46 instances, most often because of inability to manage the brace, irritation of a soft tissue wound, or progressive angulation. The speed of healing appeared to depend most obviously on the degree of soft tissue injury.

Use of prefabricated functional braces is an acceptable treatment for selected tibial shaft fractures, including many closed and open injuries with minimal associated soft tissue damage. Few open grade III fractures are suitable for bracing. The results have been cosmetically acceptable. Minimal shortening and angulation have not compromised function.

▶ This superb review is the culmination of a very long study of tibial fractures and appropriately is included in the section on fracture care rather than in Traumatology. Sarmiento's use of functional bracing has defined the limits of this treatment method. The article confirms that this technique is most appropriately applied to fractures that do not have significant shortening or major soft tissue injury, which is what distinguishes fracture care from traumatology. Fracture care encompasses the treatment of closed grades 0, 1, and possibly 2, and open grades 1 and 2. All are relatively stable isolated injuries that usually are caused by indirect force. Closed grade 2 and open grade 2 fall into a transitional zone, but closed grade 3 and open grades 3A, B, and C do not heal well with functional bracing.

This paper confirms these principles, although it does not express them in the same terminology. Functional bracing is indicated for the majority of the fractures seen in a general orthopedic practice, but it lends itself to only a few fractures that are seen in a trauma center.

Three other papers might add significantly to the reader's overall comprehension of this subject (1–3).—S.T. Hansen, Jr., M.D.

References

1. Blenman PR, et al: *J Orthop Res* 7:398, 1989.
2. Kenwright J, Goodship AE: *Clin Orthop* 241:36, 1989.
3. Henley MB: *Clin Orthop* 240:87, 1989.

The Use of a Clamp-on Plate for Forearm Fractures
Mennen U (Medical Univ of South Africa; Ga-Rankuwa Hosp, Medunsa, South Africa)
Orthopedics 12:39–43, January 1989   2–10

A clamp-on plate was developed as an alternative to conventional screw-secured plates for treating forearm fractures. The goal was to avoid the bony devascularization that occurs with the usual plates, as well as delayed fracture healing.

The clamp-on plate is made of implantable stainless steel; 12 plates of varying length and diameter are available. The central ridge has a pressed-out groove, and toothlike projections on either side embrace the bone at least halfway around its circumference. Sharpened points are pressed 1–2 mm into the bone with a crimping tool. Soft tissue dissection is minimal.

Plates were used to treat 379 forearm fractures in 266 patients. Nearly 20% of the fractures were open, and more than 38% were comminuted. Open reduction and clamp-on plating were used to treat 282 fractures. Thirty-one others were treated with conventional plates and screws, and 66 undisplaced fractures were managed nonoperatively.

Union occurred within an average of 12 weeks in patients treated with clamp-on plates. No nonunions and no late refractures or plate fractures occurred. In 6 patients osteitis developed. Eighteen had mild and acceptable deformities. Conventional plating led to healing within an average of 21 weeks.

The clamp-on plate assures reliable union of forearm fractures by providing biomechanical stability. Disruption of the periosteal and endosteal blood supply is minimal, and union occurs earlier than with screw-secured plates. This method is especially well suited to treating fractures in osteopenic bone.

▶ The authors present an innovative treatment of forearm fractures. The clamp-on plate eliminates 2 of the negative features of screwed-on plates: damage to the cortical blood supply under the plate, and stress risers caused by screw holes after the plate is removed. A third significant problem is unsightly scarring; unfortunately, this is not eliminated. This technique therefore will compete with other methods that are being devised to stabilize forearm bones. Good internal fixation of the forearm must be inserted through a small incision and must be able to control rotation. Perhaps this plate represents an evolutionary step toward a pinless external fixator or a nonreamed interlocking nail that can be used in the upper extremity and will eliminate the need for a long incision.

To further understand the reason for its development, the reader might refer to Claes (1), O'Sullivan et al. (2), and Korvick et al. (3).—S.T. Hansen, Jr., M.D.

References

1. Claes L: *J Orthop Res* 7:170, 1989.
2. O'Sullivan ME, et al: *J Bone Joint Surg [Am]* 71-A:306, 1989.
3. Korvick DL, et al: *Acta Orthop Scand* 60:611, 1989.

Displaced Intra-Articular Fractures of the Tarsal Navicular
Sangeorzan BJ, Benirschke SK, Mosca V, Mayo KA, Hansen ST Jr (Univ of Washington, Seattle)
J Bone Joint Surg [Am] 71-A:1504–1510, December 1989

Displaced fractures of the tarsal navicular are rare. Various treatments have been recommended for fractures of the body, which are the most severe. In 21 patients with displaced fractures of the body of the tarsal navicular, open reduction and internal fixation were carried out.

A classification system was developed based on the direction of the fracture line, the pattern of disruption of the surrounding joints, and the direction of displacement of the foot. Type I fractures are those with the fracture line in the coronal plane and without angulation of the forefoot; in type II fractures the primary fracture line is dorsal-lateral to plantar-medial, with the major fragment and forefoot displaced medially; type III fractures are those with comminuted fractures in the sagittal plane of the body of the tarsal navicular with the forefoot displaced laterally.

More than 60% of the joint surface in the anteroposterior and lateral planes was restored in all type I fractures treated with open reduction and internal fixation, in 67% of type II fractures, and in 50% of type III fractures. At an average of 8.5 weeks after injury, healing was evident radiographically. At an average follow-up of 44 months, 67% of the patients had good results, 19% had fair results, and 14% had poor results. The final clinical outcome was correlated directly with the type of fracture and the accuracy of operative reduction.

Overall results indicate that displaced intra-articular fractures of the tarsal navicular are difficult to treat. Only 4 patients in this series had totally asymptomatic and fully functional feet. The classification system was a good prognosticator of both the surgeon's ability to obtain a good reduction and the final clinical result.

▶ The paucity of papers concerning fractures of the tarsal navicular makes this paper somewhat unique. Tarsal navicular fractures are becoming either progressively more common or progressively more widely recognized in the past few years. They can be devastating to high-performance athletes and, like talus and os calcis fractures, can cause significant dysfunction in the hindfoot and limit subtalar motion by removing the shock absorber that is needed for gait. Fracture and trauma surgeons should have a higher index of suspicion to recognize navicular fractures. The classification presented here is functional in that it is a guide to treatment and prognosis.—S.T. Hansen, Jr., M.D.

A Comparison Between Delayed and Immediate Intramedullary Nailing in the Treatment of Comminuted and Open Fractures (Grade 1) of the Tibia
Tigani D, Sabetta E, Specchia L, Boriani S (Istituto Ortopedico Rizzoli, Bologna, Italy)
Ital J Orthop Traumaol 15:25–31, March 1989

Comminution or open fracture limits the indications for intramedullary nailing. A comparison was made between delayed and immediate intramedullary nailing in the treatment of such fractures of the tibia.

Delayed nailing was used to treat 68 closed unstable fractures of the tibial diaphysis. The patients underwent 5 to 6 days of transkeletal traction, followed by application of a plaster cast and nailing after 4 to 5 weeks. Active movement was begun immediately after nailing, and weight-bearing was allowed within 2 weeks. Fifty-eight unstable fractures were treated with early intramedullary osteosynthesis with Grosse-Kempf nails after skeletal traction for an average of 7 days. Rehabilitation began immediately after surgery; dynamization of the fixation was begun after 4 to 5 weeks, followed by direct weight bearing. Sixty-three grade 1 open fractures were treated by delayed osteosynthesis with Küntscher nailing using the described procedure, and 21 others received delayed synthesis with Grosse-Kempf nails. Five patients with early treatment for open fractures had immediate osteosynthesis with Grosse-Kempf nails after surgical toilet, irrigation, and closure of the wound.

In unstable fractures treated with delayed Küntscher nailing, consolidation occurred within 7 to 10 weeks, but 25% of patients had more than 25% limited ankle range of motion, with 6% having more than 50% loss. Ten patients also lost 25% or more motion in the knee. Results with early Grosse-Kempf nailing were much better: only 5% and 3% had better than 25% loss of motion in the ankle and knee, respectively. Open fractures treated with delayed osteosynthesis took longer to consolidate. Results with delayed nailing were good in terms of consolidation, but functional recovery was only fair. Immediate osteosynthesis with a screwed nail produced better results overall.

The criteria for delaying intramedullary nailing in grade 1 open fractures are valid, particularly when fractures cannot be treated within 8 hours; however, immediate treatment is essential in fractures associated with vascular lesions or multiple injuries. Intramedullary nailing is preferable to external fixation in open fractures with limited exposure.

▶ Because the fractures discussed here are only closed or open grade 1 fractures, this paper falls into the "fracture care" group. Their location in the tibia and mild complications with either comminution or open soft tissue injury make these injuries somewhat difficult to treat. The authors indicate that, although delayed nailing often is done because of concern about infection in an open fracture, immediate treatment is associated with better rehabilitation, a good union rate, and speedy healing. They also point out that a locked nail works well to control rotation in a comminuted fracture. The need exists for a nonreamed interlocked nail that ensures anatomical stabilization and controls length and rotation without significantly damaging the intramedullary blood supply to the tibia by reaming.—S.T. Hansen, Jr., M.D.

Fractures of the Coronoid Process of the Ulna
Regan W, Morrey B (Mayo Clinic; Mayo Found, Rochester, Minn)
J Bone Joint Surg [Am] 71-A:1348–1354, October 1989   2–13

The records of 35 patients with fractures of the coronoid process of the ulna in 1970 through 1987 showed that 3 types of fractures were seen on initial radiographs (Fig 2–3). Fourteen patients had type I fractures, which involved avulsion of the tip of the coronoid process; 16 had type II fractures, in which a single or comminuted fragment involved 50% or

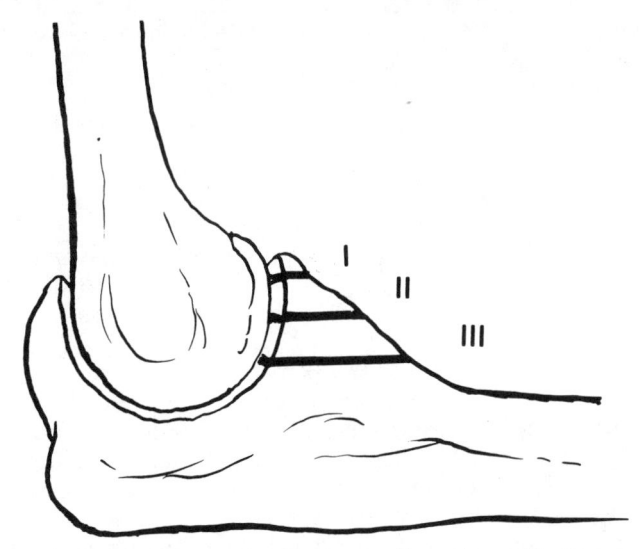

Fig 2–3.—Classification of fractures into 3 types, according to degree of involvement of coronoid process. (Courtesy of Regan W, Morrey B: *J Bone Joint Surg [Am]* 71-A:1348–1354, October 1989.)

less of the process; and 5 had type III fractures, in which a fragment involved more than 50% of the process. A concurrent dislocation or associated fracture was present in 14%, 56%, and 80% of these patients, respectively.

Open reduction and internal fixation was performed for 1 type II and 2 type III fractures. Type I, type II, and type III fractures were immobilized for a mean of 13, 20, and 28 days, respectively. Mean follow-up for 32 patients was 50.4 months (range, 12 to 103 months).

The final outcome, based on the elbow-performance index, was correlated well with the type of fracture. Satisfactory results were achieved in 92% of type I fractures, 73% of type II, and 20% of type III. Residual stiffness of the joint was common in patients with a type-III fracture; 3 of 4 patients had associated dislocation of the elbow or periarticular fracture of the radial head or olecranon, or both. There was a direct correlation between loss of motion and duration of immobilization.

Type I or type II fractures of the coronoid process of the ulna should be managed with immobilization for 3 weeks or less, followed by active-motion exercises. Type III fractures can be treated with reduction and fixation followed by early motion, when possible.

▶ The authors stress the importance of anatomical reduction when treating fractures of the coronoid process of the ulna. Grade III fractures, which cause instability of the radioulnar joint, have a particularly poor prognosis and should be treated with anatomical and rigid internal fixation followed by early motion. Our experience agrees with this and with the poor prognosis for ulnar injuries that are associated with dislocations.

Another paper published this past year addresses a different type of fracture in the same region that depends on an intact coronoid process (1).—S.T. Hansen, Jr., M.D.

Reference

1. Compton R, Bucknell A: *Orthop Rev* 18:189, 1989.

Lower Extremity Fractures: Relationship to Reaction Time and Coordination Time

Adelsberg S, Pitman M, Alexander H (Hosp for Joint Diseases Orthopaedic Inst, New York)
Arch Phys Med Rehabil 70:737–739, October 1989   2–14

Fall injury rates decrease from early childhood until about age 60 years, and increase steadily thereafter. A study was undertaken to determine the possible relationship between delayed reaction time and slow coordination time as causative factors in lower extremity fracture. A total of 105 persons aged 6 to 85 years, including 20 with fractures of the lower extremity, were tested with a 2-hand coordination tester and a reaction time apparatus. Daily activity levels also were assessed.

Slower reaction times were observed in the older age group (55 to 85 years) and in persons with fractures. Coordination times increased with increasing age, with or without fractures. Shorter reaction times and coordination times were observed in persons with higher activity levels. Multiple linear regression analysis showed a statistically significant association between fracture status and reaction time, after controlling for age.

Subjects with longer reaction times are at higher risk for fractures. A routine of therapeutic exercise designed to improve reaction and coordination time may help reduce the incidence of certain fractures in the elderly.

▶ A somewhat different slant on the causes of fractures is presented by Adelsberg and Alexander. An enormous number of fractures occur from a lack of coordination and delayed reaction time at great financial and social cost. This paper suggests that routine therapeutic exercises might prevent many medical disorders in the elderly.—S.T. Hansen, Jr., M.D.

Other papers about similar subjects are:

References

1. Nevitt MC, et al: *J Am Med Assoc* 261:2663, 1989.
2. Hornby R, et al: *J Bone Joint Surg [Br]* 71-B:619, 1989.
3. DeGroof E, et al: *Acta Orthop Belg* 54:458, 1989.
4. Herrlin K, et al: *Arch Orthop Trauma Surg* 108:36, 1989.

Traumatology

Early Versus Delayed Stabilization of Femoral Fractures: A Prospective Randomized Study
Bone LB, Johnson KD, Weigelt J, Scheinberg R (Univ of Texas; Parkland Mem Hosp, Dallas)
J Bone Joint Surg [Am] 71-A:336–340, March 1989   2–15

Immediate stabilization of femoral fractures in multiply injured patients has been shown to drastically reduce the incidence of pulmonary failure, late septic complications, and the total cost of hospital care. The effects of early and delayed treatment of femoral fractures were compared in 178 patients aged 16–75 years admitted during a 2-year study period with an acute femoral fracture. The patients were assigned randomly to early stabilization within the first 24 hours after injury or late stabilization more than 48 hours after injury. In the delayed-treatment group, fractured limbs were placed in traction for 48 hours. All other urgent surgical procedures were performed as indicated. On admission, each patient received a determination of arterial blood gases, chest radiography, and assignment to an injury-severity score. Arterial blood-gas evaluations were repeated on a daily basis thereafter.

None of the patients with isolated femoral fracture that had been treated with early or late stabilization experienced respiratory insufficiency. Three patients in the late-stabilization group and 1 in the early stabilization group had late pulmonary emboli. None of the patients with an isolated early-treated or late-treated fracture needed intubation or admission to the intensive care unit (ICU). However, 18 multiply-injured early-stabilization patients and 22 late-stabilization patients with multiple injuries needed ICU care. Three patients with multiple injuries, including 2 who had early fracture stabilization and 1 who had late stabilization, died in the hospital.

A comparison of total length of hospital stay, days in the ICU, and total cost of hospitalization showed that late stabilization added 10 days to the hospital stay, added 5 days to the ICU care, and increased the average hospital cost by approximately $13,000. Added to the finding that delay causes an increase in the incidence of pulmonary complications, the data support the recommendation for early stabilization of all acute femoral fractures in adult patients, even in those with multiple injuries.

▶ I chose this paper to introduce the section Traumatology because a femoral fracture is the prototypic orthopedic traumatology injury. Femoral fractures that occur in combination with other skeletal injuries or other system injuries are associated with secondary organ failure, particularly pulmonary decompensation. Physicians working in trauma centers have recognized for almost 15 years that when a femoral fracture is stabilized immediately or very early, fewer complications, particularly pulmonary complications, result from high-energy injuries. This paper is one of the few prospective studies that compare the effects of early and delayed treatment of femoral fractures, and it irrefutably establishes early treatment of femoral fractures as a major principle in traumatology. Cost-effectiveness and functional outcome will be the topics of studies in the next few years, and more statistics undoubtedly will be gathered to clearly show that early stabilization results in extremely functional results and significant economic savings.

Four more papers that were written on similar subjects in the past year deserve attention along with this paper (1–4).—S.T. Hansen, Jr., M.D.

References

1. Beckman SB, et al: *Am Surg* 55:356, 1989.
2. Geissler WB, et al: *J Orthop Trauma* 2:297, 1989.
3. Mize RD: *Clin Orthop* 240:77, 1989.
4. Siliski JM, et al: *J Bone Joint Surg [Am]* 71-A:95, 1989.

Plates Versus External Fixation in Severe Open Tibial Shaft Fractures: A Randomized Trial
Bach AW, Hansen ST Jr (Univ of Washington, Seattle)
Clin Orthop 241:89–94, April 1989

The proper management of severe open fractures of the tibial shaft remains uncertain. In a prospective study of 59 patients with grade II or III open fractures of this type and an average age of 37 years, débridement was carried out on a sterile basis before patients were assigned to external fixation or plate fixation of the tibial shaft. Plate fixation involved the AO principles, and external fixation involved the AO tubular frame device.

Fifty-six patients were followed up for a year or longer after injury; 30 had external fixation and 26 had plating as the primary means of stabilization. All fractures eventually were united. The average time to healing was about 5.5 months in both groups. Any loss of knee motion after either treatment was not significant. Wound infection was twice as frequent in the patients having treatment with a plate. Five of these patients and 1 with external fixation had chronic osteomyelitis. Three pin infections occurred in the external fixation group. Each group had 1 refracture. Malunion occurred in 1 patient given a plate and in 3 with external fixation.

Tibial shaft fractures healed equally well after plating and external fixation, but severe infection was significantly less frequent with external fixation. External fixation using the one-half pin technique therefore is the preferred method of primary stabilization for grades II and III open tibial shaft fractures.

▶ Methods of stabilizing tibial fractures have progressed from plates to fixators and currently to nonreamed locked nails. This paper is also a prospective study and, in fact, was written 3 or 4 years ago. It demonstrates that using the half-pin external fixation technique devised by Behrens is safer, in the hands of a trauma surgeon, than plating an open tibial fracture. The fine points of indirect reduction are technically demanding and not always were used with the plate technique in this series. Both techniques had similar final results, and although external fixation resulted in fewer overall complications, many complications still occurred with external fixation.—S.T. Hansen, Jr., M.D.

Treatment of Open Fractures of the Tibial Shaft: Ender Nailing Versus External Fixation: A Randomized, Prospective Comparison
Holbrook JL, Swiontkowski MF, Sanders R (Vanderbilt Unit Med Ctr, Nashville, Tenn)
J Bone Joint Surg 71-A:1231–1238, September 1989   2–17

In a prospective randomized study, Ender nailing was compared with external fixation in 60 patients having 63 open tibial shaft fractures. Patients with extensively comminuted fractures were excluded from the study. Anterior and anteromedial half-pin frames were used for external fixation. For Ender nailing, as many nails as could be inserted easily were placed in the canal.

Ender nailing was at least as effective as external fixation with regard to the time to union and tibial alignment. Time to union averaged about 6.5 months after external fixation and about 6 months after Ender nailing. Fewer operations, on average, were required with Ender nailing. More patients having fixation had less than 110 degrees of knee flexion. There were 4 deep infections after external fixation and 2 after Ender nailing. Three patients in the former group and 1 in the latter had loss of reduction.

Ender nailing appears to offer several advantages over external fixation, including the need for fewer operations and fewer serious complications. Some cortical apposition of the major fragments may occur if Ender nailing is to control shortening. The nails should be seated flush with the proximal metaphyseal bone to minimize irritation of the knee.

▶ Concern about complications associated with external fixation, such as pin tract infections and delayed unions, motivated this more recent prospective study. The relatively modern half-pin technique was compared with the Ender, or nonreamed nail, in grade I and II open tibial fractures. Ender nailing, which does not significantly damage the intramedullary blood supply, was found to be as safe and effective as external fixation in grades I and II open tibial fractures with stable fracture patterns.—S.T. Hansen, Jr., M.D.

Other papers that were published in 1989 on related topics include:

References

1. DeLong WG, et al: *J Trauma* 29:571, 1989.
2. Mercer NSG, Moss ALH: *Injury* 20:114, 1989.
3. Rommens P, et al: *J Trauma* 29:630, 1989.

Soft-Tissue Reconstruction in Severe Lower Extremity Trauma: A Review
Gorman PW, Barnes CL, Fischer TJ, McAndrew MP, Moore MM (Univ of Arkansas for Medical Sciences, Little Rock; Hand Surgery Associates of Indiana, Indianapolis; Hand Surgery Consultants, Little Rock, Ark)
Clin Orthop 243:57-64, June 1989   2-18

Many local rotation flaps for reconstructing the leg and foot have been described. Loss of a small area of skin from the leg often can be managed with skin grafting or local random skin flaps. Muscle transposition flaps are extremely useful. Many free-flap donor sites have been described for use in the leg. Common free flaps include those of muscle such as the gracilis or rectus abdominis, skin, and muscle or skin and underlying subcutaneous fat and fascia.

Extensive foot and leg wounds often need free tissue transfer or a free flap supported by microvascular anastomoses to native vessels. Indications for free tissue transfer include failure of local flaps, coverage of a large chronically infected wound, obliteration of dead space, and creation of a well-vascularized bed for future skeletal reconstruction. Flap timing has become more aggressive in recent years.

With current microsurgical techniques, success rates for flaps have exceeded 90%. The outcome is dependent in part on the timing of soft tissue coverage and on wound characteristics. Poor results are more frequent in patients having infected wounds with massive loss of bone and skin.

▶ Several excellent papers appeared in this symposium on salvage problems in the lower extremity. This article is valuable for comparing the various classifications of open wounds and describing the kinds of soft tissue reconstructions that might be needed in severe open tibial fractures. Microvascular surgery has progressed to a high technical level, but selecting patients to undergo these procedures is still an inexact science.—S.T. Hansen, Jr., M.D.

Reconstruction of the Lower Extremity With Microvascular Free Flaps: A 10-Year Experience With 304 Consecutive Cases
Khouri RK, Shaw WW (New York Univ; Bellevue Hosps, New York)
J Trauma 29:1086-1094, August 1989   2-19

Transfer of microvascular free tissue to reconstruct soft tissue defects has improved greatly the rate of leg salvage. However, complications, vascular thrombosis, and flap failure cast doubt about the indication to attempt the salvage of massively injured limbs. In a review of 304 consecutive reconstructions of lower extremities involving microvascular free flaps, 72 variables were recorded for each free flap to identify the patterns of usage, results, and problems.

Of 277 patients, 260 sustained trauma, the majority in motor vehicle accidents. These patients received 287 flaps. In contrast, nontrauma pa-

Timing of Lower Extremity Free Flaps

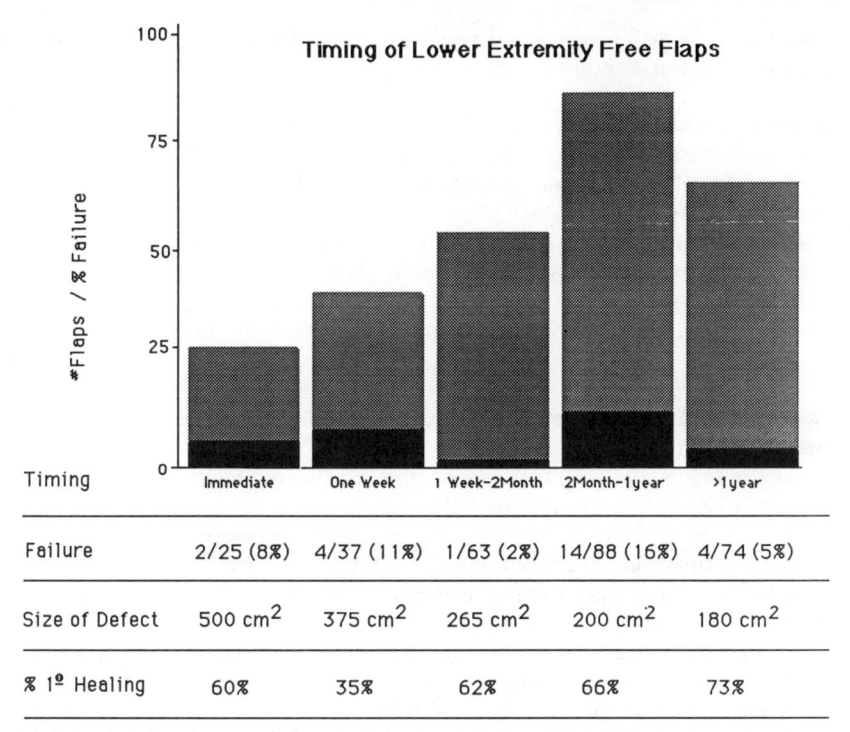

Timing	Immediate	One Week	1 Week–2 Month	2 Month–1 year	>1 year
Failure	2/25 (8%)	4/37 (11%)	1/63 (2%)	14/88 (16%)	4/74 (5%)
Size of Defect	500 cm^2	375 cm^2	265 cm^2	200 cm^2	180 cm^2
% 1° Healing	60%	35%	62%	66%	73%

Fig 2–4.—Timing. (Courtesy of Khouri RK, Shaw WW: *J Trauma* 29:1086–1094, August 1989.)

tients received only 17 flaps. The principal flaps used were rectus abdominis, parascapular, and latissimus dorsi. Seventy-three percent of defects were below the midtibia; 33% of flaps were used to provide coverage of foot and ankle defects to salvage a useful foot. Associated compound fractures were chiefly Gustilo types IIIb and IIIc. The late subacute group of patients was the largest group in the series (Fig 2–4).

The overall rate of flap failure was 8%. Most failures were in the mid to distal leg. Not counting 20 patients in whom salvage of a below-knee amputation stump was attempted, 6% of patients in whom leg salvage was attempted needed amputation within the first 3 months. In 71% of these patients, microvascular failure of the free flap was responsible. Ninety-one percent of patients followed for more than 1 year had normal leg function, a completely healed surface wound, and satisfactory bony union. The remaining patients either had undergone amputation or had poor leg function. Factors associated with thrombosis were the need for a vein graft, type IIIc injuries, end-to-side anastomosis, bone gap larger than 4 cm, larger skin defects, and an abnormal preoperative angiogram. Later cases had a higher success rate, indicating that experience is important in reducing complications.

Indications for salvage versus amputation should be redefined in light of the ability to perform early definitive reconstruction with free flaps.

The ability to add healthy and well-vascularized tissue to a traumatized limb is critical for success.

▶ A very large experience with microvascular free flaps, the most aggressive of the soft tissue reconstructive procedures, is presented in this retrospective review. The technique requires a high level of expertise. When failures occur, they usually are located in the mid to distal leg. Type IIIc injuries presented the greatest difficulties, requiring vein grafts or large bone grafts, and often presenting abnormal preoperative angiograms. The authors stress the need for better criteria to determine which patients should have salvage attempted and which should undergo early amputation.—S.T. Hansen, Jr., M.D.

Outcome of Treatment of Combined Orthopedic and Arterial Trauma to the Lower Extremity
Drost TF, Rosemurgy AS, Proctor D, Kearney RE (Univ of South Florida, Tampa)
J Trauma 29:1331–1334, October 1989   2–20

The treatment goal for combined orthopedic and arterial injuries of the lower extremity is limb salvage. More than 10,000 patients admitted for trauma treatment were evaluated to assess the morbidity and functional outcome associated with aggressive attempts at salvage of lower extremities with orthoarterial trauma.

Twenty-two patients (0.2%) sustained major concomitant orthopedic and arterial injuries of their lower extremities; 14 had blunt trauma and 8, penetrating injuries. The patients underwent more than 90 salvage operations within 30 days of admission. Eight patients (36%) eventually underwent amputation. Sixteen (76%) of 21 patients who had initially successful limb salvage underwent 43 additional extremity operations, including 7 amputations. Of the 14 patients with salvaged limbs, 7 (50%) had major long-term complications such as nonunion, chronic osteomyelitis, and nonhealing soft-tissue wounds; 2 continued to experience foot drop; and 4 had disabilities. In contrast, those who underwent extremity amputations suffered only minor stump complications and had lesser rates of disability.

The presence of neurosensory and motor impairment or serious loss of soft tissue and injuries at or distal to the popliteal artery were associated with a high frequency of disability and amputation. The mechanism of injury, the injury severity score, sequence of orthopedic and vascular procedures, use of temporary arterial shunts, the nature of the arterial reconstruction, length of ischemic time, and the presence of open fractures did not influence limb salvage or outcome.

The findings challenge the concept that limb salvage is the only acceptable goal of treatment after concomitant orthopedic and arterial injuries to the lower extremity. Although limb salvage can be achieved in most patients, the majority will have disability and significant complications needing operative intervention and prolonged hospitalizations. Patients with orthoarterial injuries of the distal lower extremity associated with neurologic impairment or major soft tissue loss may be treated best with timely amputation.

▶ Vascular surgeons provide a somewhat different look at salvage of lower extremities. Of the 10,000 trauma patients reviewed for this study, only 0.2% had combined lower extremity orthopedic and arterial injuries. Vascular injuries below the popliteal level that were associated with serious soft tissue injuries posed the most difficult problems. The authors question the value of limb salvage in these patients as "a triumph of technique and technology over reason."—S.T. Hansen, Jr., M.D.

Reconstruction of Large Diaphyseal Defects, Without Free Fibular Transfer, in Grade IIIB Tibial Fractures
Christian EP, Bosse MJ, Robb G (Naval Hosp, Portsmouth, Va)
J Bone Joint Surg [Am] 71-A:994–1004, August 1989   2–21

Eight grade IIIB tibial fractures associated with large soft tissue and segmental diaphyseal defects were reconstructed effectively without free fibular transfer. The defects averaged 10 cm in length. Soft tissue coverage involved local myoplasty for defects in the proximal tibia, but most patients need free tissue transfer. Beads impregnated with antibiotic were placed in the wound, and later the defect was filled with a massive amount of autogenous cancellous bone.

Follow-up averaged 27 months. All the tibias healed, in an average of 9 months. The average time of external fixation was 5.5 months. Two patients had deep infection that resolved after débridement, antibiotic therapy, and, in 1 case, grafting. All patients had some functional deficit or permanent partial disability at follow-up, but half had sustained many other injuries.

Coverage with free tissue is more reliable and more versatile than use of a local muscle flap in these cases. The procedure is a viable alternative to free fibular transfer for large segmental diaphyseal defects, especially if there is a large soft tissue defect and either a single remaining vessel or bilateral lower limb injury. The antibiotic beads also serve to preserve the volume of the diaphyseal defect for later receipt of a cancellous bone graft, and to keep the soft tissue flap from adhering to the defect site.

▶ Vascular injury was not a factor in this study about reconstruction of large diaphyseal defects in open grade IIIB tibial fractures (Gustilo's classification), and general surgery principles were successful with intact vascular system. The surgical technique used here is a modern variant of the Papineau technique, involving massive autogenous cancellous grafting followed by immediate coverage with free tissue transfers. Muscle flaps were used only in the proximal third. A relatively modern technique of maintaining space with antibiotic-impregnated beads was cleverly employed.

This study has several limitations if the results are to be applied to the general population and not just to young healthy males with an average age of 22 years. External fixators were applied for 4 to 10 months (average, 5.5 months), and further support was needed for 2.5 months more. Because most of the patients had multiple injuries and not isolated tibial fractures, their functional results were difficult to assess. A proven disadvantage of the Papineau graft, which makes a diaphyseal bone from cancellous bone graft, is that it remains susceptible to secondary fracture for several years. The main advantage of this study is that it will provide a basis for comparison with the Ilizarov technique, which fills in similar bone defects by diaphyseal translocation.—S.T. Hansen, Jr., M.D.

Limb Reconstruction Versus Amputation Decision Making in Massive Lower Extremity Trauma
Lange RH (Univ of Wisconsin, Madison)
Clin Orthop 243:92–99, June 1989

Massive lower limb trauma, especially open tibial fractures with associated vascular injury, poses the question of attempting limb salvage or performing primary amputation. Available data fail to provide defensible guidelines for primary amputation. Type IIIC tibial fractures are the most difficult type of case to decide. Considerations in attempting limb salvage include the need for prolonged hospitalization and multiple operations, a high rate of failure, increased mortality, and prolonged disability. In addition, significant dysfunction is frequent and the infection rate is high.

The prognosis for limb salvage is relatively poor if massive crush injuries or other high-energy soft tissue injuries are present or the warm ischemia time exceeds 6 hours. Severely comminuted or segmental fractures and infrapopliteal arterial injury also worsens the outlook, as does prolonged, severe hypovolemic shock. Patients aged more than 50 years have a poorer outlook than younger patients. Occupational demands should be taken into account, and the presence of underlying disease is an important factor. In patients with multiple injuries, it may be necessary to amputate a massively injured limb even if it appears salvageable.

A decision-making team and a tertiary-care facility are important for those patients—the majority—whose prognosis is indeterminate. A grading system for assessing cumulative injury to the extremity would be helpful.

▶ Lange's excellent article, which also appeared in the symposium dedicated to lower extremity salvages, clearly summarizes the difficulties in making good decisions about amputation. The author points out the tragedy of misguided salvage attempts as well as the extreme difficulty of being sure that one has assessed all the parameters accurately enough to go directly to amputation. Even when all the criteria are evaluated and all the problems are recognized, making this decision requires experience and ideally is made by an experienced team. Third-party payers, hospital directors, deans, and chairmen must be induced to make the life of traumatologists more attractive to keep them working in trauma centers long enough to gain the necessary experience to make these crucial decisions.—S.T. Hansen, Jr., M.D.

Reference

1. McNutt R, et al: *J Trauma* 29:1624, 1989.

Immediate Internal Fixation of Open Ankle Fractures
Wiss DA, Gilbert P, Merritt PO, Sarmiento A (Los Angeles County–Univ of Southern California)
J Orthop Trauma 2:265–271, 1989   2–23

Open ankle fractures often require urgent intervention to minimize the risks of skin necrosis and wound infection. Experience with this intervention was reviewed in 62 patients who had immediate internal fixation of open ankle fracture. Of these patients, 22 had significant associated injuries. Open fracture wounds were cultured and dressed, and the legs were splinted. Radiographic studies of the ankle were obtained. In large wounds, reduction and fixation of the medial malleolus was accomplished through the open wound. An incision was required for smaller wounds to allow visualization and fixation without tension on the surrounding soft tissues. When possible, exposed joint surfaces were closed and subcutaneous tissue was closed when tension could be avoided, but traumatic wounds were left open. The foot was splinted at 90 degrees. Grade I and grade II wounds were allowed to heal by secondary intension. Grade III wounds were redébrided at 48 to 72 hours. Ten patients had a delayed primary closure, whereas in 18 the wounds were partially closed or left open.

Patients were followed for an average of 16.4 months. Fractures healed in an average of 8 weeks in all patients. Average duration of cast immobilization was 8 weeks. Excellent results were achieved in 25 patients; results were good in 20, fair in 5, and poor in 12 patients. Fewer than half the patients had no pain at follow-up, and only 47% could walk as far as they liked without a limp or pain. Thirty-nine percent experienced mild pain with strenuous activities or daily activities; 17% had pain with weight bearing. Only 18% could return to preinjury recreation levels, but 81% could work at their jobs. Late ankle arthrodesis was required in 8% of patients.

Immediate internal fixation is recommended as treatment for displaced open ankle fractures; however, a significant rate of complications may result. Poor results are mainly caused by articular surface damage, deep infection, or nonanatomical reductions.

▶ The conclusions that this paper draws on open ankle fractures are similar to those of the 2 previously mentioned retrospective papers from trauma centers on the west coast. Like the paper on immediate stabilization of femoral fractures, this article points out a major principle in traumatology: that open joint fractures are best fixed internally and immediately. Complications in these injuries are not uncommon because they often involve significant direct damage to articular surfaces and may occur in conjunction with other injuries. However, the best time to restore a reasonable articular surface, to provide some protection to the local soft tissues, and to make overall patient management easier without increasing the infection rate that is attributed to the open injury itself is immediately after the injury.—S.T. Hansen, Jr., M.D.

MAST-associated Compartment Syndrome (MACS): A Review
Aprahamian C, Gessert G, Bandyk DF, Sell L, Stiehl J, Olson DW (Med College of Wisconsin, Milwaukee)
J Trauma 29:549–555, May 1989

The use of pneumatic antishock trousers (MAST) has been implicated in the development of MAST-associated compartment syndrome (MACS), which has contributed to amputation and mortality in patients both with and without lower extremity trauma. To determine whether compartment syndromes develop as a consequence of the trauma that leads to the use of MAST or from the extrinsic compression and ischemia produced by the inflated MAST, data on 15 patients who received treatment for vascular injuries at 1 institution during an 8-year study period and on 12 previously reported cases were reviewed.

Duration of MAST use varied between the 2 groups: MAST was used for 60 minutes or less in 5 (33.3%) of the 15 hospital cases and for a mean of 16 hours in 10 of the 12 literature cases. In the other 10 hospital cases and 2 literature cases, the MAST had been removed during or at the completion of surgery.

Five of the 15 hospital patients and 5 of the 12 literature patients died of multiple organ failure. Three hospital patients and 4 literature patients needed amputation. Two of the 5 hospital patients who died may have had ischemic and infected limbs that contributed to their deaths. The other 3 patients all had viable limbs at the time of their deaths.

Thus, lower extremity trauma and systemic hypotension appear to be cofactors responsible for the development of compartment syndromes. However, MAST use contributes to this process by prolonging muscle ischemia. It is suggested that complications of lower limb compartment hypertension may be avoided with early diagnosis and fasciotomy.

▶ Pneumatic antishock trousers (MAST) were thought to be an important part of immediate patient stabilization several years ago, but concerns have been raised about the safety of this technique. This paper indicates that, although the severity of the injury that indicates the use of MAST trousers may be the greatest contributor to major complications, using MAST may contribute to complications by prolonging muscle ischemia. The trousers therefore must be used briefly and carefully, if at all. If they are used, a surgeon must watch carefully for lower limb compartment syndrome and perform an early fasciotomy if compartment syndrome is noted.

A companion paper written by Wright and colleagues suggests that these secondary complications may be ameliorated by hypothermia (1).—S.T. Hansen, Jr., M.D.

Reference

1. Wright JG, et al: *J Surg Res* 47:389, 1989.

Split-Thickness Skin Excision: Its Use for Immediate Wound Care in Crush Injuries of the Foot
Myerson M (Union Mem Hosp, Baltimore)
Foot Ankle 10:54–60, October 1989
2–25

The management of crushing injuries to the foot depends on successful handling of the soft tissues. Split-thickness skin excision (STSE) was used in the treatment of 8 crush injuries of the foot associated with shearing and degloving of skin, which were treated at 1 hospital.

The compartment syndromes seen in 4 feet were treated with fasciotomy. All wounds were débrided thoroughly and fractures and fracture-dislocations were stabilized with internal fixation techniques. The avulsed flaps were treated with the STSE technique by using dermal capillary bleeding as the indicator of skin viability.

A split-thickness graft 0.010 to 0.015 in. thick was obtained from the potentially nonviable skin flap as well as the adjacent normal skin. The nonviable skin flap was excised, and the graft was meshed 1:1.5 or 1:3 and reapplied to the denuded area.

All flaps survived, and all the degloved STSE grafts healed. Additional procedures were performed in 4 patients (2 free flaps and 2 split-thickness grafts) adjacent to the débrided flap for complete coverage. No delayed wound sloughs occurred with either the STSE grafts or the split-thickness grafts. Functional and cosmetic outcomes were satisfactory in all patients.

The STSE is an effective technique for skin coverage in crush injuries of the feet associated with degloving of the skin.

▶ Crush injuries to the foot are extremely difficult injuries to treat, particularly because the dorsum of the foot has very poor soft tissue coverage. Myerson describes an elegant technique, which was originated by Ziv in 1988, to manage these devastating foot injuries. It is effective, both for delineating viable skin from nonviable skin and for securing an immediate split-thickness skin graft to cover the exposed area. As in the tibia, the criteria determining whether salvage of the foot should be attempted or whether it should be amputated immediately are extremely difficult to define and were not discussed thoroughly.

Two related papers should be read along with this article, the first by the originator of the skin graft technique (1, 2).—S.T. Hansen, Jr., M.D.

References

1. Ziv I, et al: *Foot Ankle* 9:185, 1989.
2. Hoogeboom JE, et al: *JAOA* 89:1066, 1989.

Stimulation of the Healing Response

Morbidity at Bone Graft Donor Sites
Younger EM, Chapman MW (Univ of California, Davis)
J Orthop Trauma 3:192–195, 1989
2–26

The morbidity resulting from harvesting autogenous bone grafts was studied using data for 239 patients who had had 243 grafts in a 2-year period. The procedures had been carried out by orthopedic, neurosurgery, and maxillofacial services. Rib grafts and grafts taken from near the recipient site were excluded. The mean follow-up was 11 months. The iliac crest served as the donor site in 90% of cases. A suction drain was used in 73% of donor sites.

Major complications occurred at a rate of 8.6%, whereas the minor complication rate was 20.6%. Early major complications included 6 wound infections and 3 hematomas requiring operative removal. Six patients had prolonged pain, 3 had sensory loss, and 1 had osteomyelitis. Complications were fewer for grafts taken through a separate incision rather than through the primary incision. Complications were relatively frequent when the inner table of the anterior iliac crest served as the donor site. Patients with significant medical illness had an increased rate of major complications.

Bone graft harvesting entails definite morbidity, and some complications are unavoidable. The use of other materials such as banked bone or synthetic bone might be necessary to avoid complications altogether. Limiting the incision inferior to iliac crest will lessen the risk of damaging the lateral femoral cutaneous nerve.

▶ Many surgeons believe that autogenous bone grafting from a patient's pelvis is not without risk, and this unique paper verifies this belief. Patients often have more pain from a graft donor site than from the operative site itself; we should perfect our techniques of harvesting bone grafts and look for sources of substitute bone.

Bone grafting was discussed in 2 other papers published in 1989 (1, 2).—S.T. Hansen, Jr., M.D.

References

1. Sanders R, DiPasquale T: *J Orthop Trauma* 3:287, 1989.
2. Mauerhan DR: *Orthop Rev* 18:239, 1989.

Interporous Hydroxyapatite as a Bone Graft Substitute in Tibial Plateau Fractures
Bucholz RW, Carlton A, Holmes R (Univ of Texas Southwestern Med Ctr, Dallas; Univ of California, San Diego, Med Ctr)
Clin Orthop 240:53-62, March 1989
2-27

Porous mineral materials such as interporous hydroxyapatite offer an alternative to traditional filling agents such as cancellous or cortical autograft. Interporous hydroxyapatite was compared with cancellous autograft in a study of 40 patients with displaced tibial plateau fractures that needed surgical repair. The metaphyseal defects were filled with either cancellous autograft from the iliac crest or interporous hydroxyapatite, and patients were followed up for 15 or 34.5 months, respectively, on average.

Any clinical or radiographic differences between the 2 treatment groups were not significant at follow-up. Satisfactory reduction was achieved in all patients except 2 who had autografts. Articular surfaces were less depressed in hydroxyapatite cases. Complications were more numerous in cases of autografting. The autograft group had 2 deep wound infections; the hydroxyapatite group had 1.

Interporous hydroxyapatite is an effective and safe alternative to autogenous cancellous bone for filling metaphyseal defects associated with tibial plateau fractures. The material has been used successfully in other long bones with metaphyseal defects, but its properties must be improved before it can be used to treat diaphyseal defects, delayed union, or nonunion.

▶ This excellent prospective study compares the effectiveness of bone substitutes and autogenous grafts in tibial plateau fractures. A tibial plateau fracture makes a good subject for investigation because it occurs fairly often and virtually always needs grafting. The study has encouraging results; it should be continued or repeated with larger numbers.—S.T. Hansen, Jr., M.D.

This technique should be compared with those described in the following papers:

References

1. Aspenberg P, et al: *Acta Orthop Scand* 60:607, 1989.
2. Tajana GF, et al: *Orthopedics* 12:515, 1989.
3. Aronson J, et al: *Clin Orthop* 241:106, 1989.
4. Connolly J, et al: *J Bone Joint Surg [Am]* 71-A:684, 1989.
5. Connolly JF, et al: *J Orthop Trauma* 4:276, 1989.

Early Prophylactic Bone Grafting of High-Energy Tibial Fractures
Blick SS, Brumback RJ, Lakatos R, Poka A, Burgess AR (Univ of Maryland Med System, Baltimore)
Clin Orthop 240:21–41, March 1989   2–28

Fifty-three tibial fractures made by high-energy force were managed with prophylactic posterolateral bone grafting, done a mean of 10 weeks after injury and 8 weeks after soft tissue coverage. All patients had grafting within 16 weeks after injury or wound closure. Fifty-three fractures in 47 patients were evaluated. Myoplasty was necessary for wound closure in nearly one third of cases. All the fractures initially were stabilized with Hoffmann external fixation. Thirteen patients needed decompression for compartment syndrome.

External fixators were removed an average of 23 weeks after injury. The mean time without weight bearing was 29 weeks. All but 4% of the fractures healed in an average of 43 weeks. Seven fractures needed second bone grafts to unite. Treatment failed in 2 cases. Two thirds of patients had complications, the most frequent being pin tract infection. Four patients had infection at their fracture sites, and 4 had later tibial or fibular fractures.

Time to union was reduced by about 12 weeks with this approach, compared with historical controls not given early bone grafts. A 6-week delay after coverage with freely vascularized soft tissue is proposed. Bone grafting may be done 2 weeks after delayed primary wound closure, skin grafting, or local rotational myoplasty.

▶ Early prophylactic posterolateral bone grafting was compared retrospectively with historical controls. This approach normally would pose some difficulties, but the differences were not meaningful. Because the authors have a long experience with severe injuries, many of the practical points they discuss here are valid. For example, they advocate early soft tissue coverage by modern methods, including free tissue transfer before grafting, instead of open methods. They prefer the posterolateral approach, which preserves the blood supply going to the graft. The time necessary for these serious fractures to heal was still long: the healing period was 10 months, and some patients needed several grafts and even longer healing times. External fixators were kept in place for long periods, and the authors advised against converting from external to internal fixation. The main deficiency of the paper is the lack of a functional outcome study. Some comments about cost-benefit analysis and the benefits at least some of these patients would have received from early amputation would have been helpful.

Two other papers published in 1989 are pertinent to the topic of bone grafting in the tibia (1, 2).—S.T. Hansen, Jr., M.D.

References

1. Hulth A: *Clin Orthop* 249:265, 1989.
2. Aebi M, et al: *Int Orthop* 13:101, 1989.

The Effects of Drilling on Revascularization and New Bone Formation in Canine Femoral Heads With Avascular Necrosis: An Initial Study
Dahners LE, Hillsgrove DC (Univ of North Carolina, Chapel Hill; Univ of California, Los Angeles)
J Orthop Trauma 3:309-312, December 1989   2-29

Avascular necrosis (AVN) of the femoral head is a common cause of chronic hip pain. A previous histologic study of posttraumatic AVN of the femoral head showed a broad front of revascularization that rapidly progressed through the traumatically devitalized femoral head during the healing stage. In cases of late segmental collapse, the revascularization process has ceased, and collapse occurred through the dead bone beyond the halted revascularization front. Whether drilling holes in femoral heads with AVN would accelerate revascularization and promote new bone formation was investigated.

Avascular necrosis of the femoral head was induced surgically in 10 dogs. Three dogs had no holes drilled and served as controls. At the time of vascular interruption, the other 7 dogs had 2 or 3 holes varying in diameter between 2.5 and 4.5 mm from the lateral cortex of the greater trochanter to the subchondral bone of the femoral head. Vital fluorescent bone stains were injected as follows: calcein green immediately after operation, xylenol orange 6 weeks after operation, and oxytetracycline 12 weeks after operation. The dogs were killed at 13 weeks after operation. The 10 treated femoral heads as well as 3 contralateral control femoral heads were sectioned for histologic examination.

Nine of the 10 operative femoral heads had morphological changes, including flattening of the head and a narrowing of the femoral neck relative to that of nonoperative control specimens. Areas of obvious collapse of the articular surface or evidence of articular cartilage degeneration were not observed. Histologic examination of the stained sections showed a relative absence of calcein green, confirming the successful production of AVN. In all specimens oxytetracycline uptake was evident, indicating complete revascularization within 12 weeks after surgery. Xylenol orange was found throughout the femoral head in 6 of the 7 drilled heads, indicating complete revascularization within 6 weeks after operation. Calcein green was observed along the full length of the drill tracts, indicating very early new bone deposition.

Drilling holes in femoral heads with AVN appears to accelerate the normal process of revascularization. Early vascular invasion of the drill tracts provides a larger area from which a blood supply may spread to revitalize avascular sections of the femoral head.

▶ Like some earlier studies, this article confirms that perforating the fracture site accelerates revascularization in avascular necrosis. It also points out that a study of dogs is not necessarily pertinent to the human condition.
Another pertinent study done in 1989 was written by Celebi and associates (1).—S.T. Hansen, Jr., M.D.

Reference

1. Celebi MC, et al: *Eur J Plast Surg* 12:29, 1989.

The Fate of Articular Cartilage After Transplantation of Fresh and Cryopreserved Tissue-Antigen-Matched and Mismatched Osteochondral Allografts in Dogs

Stevenson S, Dannucci GA, Sharkey NA, Pool RR (Univ of California, Davis)
J Bone Joint Surg [Am] 71-A:1297–1307, October 1989   2–30

The long-term success of large osteochondral allografts is dependent on the incorporation of the bony portion of the graft as well as on the integrity of the transplanted articular cartilage. Intact cartilage is considered nonimmunogenic in human beings, but chondrocytes are immunogenic. Stimulation of the immune response in allograft recipients renders the implanted cartilage vulnerable to direct injury by cytotoxic antibodies or lymphocytes, or to indirect injury by inflammatory mediators and enzymes induced by the immune response. The utility of histocompatibility antigen-matching when using transplanted articular cartilage was assessed.

Four groups of dogs underwent operation in which the proximal 3 cm of the radius were transplanted. All dogs were tissue-typed. Transplanted were canine leukocyte antigen-mismatched frozen articular cartilage allografts, leukocyte antigen-mismatched fresh allografts, leukocyte antigen-matched fresh allografts, or leukocyte antigen-matched frozen allografts. All animals were observed for 11 months after operation before being killed. Sham operations were performed in the contralateral legs of 12 dogs, and autogenous grafts were placed in the contralateral legs of 10 dogs.

During follow-up, none of the dogs had obvious gross clinical abnormalities. All host-graft interfaces healed; no joints dislocated. At autopsy, synovial membrane of all joints was mildly fibrotic and hyperplastic. However, only dogs that received allografts had severely fibrotic and hyperplastic synovial membranes, showing signs of an inflammatory response. Reaction was most severe in joints treated with fresh canine leukocyte antigen-mismatched allografts. Frozen grafts had significantly poorer histologic scores than did fresh grafts. The deleterious effects of antigen mismatch and freezing were cumulative. Only fresh antigen-matched grafts did as well as autogenous grafts or segments subjected to sham operation.

Osteochondral allografts matched for tissue antigens fare much better than mismatched allografts. Cryopreservation is deleterious to osteochondral allografts as few chondrocytes survived freezing. Because the host response to osteochondral allografts is not innocuous to articular cartilage and current technology of cryopreservation is harmful to allografts, fresh osteochondral allografts matched for tissue antigens will cause the fewest long-term joint-related complications.

▶ This study should generate significant interest among traumatologists and oncologists because orthopedic tumors and trauma can destroy joints in young patients. As might be expected, fresh osteochondral allografts with matching tissue antigens were more successful than frozen allografts. Cryopreservation was associated with significant cartilage damage, but a certain amount of articular damage occurred even in the fresh joints.—S.T. Hansen, Jr., M.D.

Complications and Their Management

The Ilizarov Technique in the Treatment of Infected Tibial Nonunions
Pearson RL, Perry CR (Washington Univ, St Louis)
Orthop Rev 18:609–613, May 1989   2–31

The Ilizarov method of distraction osteogenesis involves placement of a circular small-wire external fixator, corticotomy at a site removed from the bone defect, and advancement of a free bone segment inside its periosteal sleeve into the area of the defect. The segment is moved at a rate of 1 mm/day. The need for large amounts of autologous bone graft is avoided, and the vascular bed of the bone is well preserved. Early weight-bearing ambulation is feasible with this approach.

Infected tibial nonunion was managed in this way in 11 patients since early 1988, and 5 have had adequate follow-up. Four patients had excellent clinical and radiographic bone regeneration at their distraction sites, but 1 had no evidence of new bone, possibly because of compromise of the endosteum after previous treatment. The mean distraction time was 2.4 months, and the mean consolidation time was 5.3 months. One patient needed a second corticotomy. Three patients had superficial pin tract infection, and 4 needed revision of their frames because of a broken pin or improper pin placement. No deep infections occurred, and no patient had prolonged knee stiffness.

The Ilizarov technique is a significant advance in the treatment of infected tibial nonunions, especially those with segmental defects.

▶ Although only half the patients in this recent retrospective study actually had treatment with the Ilizarov method, the principles of treating infected tibial nonunions are well pointed out. The dead and infected bone in the region must be débrided completely before the bone transport method may be used to fill the defect with live bone. It is a slow process that generally works well, although it is subject to virtually guaranteed minor complications. It is interesting that 1 patient showed no new bone with transportation. Most cases required internal fixation and bone grafting at the end of the transport period, but this technique still was considered successful because no dead bone remained.—S.T. Hansen, Jr., M.D.

Infected Tibial Pseudarthrosis: A 2-Year Follow-up on Patients Treated by the Ilizarov Technique

Morandi M, Zembo MM, Ciotti M (Louisiana State Univ Med Ctr, New Orleans; Istituti "Codivilla-Putti," Cortina d'Ampezzo, Italy)
Orthopedics 12:497–508, April 1989

Ilizarov described a method of distraction osteogenesis in which bone regenerates when tensile stress is applied to it. The method requires good limb stability and preservation of the blood supply to the bone. Bone is interrupted only in the cortical layer, and stability is maintained with a circular external fixator. A distraction force of 1 mm per day is applied across the corticotomy gap. Transport of a bone fragment avoids the need for a bone graft. This approach can serve to treat an infected pseudarthrosis in a single stage.

Sixteen patients with infected tibial nonunion underwent transosseous compression distraction osteosynthesis by the Ilizarov technique. Thirteen patients had follow-up for an average of 26 months after removal of the fixator. Ten patients had bone defects averaging 2.6 cm in size. Ten patients had leg length discrepancies averaging 3.2 cm. All patients were able to walk on their affected legs throughout treatment, and all had healing of their tibial pseudarthroses. All were able to walk without crutches. Infection remitted totally in all cases. Only 1 patient had a leg length discrepancy of more than 2 cm at follow-up. Four patients had knee flexion contractures, and a stress fracture developed in 1 at the site of the pseudarthrosis. Problems associated with K-wires were many.

The Ilizarov method is an effective approach to the infected tibial pseudarthrosis and to associated problems without the need for additional surgery. All patients described above previously had undergone conventional treatment.

▶ A large group of patients had follow-up an average of 26 months after their external fixators were removed following treatment with the Ilizarov technique for infected nonunions of the tibia in this somewhat longer and better study. Patients were encouraged to walk during treatment, and all transported bone fragments healed without bone grafting. Infection remitted totally in all cases, but several other complications were noted. A discrepancy in leg length of more than 2 cm remained in 1 patient, knee flexion contractures were noted in 4 patients, and 1 stress fracture occurred through the previous site of pseudarthrosis. Many minor problems were associated with the use of Kirschner wires. Clearly, sophisticated use of this interesting technique may be successful in patients with severe problems and those with previously failed treatment of infected pseudarthroses. The compression-distraction technique described in this paper precluded the use of skin grafts, rotational flaps, or free muscle flaps by virtue of the accompanying vascular neogenesis and its positive effect on the regional soft tissues.—S.T. Hansen, Jr., M.D.

Infection After Intramedullary Nailing of Severe Open Tibial Fractures Initially Treated With External Fixation
Maurer DJ, Merkow RL, Gustilo RB (Hennepin County Med Ctr, Minneapolis)
J Bone Joint Surg 71-A:835–838, July 1989   2–33

External fixation and reamed intramedullary nailing have become standard methods of treatment for open tibial fractures even though external fixation is associated with risks of both pin tract infection and delayed union or nonunion. Twenty-four patients with such fractures were examined for the incidence of pin site infection, nail infection, and factors contributing to these complications.

All but 1 of the fractures were sustained in motor vehicle accidents. The patients' average age was 27.8 years, and all but 3 were male. An average of 5.5 pins had been used, and external fixation had been maintained for an average of 52 days. When an external fixator was removed, a cast or brace was worn for an average of 65 days before intramedullary nailing was performed.

Seven patients (29%) had a proved infection at 1 or more pin sites. Five of these patients subsequently had deep infection around their intramedullary nails. In contrast, only 1 patient without a previous pin tract infection had a nail infection. Pin site infection was not related significantly to the duration of external fixation, number of pins used, patient age, or type of fracture.

The overall risk of infection in reamed intramedullary nailing after initial external fixation was approximately 25%. However, when divided into groups of (1) those with no evident pin tract infection during the course of external fixation and (2) those with clinical pin tract infection, the infection rates were 71% vs. 6%. Clearly, reamed intramedullary nailing is unacceptably risky after external fixation of an open tibia fracture if there has been a clinically evident pin tract infection.

▶ Treating delayed tibial unions that result from external fixation with intramedullary nailing is a topic of continuing interest. The authors point out that the criterion that indicates intramedullary nailing after an external fixator is removed is absence of a clinical pin tract infection. Because pin tract infections occur commonly in fractures treated with external fixators, this paper provides evidence that nonreamed locked intramedullary nails should be evaluated for treatment of open tibial fractures that have been treated with external fixators in the previous 5 to 10 years.— S.T. Hansen, Jr., M.D.

Severe Trauma to the Lower Extremity: Long-term Sequelae
Moore TJ, Green SA, Garland DE (Rancho Los Amigos Med Ctr, Downey, Calif)
South Med J 82:843–844, July 1989   2–34

Despite advances in emergency medicine and orthopedic surgery, salvaged lower limbs often lack normal function. Management and outcome were reviewed in a series of patients with severe trauma to the lower extremities that needed long-term reconstruction.

Of 121 patients referred to a tertiary level hospital over a 15-year period, most had injuries caused by motor vehicle or motorcycle accidents. Limb salvage was achieved in 109 patients after 224 surgical procedures and an average of 3 years of treatment. Seventy patients had 72 tibial nonunions. Septic tibial nonunion resulted in 9 amputations, 2 after failure of attempted reconstruction. Thirty patients were admitted with complications after surgery for supracondylar fractures of the femur. Two of 3 patients needing amputation died of systemic sepsis. Approximately half of the patients returned to preinjury ambulatory level. Nine of 12 patients given treatment for chronic sepsis after intramedullary nailing of femoral fractures had clinical success, but had persistent knee symptoms; 8 of 9 patients with impaired knee function resulting from severe femoral fractures had satisfactory knee flexion after quadricepsplasty.

Success was measured by fracture healing, satisfactory joint motion, and eradication of infection; most patients continued to have significant disability. After a lengthy and expensive process, severely traumatized limbs that are salvaged generally do not return to preinjury function and appearance.

▶ The authors of this paper have extensive experience in salvage procedures of the lower limb. They present a moderately depressing picture of difficult long-term limb salvage, listing complications that range from multiple operations that result in a dysfunctional limb to delayed amputation and even sepsis and death. Experienced surgeons who deal with severe injuries in the immediate phases are required to make appropriate decisions about amputation or salvage and to carry them out extremely well. The paper also points out the need to evaluate the results of salvage procedures in terms of function and cost-effectiveness.—S.T. Hansen, Jr., M.D.

References

1. Sledge SL, et al: *J Bone Joint Surg [Am]* 71-A:1004, 1989.
2. Miller ME, et al: *Clin Orthop* 245:233, 1989.

Compartment Syndrome: A Complication of Intravenous Regional Anesthesia in the Reduction of Lower Leg Shaft Fractures
Maletis GB, Watson RC, Scott S (Tahoe Fracture and Orthopedic Med Clinic, South Lake Tahoe, Calif)
Orthopedics 12:841–846, June 1989

Compartment syndrome is a known complication of lower leg fractures. It has been suggested that applying a tourniquet above a fracture site sets up a condition of ischemia in an area that is already a prime target for compartment syndrome, and that intravenous (IV) regional anesthesia compounds the situation and increases the chances of compartment syndrome. The incidence of compartment syndrome after IV regional anesthesia for the reduction of a lower leg fracture was compared with that in a control group of patients who underwent general anesthesia or IV analgesia alone.

The study included 41 patients who underwent closed reduction of displaced lower leg shaft fractures under IV regional anesthesia and 39 patients who underwent reduction of lower leg shaft fractures under IV analgesia or general anesthesia. After operation, 4 of the 41 patients who underwent closed reduction under regional anesthesia were graded as having mild compartment syndrome, 2 had moderate cases, and 5 had severe cases, yielding a 27% overall incidence rate of compartment syndrome. Of the 39 control patients, 3 were graded as having mild compartment syndrome and 2 were graded as severe, yielding an overall compartment syndrome incidence rate of 13%. Because acceptable alternative methods of pain control are available, it is suggested that IV regional anesthesia not be used in the management of lower leg shaft fractures.

▶ Regional anesthesia, especially the intravenous regional technique or so-called Bier block that is used in the lower extremity after trauma, potentially may cause compartment syndromes. Many people regard unusual pain as the most reliable symptom of compartment syndrome, and this type of intravenous analgesia has the potential to mask the pain caused by compartment pressure, leaving a patient completely free of pain while mild necrosis advances. Compartment syndromes are completely preventable, and their medical-legal ramifications can be devastating. Traumatologists must learn to recognize the conditions that predispose a patient to compartment syndrome.

Several other papers about compartment syndrome should be read along with this article (1–5).—S.T. Hansen, Jr., M.D.

References

1. Younge D: *J Hand Surg [Br]* 14-B:194, 1989.
2. Smith MD: *Orthop Rev* 18:1316, 1989.
3. Shah PM, et al: *Am J Surg* 158:136, 1989.
4. Jones WG, et al: *Arch Surg* 124:801, 1989.
5. Strauss MB, Hart GB: *Contemp Orthop* 18:167, 1989.

Acute Compartment Syndrome of the Thigh: A Spectrum of Injury
Schwartz JT Jr, Brumback RJ, Lakatos R, Poka A, Bathon GH, Burgess AR (Maryland Inst for Emergency Med Services Systems, Baltimore; Univ of Maryland)
J Bone Joint Surg 71-A:392–400, March 1989

2–36

Compartment syndrome of the thigh is a rare condition. A retrospective study was made of 21 cases of compartment syndrome of the thigh in 17 patients seen from 1983 to 1987.

Patients who were awake and alert at the time of examination reported severe pain in the thigh, and they had neuromuscular deficits. The presence of tension and swelling in the thigh raised the suspicion of compartment syndrome. Among patients who could not cooperate because they were under general anesthesia or because of associated injuries, measurement of the intracompartmental pressure was essential to the diagnosis. All patients had tense swelling in the involved thigh.

Average injury severity score for the entire group was 32.5 points (range, 17–57). Average Glasgow coma score was 11.4 (range, 4–15). Ten compartment syndromes were associated with an ipsilateral femoral fracture, including 5 open fractures. Compartment syndrome occurred after intramedullary stabilization in 5 patients. The remaining 11 syndromes occurred after blunt trauma to the thigh, prolonged compression by the body weight, and vascular injury. The incidence of predisposing factors to the development of compartment syndrome of the thigh was high among these patients. These factors included systemic hypotension, history of external compression of the thigh, use of military trousers, coagulopathy, vascular injury, and trauma to the thigh, with or without a fracture of the femur. Crush syndrome, consisting of myoglobinuria, acute renal failure, and multiple organ system collapse, developed in 7 patients.

Decompressive fasciotomy was undertaken an average of 4 hours (range, less than 1 hour to 16.3 hours) after diagnosis. Eight patients died of multiple injuries. Of the 9 survivors, infection developed at the site of fasciotomy in 6 and follow-up showed marked morbidity, including sensory deficit and motor weakness of the lower extremity.

Compartment syndrome of the thigh, although rare as an isolated injury, occurs frequently in patients with multiple trauma. Early diagnosis, followed by immediate fasciotomy of the thigh, is necessary.

▶ Compartment syndromes may occur in the thigh after high-energy trauma. Such syndromes usually are caused by injury of very high energy and is almost always accompanied by a high injury severity score and the potential for major complications, including adult respiratory distress syndrome. Fasciotomy is needed as soon as compartment syndrome is diagnosed to prevent mild necrosis, even though it may introduce new problems. Rehabilitation after fasciotomy in the thigh may be prolonged, but appropriate treatment of the thigh compartment facilitates functional recovery.

An article written by Forrest and colleagues may be helpful in understanding compartment syndrome and the reperfusion syndrome (1).—S.T. Hansen, Jr., M.D.

Reference

1. Forrest I, et al: *J Vasc Surg* 10:83, 1989.

Amputation

How Successful Is Below-knee Amputation for Injury?
Purry NA, Hannon MA (DSA Artificial Limb and Appliance Centre, Bristol, England)
Injury 20:32–36, January 1989   2–37

Although limb preservation after severe below-the-knee leg injury in young adults always is considered the first approach, a patient's interests sometimes may be better served by amputation. Because rehabilitation results after below-the knee amputation have not been well studied, data for 25 patients aged less than 45 years at the time of amputation were reviewed to determine how successfully they had rehabilitated.

All patients were healthy young adults aged 4–43 years at the time of the accident. At evaluation 2–12 years after amputation, 21 patients were wearing patellar tendon bearing (PTB) prostheses; unable to tolerate the PTB prosthesis because of stump problems, 4 were wearing other prostheses. Most (84%) were wearing their prostheses for 13 hours a day or longer. Eighteen of the 25 patients were able to participate in 1 or more sports. Eighteen patients could walk 1 mile or more on flat surfaces without problems, 6 could walk on slopes, and 10 were able to walk upstairs without problems. Only 4 patients were using canes, and 2 sometimes used crutches. Twenty-one patients owned and drove cars, 4 of whom also owned and rode motorcycles.

Present level of activity was reached in 7 patients in 6 months or less, in 7 within 1 year, and in 11 about 1 year. None of the patients considered themselves very disabled, and 17 patients thought they lived lives similar to those of noninjured patients. However, phantom or stump pain remained a problem for many patients. Four patients were having constant stump pain, and 3 had frequent pain. Despite persistent phantom or stump pain, 7 patients were able to go back to the same type of work they had before their accidents and 15 found different work. Two patients were housewives, and only 1 patient was unemployed. Thus, most young, healthy adults who undergo below-the-knee amputation will do extremely well.

▶ An extremely interesting view of the trend toward amputation of severely injured tibias, particularly grade IIIC injuries, is presented here. Grade IIIC injuries are generally severe, high-energy fractures that often have accompanying vascular injuries and usually require repair of a large zone of injury. This paper shows that patients aged as much as 43 years at the time of accident can be rehabilitated successfully after amputation.

I analyzed the authors' data and found that, although many aspects of rehabilitation were the same for both the immediate and delayed groups, how soon a patient returned to work after injury was significantly different. Delays in amputation averaged a little more than 2 years—even without including 1 patient who had a delay of 15 years—and 2 more years before such patients actually returned to work. In comparison, patients who had immediate amputations, probably because their injuries were more severe, returned to work after just more than 1 year. Thus, if the need for an amputation could be predicted, approximately 3 years could be saved in productive work time by performing an amputation immediately.—S.T. Hansen, Jr., M.D.

Relief of Persistent Postamputation Stump and Phantom Limb Pain With Intrathecal Fentanyl
Jacobson L, Chabal C, Brody MC (Univ of Washington; VA Med Ctr, Seattle)
Pain 37:317–322, June 1989   2–38

Two patients obtained temporary relief of postamputation stump pain and phantom limb pain after treatment with intrathecal fentanyl.

Case 1.—Man, 35, had undergone a left above-knee amputation 3 months earlier because of intractable osteomyelitis after a motorcycle accident 3 years previously that severely injured his left leg. He reported left phantom limb pain that felt as if hot electric needles were repeatedly sticking him. There also seemed to be an electric current running through the left phantom foot. Amitriptyline given at night and a pain cocktail of methadone, hydroxyzine, and acetaminophen given every 6 hours had not been effective. After an intravenous cannula was inserted and monitoring was established, fentanyl, 25 µg, was injected at the L2–L3 interspace. Within 1 minute of injection, the patient felt a warmth in the lower trunk that ran down his leg into the phantom foot; by 3 minutes, all pain was gone. The feelings of warmth and euphoria reached a peak at 5 minutes, persisted for 15 minutes, but gradually receded until they disappeared by 90 minutes. The complete pain relief lasted for 2 hours, when sensations of pins and needles returned.

Case 2.—Man, 45, with a left below-knee amputation after a parachuting mishap had had persistent stump pain since 1979. He had undergone 3 neuroma excisions with no relief. Meperidine and codeine had been ineffective. He also was given subarachnoid fentanyl, which relieved the stump pain within 1 minute of injection. The intense feelings of warmth and euphoria subsided after 1–2 hours, but some degree of warmth persisted for 18 hours, and he remained pain free for 9 days after the intrathecal injection of fentanyl. He subsequently was given a series of other injections, including intrathecal, extradural, and intravenous fentanyl and an intrathecal lidocaine injection. Whereas intrathecal and epidural fentanyl injections temporarily abolished the pain, intravenous fentanyl and intrathecal lidocaine injections did not.

These data indicate that lumbar neuraxial fentanyl administration can produce dramatic pain relief and euphoria in patients with postamputation stump pain and phantom limb pain.

▶ The previous papers indicated that one of the major complications seen in amputations is postamputation stump and phantom limb pain. Anesthesiologists are becoming interested in managing postoperative pain, and many centers are developing divisions or specialists within their departments to deal with these problems. This paper reports an early step in that direction.—S.T. Hansen, Jr., M.D.

Reference

1. Katz J, et al: *Pain* 36:367, 1989.

Estimation of Amputation Level With a Laser Doppler Flowmeter
Gebuhr P, Jørgensen JP, Vollmer-Larsen B, Nielsen SL, Alsbjørn B (Hvidovre and Bispebjerg Hosps, Denmark)
J Bone Joint Surg [Br] 71-B:514–517, May 1989   2–39

Available methods of selecting an amputation level for atherosclerotic disease are invasive, costly, and painful. Laser Doppler flowmetry (LDF), a noninvasive alternative that records microperfusion of the tissues continuously (Fig 2–5), was compared with isotopic clearance studies and segmental systolic blood pressure testing in 24 consecutively seen patients who underwent amputation for atherosclerotic gangrene or rest pain.

Laser Doppler flowmetry was very sensitive to altered blood flow or any outside disturbance; fixing the measuring head to the skin with adhesive rings produced the most steady recordings. The increase in flow that occurred promptly after local heating was correlated directly with heal-

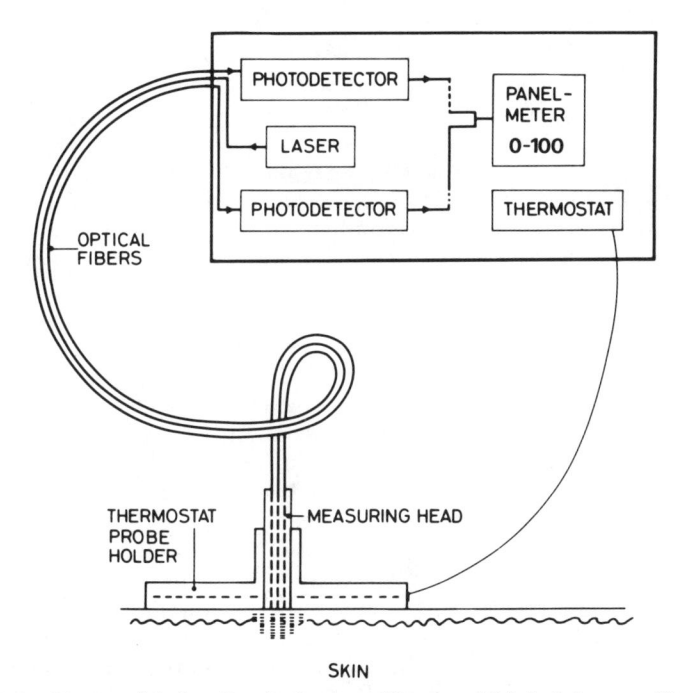

Fig 2–5.—Diagram of the laser Doppler flowmeter. (Courtesy of Gebuhr P, Jørgensen JP, Vollmer-Larsen, et al: *J Bone Joint Surg [Br]* 71-B:514–517, May 1989.)

ing. Baseline flow, however, was not correlated with the level of amputation.

A useful means of predicting healing after amputation, LDF may be used at the bedside and entails no discomfort for the patient. The level of successful amputation is correlated closely with maximal blood perfusion of the skin. A positive "local heat test" implies the presence of microcirculatory reserve that is needed to ensure healing.

▶ Laser Doppler flowmetry is one of the exciting new techniques being applied to orthopedic problems and has been used successfully in débriding osteomyelitis. The technique is somewhat difficult to master, but this group achieved excellent results with local heating and by measuring flow changes with the laser Doppler flowmeter. This technique offers a major advance in predicting primary healing after amputation.
Several other studies about lowering the risks of complications after amputation were published last year (1–4).—S.T. Hansen, Jr., M.D.

References

1. Kram HB, et al: *Am J Surg* 158:29, 1989.
2. Falstie-Jensen N, et al: *Acta Orthop Scand* 60:483, 1989.
3. Falstie-Jensen N, et al: *J Bone Joint Surg [Br]* 71-B:102, 1989.
4. Au KK: *J Bone Joint Surg [Br]* 71-B:597, 1989.

Comparison of CAD-CAM and Hand Made Sockets for PTB Prostheses
Köhler P, Lindh L, Netz P (Karolinska Hosp, Stockholm)
Prosthet Orthot Int 13:19–24, April 1989
2–40

In the 1970s a computer-aided design and computer-aided manufacturing (CAD-CAM) system was developed at the University of British Columbia. The shape of a socket for a below-knee prosthesis is defined by a computer from manual measurements of the stump. Another CAD-CAM system developed at University College London involves a plaster wrap of the undeformed stump made for probe measurements, which are transferred digitally into a computer. The computer makes the average rectifications of a skilled prosthetist at standard areas. Both systems reportedly have provided well-tolerated sockets for below-knee amputees.

Sockets made with CAD-CAM were compared with handmade sockets in 8 unilateral below-knee amputees who used their prostheses all day. Apart from the sockets, the prostheses were identical. Only 2 of the manually made sockets but all except 1 of the CAD-CAM sockets had to be changed. The 2 types of socket were equally comfortable, and both types were accepted well by all the patients. Nevertheless, sockets obviously differed in width, trim line, and configuration of inner surface.

This series is a small one, but the patients served as their own controls, and it is apparent that CAD-CAM sockets are not significantly more or less comfortable than their handmade counterparts in below-knee amputees. The computerized approach can provide sockets of uniformly high quality. Stump forms are easily stored. In addition, the method will aid the teaching of prosthetists.

▶ The technology is available to make excellent prosthetics not only very quickly but also very inexpensively. Many amputees in the third-world war zones, including Afghanistan, southeast Asia, Central America, and South America, could benefit from this technology, which is easily transportable and could be adopted successfully by many of these countries.—S.T. Hansen, Jr., M.D.

Other pertinent papers published in 1989 about the manufacture of prosthetic sockets include:

References

1. Krouskop TA, et al: *J Prosthet Orthop* 1:131, 1989.
Note the different terminology in the paper by:
2. Flandry F, et al: *Clin Orthop* 239:249, 1989.
3. Gottschalk FA, et al: *J Prosthet Orthop* 2:94, 1989.
4. Ozyalcin H, Sesli E: *Prosthet Orthop Int* 13:86, 1989.

Imaging

Preoperative Angiographic Assessment of the Superior Gluteal Artery in Acetabular Fractures Requiring Extensile Surgical Exposures
Bosse MJ, Poka A, Reinert CM, Brumback RJ, Bathon H, Burgess AR (US Naval Hosp, Portsmouth, Va; Maryland Inst of Emergency Med Services, Baltimore)
J Orthop Trauma 2:303–307, 1989   2–41

Complex acetabular fractures often are treated by constructing an abductor muscle flap that is pedicled solely on the superior gluteal artery. However, a potential risk exists for ischemic necrosis of this muscle flap if the superior gluteal artery is injured either before or during operation.

Preoperative arteriographic evaluation of the superior gluteal artery was assessed in 8 patients with complex acetabular fractures displaced into the sciatic notch. In 5 patients, arteriograph examinations and findings at operation were normal. One arteriogram showed entrapment of the superior gluteal artery by the displaced fracture fragments that was confirmed at operation. The artery was carefully dissected from the fracture site, and the surgery was concluded without complications. Arteriography studies in 2 other patients showed active bleeding and occlusion of the superior gluteal artery. Because of their arterial injuries, these 2 patients were not eligible for undergoing the abductor flap operation. One patient died of associated injuries before hip surgery could be performed. The other patient had temporary medical treatment, keeping open the option for later total hip replacement if degenerative arthritis develops.

The successful completion of extented iliofemoral surgical dissection in the reconstruction of complex acetabular fractures requires a patent superior gluteal artery. All patients with fracture displacement into the sciatic notch should undergo arteriography before surgery to assess the status of the superior gluteal artery. Those in whom superior gluteal artery injury is shown on the arteriogram examination are at risk for ischemic necrosis of the abductor muscles and should be treated with alternate approaches.

▶ This paper also could have been included in the section Traumatology because it illustrates the extremely sophisticated surgical and imaging techniques that are needed for very severe injuries. Preoperative angiographic assessment of the superior gluteal artery, a major artery that must be protected in complex acetabular operations, is essential for successful acetabular fracture reconstruction. Using Dopplers to duplicate scans of the venous system after major pelvic injury may be helpful in averting fatal postoperative pulmonary embolism by the occasional use of prophylactic filters in the inferior vena cava.
Imaging also was used to detect an abnormality, as reported by Catsikis and associates (1).—S.T. Hansen, Jr., M.D.

Reference

1. Catsikis BD, et al: *J Comput Assist Tomogr* 13:148, 1989.

Occult Intraosseous Fracture: Magnetic Resonance Appearance Versus Age of Injury
Lee JK, Yao L (Albany Med College; Albany Med Ctr Hosp, Albany, NY)
Am J Sports Med 17:620–623, September–October 1989   2-42

The diagnosis of occult intraosseous fracture is based on typically located findings on magnetic resonance imaging (MRI) with a history of recent injury and normal radiographic appearance. To correlate the MRI findings with the age of injury, data on 22 patients were reviewed.

The history always included a solitary injury to the knee, but the mechanism varied. Magnetic resonance imaging revealed bandlike or speckled areas of decreased intensity of signal in the epiphysis, especially in T_1-weighted or proton density images. The T_2-weighted images of corresponding regions showed signal intensities ranging as follows: rare or absent high signal, graded as 0; increased intensity of signal in an area slightly smaller or equal in size, grade 1; high signal findings in a more extensive area, grade 2. Generally, as the area of high signal findings on the T_2-weighted images increased, the duration of injury decreased, but the groups varied considerably.

The T_2-weighted images showing high signal intensity apparently change more quickly than the low signal intensity on T_1-weighted images, but the age of the lesion cannot be predicted only on the basis of the image. The fracture seems to be caused by direct impact or axial overloading. Diagnosis requires interpretation of the MRI appearance in light of the clinical setting of pain persisting after injury in the absence of other knee lesions.

▶ Magnetic resonance imaging is potentially very useful in cases of trauma; for example, grade 1 osteochondral lesions in the ankle may be visible only with MRI. This paper indicates that only T_1-weighted images revealed otherwise unapparent intraosseous fractures after trauma in the metaphyseal area. The relative usefulness and cost-effectiveness of MRI must be compared with those of standard roentgenography, CT, and scintigraphy in the next several years.—S.T. Hansen, Jr., M.D.

References

    1. Laasonen EM, et al: *Arch Orthop Trauma Surg* 108:40, 1989.
    2. Tawn DJ, Watt I: *Br J Radiol* 62:790, 1989.

Miscellaneous

The Mechanical Performance of Ambulation Using Spring-Loaded Axillary Crutches: A Preliminary Report
Parziale JR, Daniels JD (Brown Univ; Rhode Island Hosp, Providence, RI)
Am J Phys Med Rehabil 68:192–195, August 1989   2–43

    Can upper limb stress be reduced during crutch-aided ambulation? A study of gait involved both standard axillary crutches and axillary crutches having the extension post replaced by a spring-loaded post. Of the 7 experienced crutch users studied, 6 were physical therapists. They ambulated for 100 feet using a swing-through gait pattern at a comfortable rate. Both high and lower spring constants were tried.
    Speed of ambulation was nearly identical with each of the crutch pairs, and time to maximal stress also was similar. The shock wave amplitude was 22% less with spring-loaded crutches than with the wooden crutch. Maximal stress was 24% less when spring-loaded crutches were used. Slow-motion videotapes showed that down-directed weight was borne by the crutches.
    Spring-loaded crutches significantly reduce peak stress when normal subjects use them. The energy-storing ability of these crutches, along with reduced shock wave amplitude and lower peak stress at the hand and wrist, could minimize fatigue and upper limb pain in crutch users.

▶ Impact-loading can result in arthrosis; its effects can be neutralized by spring-loaded ambulation aids. This principle has been applied in prosthetics made for amputees who attempt to run. Arthrosis is also much more common in limbs that have lost the subtalar joint, which is the major shock absorber in the lower extremity. It is hoped we will hear much more about this basic principle in the coming years.
    A particularly good companion paper was written by Di Angelo and co-workers (1).—S.T. Hansen, Jr., M.D.

Reference

1. Di Angelo DJ, et al: *J Biomechanics* 22:543, 1989.

A Biomechanical Analysis of the Ilizarov External Fixator
Fleming B, Paley D, Kristiansen T, Pope M (Univ of Vermont, Burlington; Univ of Maryland, Baltimore)
Clin Orthop 241:95–105, April 1989   2–44

The Ilizarov system consists of a modular ring fixator that uses K wires to hold the bone fragments in place and a calibrated tensioning device that transforms the flexible wires into relatively stiff pins. The goal is to hold the fragments in alignment while allowing axial dynamization at the fracture site. Stiffness and fracture gap motion of 5 configurations of the Ilizarov ring fixator were compared with 8 conventional one-half pin fixators.

The Ilizarov fixator was comparable to the one-half pin fixators with respect to overall stiffness and shear rigidity in bending and torsion. The stability of the Ilizarov fixator was dependent on bone position within the fixator rings and fixation wire tension. The use of olive stop wires increased the shear resistance of the Ilizarov system. Axial stiffness of the Ilizarov fixator was considerably less than that of the uniplanar and biplanar one-half pin fixators.

The Ilizarov fixator allows axial dynamization at the fracture site. It controls shear at the fracture site as well as conventional fixators. Differences in overall stiffness in torsion and bending seem minimal. The mechanical properties of the Ilizarov fixator appear to be ideal.

▶ The Ilizarov external fixator has generated a great deal of interest recently. The device is meant to be used in conjunction with active walking, and it allegedly produces the best results when a patient bears significant weight on the affected extremity. This paper demonstrates that the Ilizarov fixator allows significantly more axial motion at the fracture site during axial compression than other, conventional fixators that were tested. This information should be of major interest to those wanting to use the Ilizarov fixator for the advantages that it provides in correcting deformity and equalizing length, and for its unique property of stimulating osseous and vascular neogenesis.—S.T. Hansen, Jr., M.D.

Two papers that compare different aspects and properties of the Ilizarov technique are:

References

1. Zarnett R, Salter RB: *CJS* 32:171, 1989.
2. De Boer HH, Wood MB: *J Bone Joint Surg [Br]* 71-B:374, 1989.

3 Shoulder, Elbow, and Forearm

Introduction

Trauma and its sequelae are a prominent part of the literature so far as the shoulder, arm, elbow, and forearm are concerned. Proximal humeral fractures continue to be difficult to treat; attempts are being made to better understand these fractures and to offer alternative treatment methods. Instability after dislocation of the shoulder also continues to be an important and common problem. Many forms of operative treatment deal with recurrent instability, and both the benefits and limitations of these procedures are becoming understood more fully. Not much is known about sternoclavicular instability, but this year, several articles have addressed it. It is suggested that surgeons continue to adopt a conservative approach when treating this problem. The variations in fracturing about the elbow are being defined continually, and new classification systems are being offered. Internal fixation is difficult. Maintaining stability of the internally fixated fracture, yet attempting early movement, is often counterproductive. Instability associated with elbow fracturing is often extremely difficult to treat successfully. Forearm fractures have been revisited. Plate fixation is very good in terms of achieving union and a satisfactory result. When larger plates are used, refracturing is apparently all too frequent.

Developments in imaging of the shoulder, particularly the rotator cuff, have been exciting. Ultrasound was introduced a number of years ago. Success in imaging the rotator cuff initially was thought to be quite high; now, the limitations of ultrasound are recognized, and it apparently is quite difficult to image smaller tears with consistency using this modality. Magnetic resonance (MR) imaging is being improved dramatically relative to shoulder imaging; it now essentially equals arthrography in terms of effectiveness in imaging the rotator cuff. However, MR will show certain things better than arthrography and arthrography will define other things better than MR. The two methods may, in fact, be complementary tests in some instances. The importance of the frozen shoulder, whatever that might be, has been understated in the recent past. Fortunately, this year several articles exist on this subject, which is a common problem and cannot be forgotten.

Prosthetic arthroplasty has achieved a high level of acceptance for the shoulder and is bordering on the same for the elbow. The results of the unconstrained total shoulder arthroplasties are now well understood. More than 90% of patients have satisfactory pain relief. Return of movement and strength varies among diagnoses and by the extent of rotator cuff disease. However, the return of movement and strength tends to average about two thirds normal, which is not much different from total arthroplasty of other major joints. Total shoulder arthroplasty rarely requires reoperation, and the clinical results to date have, by and large, been quite good. Almost all series, though, have had significant changes at the bone–cement interface of the glenoid, which continues to be worrisome. At the elbow, the unconstrained arthroplasty historically did not loosen frequently, but had the complications of instability and ulnar nerve injury. Now, the surgical approach has been modified to deal with the latter, and more exacting technique has to some extent reduced the former. Semiconstrained total elbow replacements with hinge mechanisms have been developed to reconstruct elbows in patients for whom an unconstrained device would not be appropriate. These devices still have some difficulties, the most predominant of which is loosening or mechanical failure at the hinge. Thankfully, these complications are greatly diminished compared with what they were in the past.

Scientific activity in this anatomical region is great. Disease processes are becoming better understood. Diagnostic modalities are being increasingly refined, or new ones have been developed. Now treatment for most of the traumatic problems, for rotator cuff disease, and for arthritis of the shoulder or the elbow is effective. We are all thankful to have so many persons actively investigating problems within this region.

Robert H. Cofield, M.D.

Shoulder

TRAUMA AND RELATED CONDITIONS

The Epidemiology of Fractures of the Proximal Humerus
Lind T, Krøner K, Jensen J (Aarhus County Hosp; Aarhus Municipal Hosp, Aarhus, Denmark)
Arch Orthop Trauma Surg 108:285–287, 1989   3–1

Fractures of the neck of the humerus are common, particularly in older patients. About 5% of all humeral fractures are localized to the proximal humerus. The epidemiology of proximal fractures of the humerus were examined.

During a 5-year study period, 730 proximal fractures of the humerus were treated at the 3 hospitals in Aarhus, a community of 250,000 residents. Most of the fractures (75.8%) occurred in women; 71% of the fractures occurred in patients aged more than 60 years. When grouped by age and by sex, the incidence of proximal humeral fractures showed no significant differences among patients aged up to 50 years (Fig 3–1). However, after age 50 years, incidence rates for women were increased exponentially, reaching a maximum of 409/100,000, whereas the total incidence rate of fractures was 73/100,000 population. Only 210 of the 730 patients were hospitalized, but 75% of the hospitalized patients were aged more than 60 years. Although reduction or internal fixation was performed in only 44 (21%) hospitalized patients, most hospital admis-

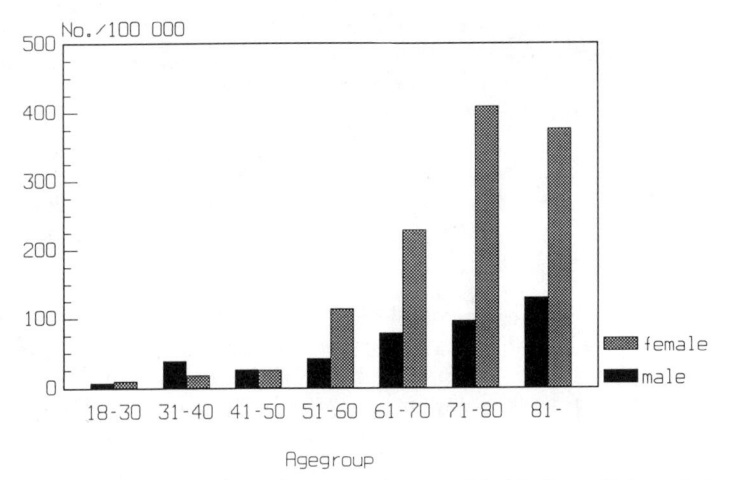

Fig 3-1.—Age- and sex-specific incidence rates. (Courtesy of Lind T, Krøner K, Jensen J: *Arch Orthop Trauma Surg* 108:285-287, 1989.)

sions were for social reasons. The average hospital stay was 13.8 days. A total of 583 bed-days/year were used for the treatment of humeral fractures.

Uncomplicated falls, mostly on level ground, caused 79% of the humeral neck fractures. Traffic accidents, including pedestrian falls, were responsible for another 14%. Only 1.5% of the fractures were caused by industrial accidents. Most accidents occurred around midday, with another peak occurring before midnight. Humeral fractures occurred most often in December and January. About half of all humeral neck fractures were 2-part fractures, whereas fractures of the greater tubercle accounted for 21%, and 3-part fractures, for 17%. Based on the current increases in the population's average life span in Denmark, it is expected that proximal fractures will increase the hospital workload significantly in the near future.

Treatment of Displaced Fractures of the Proximal Humerus: Transcutaneous Reduction and Hoffmann's External Fixation
Kristiansen B (Univ of Copenhagen)
Injury 20:195-199, July 1989   3-2

Displaced 2-, 3-, and 4-part fractures of the proximal humerus have been treated in various ways. Closed methods sometimes result in poor reduction and instability. Open reduction and internal fixation provides stability but is technically demanding and carries risk of infection. The results of an alternative treatment, transcutaneous reduction and external fixation, performed in 27 patients (28 fractures) were reviewed.

The patients' median age was 66 years. Eight fractures were 2-part, 14 were 3-part, and 6 were 4-part. Reduction is performed while a patient is under general anesthesia.

Technique.—In the 2-part fracture, a Steinmann pin is introduced into the humeral head. Reduction is then performed by manipulation of the shaft (Fig 3–2). With a 3-part fracture, the head fragment is derotated by the Steinmann pin. If present, an avulsion of the greater tuberosity can be reduced by one of the half pins in combination with manipulative extension-abduction of the shaft. Four-part fractures have depression of the articular fragment between the tuberosities. After reduction, 2 half-pins are drilled into the head and 3 pins are drilled into the shaft laterally. The Steinmann pin is removed after a neutralizing bar is applied.

Nineteen patients were available for follow-up. Results were excellent or satisfactory in 13 (68%) patients, unsatisfactory in 4 (21%), and poor in 2 (11%). Nonunion occurred in 1 patient. A major complication was loosening of the pins in 5 patients, all of whom had severe osteoporosis

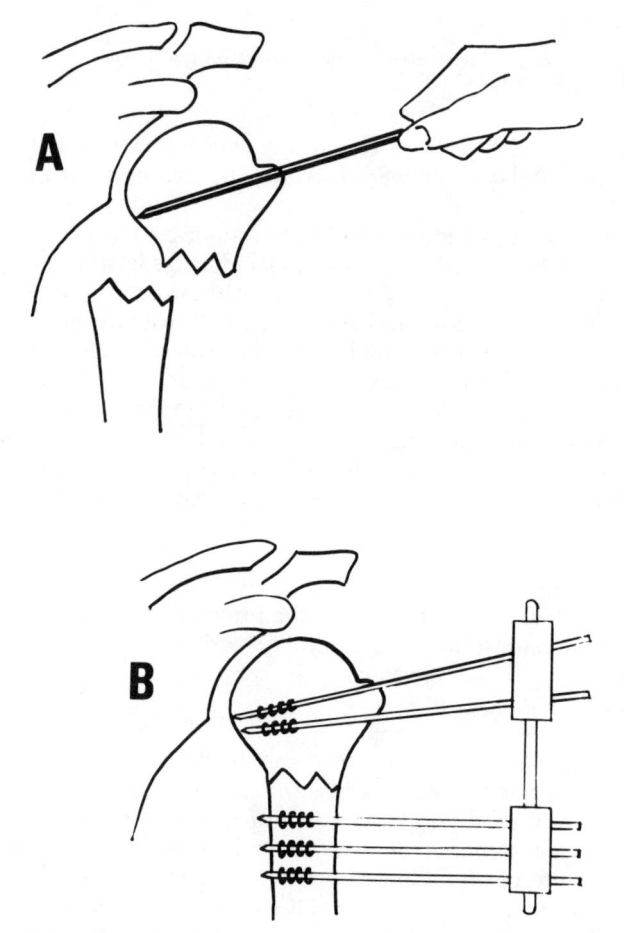

Fig 3–2.—Displaced surgical neck fracture. **A**, transcutaneous reduction using a Steinmann pin; **B**, external fixation. (Courtesy of Kristiansen B: *Injury* 20:195–199, July 1989.)

or head splitting fractures. Transcutaneous reduction and external fixation is a useful technique in certain cases. When this method fails, 2- and 3-part fractures can be treated with open reduction and internal fixation, whereas 4-part fractures may require primary arthroplasty.

▶ The author not only uses the pins and external fixator to hold a reduction but actually manipulates the fragments with a pin, creating a much better reduction than otherwise could be obtained. Most surgeons probably could not be as skilled with the use of pins for reduction as the author shows, but certainly this is another apparently quite reasonable method for the fracture surgeon to have in his treatment armamentarium for these difficult injuries.—R.H. Cofield, M.D.

A Reassessment of the Role of Arteriography in Penetrating Proximity Extremity Trauma: A Prospective Study
Frykberg ER, Crump JM, Vines FS, McLellan GL, Dennis JW, Brunner RG, Alexander RH (Univ of Florida, Jacksonville)
J Trauma 29:1041–1052, August 1989   3–3

The need for routine arteriography (AG) in patients with penetrating extremity wounds that are proximal to major blood is controversial. To clarify the role of routine arteriography, 152 penetrating proximity extremity (PPET) injuries in 135 patients were studied over a 24-month period.

The patients ranged in age from 14 to 84 years; 86% were men. Sixty-nine patients were assigned randomly to immediate AG, and 66 to AG delayed for up to 24 hours. Of the 27 AG abnormalities, 11 occurred in noncritical vessels and were not investigated further. The remaining 16 clinically occult injuries involved major blood vessels. One patient with an acute arteriovenous fistula in the superficial femoral vessels underwent immediate surgical exploration. The remaining 15 vascular injuries were treated nonsurgically. One patient who showed arteriographic enlargement of a small pseudo-aneurysm of the brachial artery after a 10-week interval underwent prompt surgical repair, even though he was asymptomatic. None of the patients died, and no extremity morbidity resulted from either delayed AG or the nonsurgical vascular injury management.

The routine AG assessment of PPET for the 135 study patients led to a charge of at least $132,840.00. The detection of each of the 16 injuries to a major extremity artery led to a charge of $8,302.50. It took $66,420.00 to detect each of the 2 injuries that ultimately required surgical repair. The natural history of clinically occult arterial injuries from PPET appeared to be predominantly benign, and AG could be safely delayed for up to 24 hours. In view of the high cost associated with routine AG screening, AG does not appear to be a cost-effective screening modality for patients with PPET.

▶ This interesting study questions the role of immediate arteriographic evaluation of vascular injuries in the upper extremities. In these authors' practice, the number of penetrating wounds was incredible. When arteriography was used routinely for assessment of an extremity at risk, a large proportion of the studies were negative. The authors seemingly have told us that when vascular injury is questionable observation followed by delayed arteriography is as effective as routine early arthrography. Thus, repeated physical examination may replace the need for this expensive diagnostic modality in many of these types of patients. The authors note that shotgun wounds may be an exception to this general rule.—R.H. Cofield, M.D.

Nonunion of the Clavicle and Thoracic Outlet Syndrome
Connolly JF, Dehne R (Univ of Nebraska and VA Med Ctrs, Omaha)
J Trauma 29:1127–1133, August 1989   3–4

Fractures of the midportion of the clavicle are common, particularly in children. Most clavicle fractures heal uneventfully with an estimated overall nonunion rate of less than 1%. Although clavicle fractures are less common in adults than in children, the potential for complications and nonunion in adults is much higher than it is in children. Data on 15 adults with clavicular nonunions were reviewed.

During a 10-year period, 9 men and 6 women aged 21–70 years had treatment for nonunion of clavicular fractures. Fourteen fractures had been treated acutely with a figure-of-8 clavicle strap, which had provided incomplete reduction. The time from injury to diagnosis of nonunion ranged from 4 to 18 months. One patient had an iatrogenic nonunion because of surgical resection of the midclavicle to repair a lacerated subclavian vessel. All patients complained of pain at the nonunion site. Seven patients had narrowing of the costoclavicular space and symptoms of obstruction of the thoracic outlet. Of the 7 patients with thoracic outlet syndrome, 4 had hypertrophic nonunions.

Six patients had hypertrophic nonunions that were treated with the transcortical interlocking Knowles pin fixation technique, which is known to be effective in the treatment of hypertrophic nonunion and unreducible acute fractures. Two patients had atrophic nonunions that were treated with plate fixation and autologous grafts taken from the pelvis. Each of 6 patients had resection of the callus and a portion of the lateral clavicle fragment. One patient with a massive hypertrophic nonunion and thoracic outlet impingement underwent resection of the callus, which was morcelled and redeposited into the periosteal bed. Most patients had excellent results. One patient, a man aged 70 years who had waited 4 years until operation, had persistent shoulder stiffness after undergoing resection of the lateral clavicle segments. Another patient had some shoulder discomfort. A third patient later needed repair of an ipsilateral torn rotator cuff. Adults with a displaced fractured clavicle should have treatment different from that of children with this fracture. The use of figure-of-8 devices on adults provides incomplete reduction and may result in nonunion.

▶ The authors quite nicely reintroduce us to thoracic outlet syndrome as a complication of malunion or nonunion in clavicle fractures in adults. The adjunctive information they supply is useful. The authors note that clavicle fractures in adults may be different from those in children and reduction should be sought with greater vigor; that fixation with Knowles' pins is usually very effective; and once again that resection of the midclavicle for this problem is not always effective and may lead to continuing significant symptoms.—R.H. Cofield, M.D.

Inferior Subluxation of the Humeral Head After Injury to the Shoulder: A Brief Note

Yosipovitch Z, Goldberg I (Beilinson Med Ctr, Petah Tikva, Israel; Tel Aviv Univ)
J Bone Joint Surg [Am] 71-A:751–753, June 1989   3-5

Inferior subluxation of the glenohumeral joint may occur after a number of traumatic or nontraumatic shoulder lesions (table). Although the occurrence of inferior subluxation after a fracture of the proximal part of the humeral head has been well studied, no consensus yet exists on what constitutes the most appropriate treatment. To assess the clinical features of inferior subluxation of the humeral head that occurred after traumatic shoulder injuries, data on 20 patients aged 10–73 years who had treatment for inferior subluxation that developed after acute trauma to the shoulder or the proximal part of the humerus, or both, were studied. Nine patients had avulsion of the greater tuberosity. Subluxation was first noted on the day after injury in 2 patients, within the first 2–4 days in 10 patients, and at the end of 1 week in 7 patients. For 1 patient, subluxation was not diagnosed until 33 days after the injury occurred. All patients underwent standard radiographic examinations, and all have conservative treatment by maintaining the involved arm in an elbow sling for about 3 weeks, followed by early physiotherapy.

Seventeen of the 20 patients had recovered completely after an average

Etiologies of Inferior Subluxation of the Glenohumeral Joint

Traumatic	Non-Traumatic
Fracture of the proximal part of the humerus[3,5,6,8,10,13-15,17,19,22,27,28]	Stroke or hemiplegia (16-66 per cent)[20,22]
Fracture of the glenoid	Poliomyelitis[14]
Tear of a capsule or ligament[27]	Ligamentous laxity[17,18]
Dislocation of the shoulder with neural injury	Apical lung tumor involving the brachial plexus[17]
Brachial plexus (see Fig. 1)	Neuralgic amyotrophy[9]
Axillary nerve[4]	Septic arthritis[1]
Suprascapular nerve[30]	Hemarthrosis (hemophilia)[26]
Postoperative (100 per cent)[21]	Rheumatoid arthritis[2]
Brachial plexus injury[16]	Aging process[2,6]

(Courtesy of Yosipovitch Z, Goldberg I: J Bone Joint Surg [Am] 71-A:751–753, June 1989.)

of 5 weeks. The remaining 3 patients had an obvious peripheral nerve injury as confirmed by electromyography, and their recovery took about 15 weeks. Inferior subluxation of the humeral head after shoulder trauma has an excellent prognosis for quick recovery, using only a simple sling to support the involved arm.

▶ The authors have reviewed quite effectively the literature on this subject and have categorized the conditions in which inferior subluxation of the humeral head occurs. They reinforce external support and physical therapy as being almost always effective in resolving this subluxation. Of course, we all should remind ourselves that the subluxation is not always resolved with these methods. The failure of resolution may be most common in situations that include significant capsule and rotator cuff tearing. When inferior subluxation is not resolved, in addition to investigating for nerve injuries, one might wish also to investigate for tearing of these structures.—R.H. Cofield, M.D.

An Anatomic Study of the Musculocutaneous Nerve and Its Relationship to the Coracoid Process
Flatow EL, Bigliani LU, April EW (Columbia Univ; Columbia-Presbyterian Med Ctr, New York)
Clin Orthop 244:166–171, July 1989   3–6

Injury to the musculocutaneous nerve is a well-known complication of anterior shoulder surgery. An abnormally high penetration of the musculocutaneous nerve into the coracobrachialis muscle has been considered a factor leading to nerve injury. An autopsy study of 93 shoulders assessed the anatomy of the musculocutaneous nerve and its relationship to the coracoid process.

The main trunk of the musculocutaneous nerve entered the coracobrachialis muscle in 92% of shoulders. In each of these 86 shoulders, the nerve sent twigs to the muscle before the main nerve trunk penetrated the muscle (Fig 3–3). The mean distance from the coracoid to the point of entrance of the main nerve trunk into the coracobrachialis muscle was 56 mm (range, 31–82 mm). The small proximal twigs entered the muscles as close as 17 mm below the coracoid (mean, 31 mm). Twenty-nine percent of the musculocutaneous nerves entered the coracobrachialis muscle proximal to 5 cm below the coracoid. This increased to 74% if the proximal twigs were counted.

The frequently cited range of 5–8 cm below the coracoid for the level of penetration of the coracobrachialis muscle cannot be relied on to describe a safe zone for coracoid mobilization in anterior shoulder surgery.

▶ The authors restate for us in relation to the musculocutaneous nerve the anatomical principle that the courses of nerves are usually rather uniform, but the position at which the nerve will enter a muscle along its course is somewhat variable. Thus, surgeons should not be surprised that the musculocutaneous nerve will on occasion enter the coracobrachialis quite a bit more proximal than

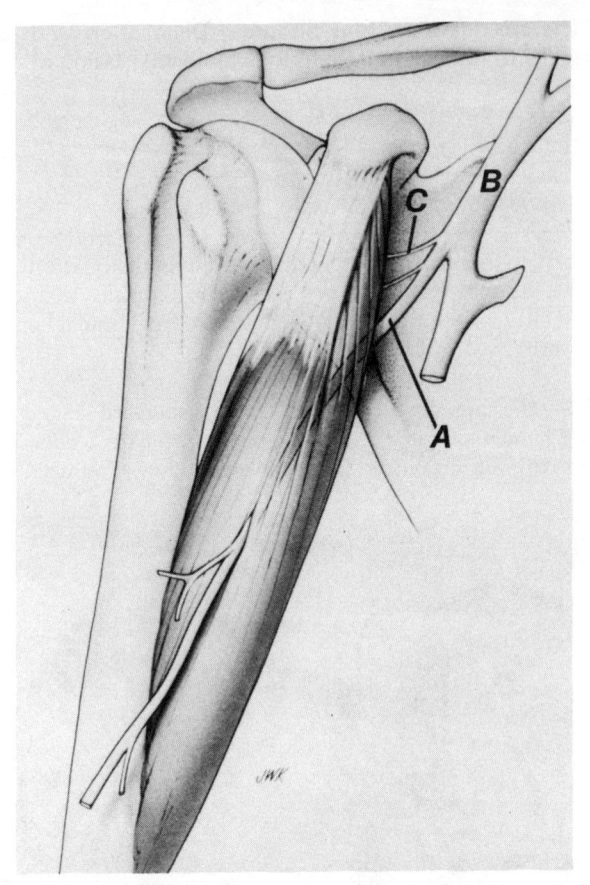

Fig 3-3.—Usual course of the nerve. The musculocutaneous nerve, A, is a terminal branch of the lateral cord, B, of the brachial plexus. It (or the lateral cord) sends twigs, C, to the coracobrachialis before entering it. (Courtesy of Flatow EL, Bigliani LU, April EW: *Clin Orthop* 244:166–171, July 1989.)

is typically described. The investigators also note the presence of proximal twigs from the musculocutaneous nerve to the coracobrachialis, and in some of their specimens these branches enter the coracobrachialis less than 2 cm from the coracoid. Surgery in this anatomical region is difficult. One of the major reasons for this difficulty is the proximity to neural structures. The authors suggest that if coracoid mobilization is a part of the procedure, the musculocutaneous nerve and its branches should be identified and carefully protected.— R.H. Cofield, M.D.

Operative Therapy for Recurrent Shoulder Dislocation With Special Regard to Long-Term Clinical and Radiological Results Using M. Lange Technique

Melzer C, Manz P, Krödel A, Stürz H (Medizinische Hochschule im Annastift, Postfach, Hannover; Allgemeines Krankenhaus, Celle; Ludwig-Maximilians Universität, München, West Germany)
Arch Orthop Trauma Surg 108:107–111, February 1989   3–7

The operative treatment of recurrent shoulder dislocation remains difficult. The M. Lange procedure for recurrent shoulder dislocation is described, as well as its limitations with regard to clinical and radiologic long-term results.

Technique.—The shoulder is exposed through a standard deltoid-pectoral incision. With the humerus rotated externally, the subcapularis tendon is divided 2.5 cm medial to its insertion on the lesser tuberosity and is retracted medially. At

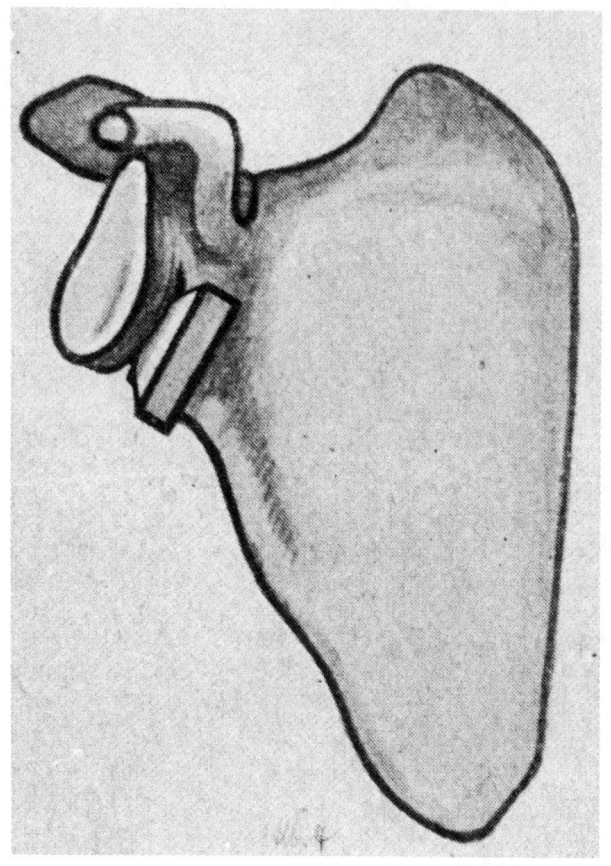

Fig 3–4.—Correct position of tibial graft (from Lange). (Courtesy of Melzer C, Manz P, Krödel A, et al: *Arch Orthop Trauma Surg* 108:107–111, February 1989.)

about 0.5 cm medial to the lower anterior glenoid rim, a 2.5-cm chisel is driven in, elevating the glenoid rim laterally. A wedge of bone from the tibia, measuring 2.5–3.5 cm, is driven into the osteotomy defect, with the periosteal side of the splinter directed anteriorly (Fig 3–4). The subscapularis tendon is sutured to the joint capsule with the humerus rotated internally. The arm is immobilized in 70 degrees abduction and 40 degrees anteversion for 3–4 weeks.

A total of 20 shoulders in 20 patients had treatment. After an average postoperative period of 13.5 years, 19 patients reported outstanding-to-satisfying results, but only 12 remained pain free. Striking radiologic signs of osteoarthritis were present in 57% of patients. Degenerative changes occurred in 81% of patients with radiologically significant glenoid augmentation compared with only 30% of patients without glenoid augmentation. Real postoperative redislocation was evident in only 1 patient. Measurable limitation of external rotation was evident in more than 50% of patients.

In this method, the tibial splinter not only is added to the anterior glenoid rim but also is driven into an osteotomy defect medially at the scapular neck. Despite the lack of comparable studies, these results, including pain, limitation of motion, and osteoarthritic changes, should be taken into consideration when choosing an operative procedure for recurrent shoulder dislocation.

▶ This procedure may well eliminate instability, but the cost may be too high, for glenoid arthritis developed in a third to half of the patients. This development was particularly common when the bone graft was used as an extension of glenoid surface. Here is another series that seemingly would indicate that the use of bone grafts on the glenoid to correct shoulder instability may be effective in correcting the instability but may also result in glenohumeral arthritis. The reader might well ask, why use bone block techniques that have the potential to cause arthritis when other techniques involving soft tissue repair are equally, if not more, effective and are not associated with this high frequency of subsequent shoulder arthritis.—R.H. Cofield, M.D.

Reconsideration of the Putti-Platt Procedure and Its Mode of Action in Recurrent Traumatic Anterior Dislocation of the Shoulder
Symeonides PP (Aristotelion Univ of Thessaloniki, Thessaloniki, Greece)
Clin Orthop 246:8–15, September 1989   3–8

A modification of the Putti-Platt procedure deletes suturing the lateral stump of the subscapularis to the anterior rim of the glenoid cavity (Fig 3–5). The results of both original and modified operations in patients with recurrent anterior traumatic dislocation of the shoulder were compared, and the mode of action of the classic procedure by clinical and anatomical study was investigated.

Of 65 patients who underwent the classic operation in 1961–1986, 2 had recurrences. Lateral rotation of the arm was restored in 19 patients.

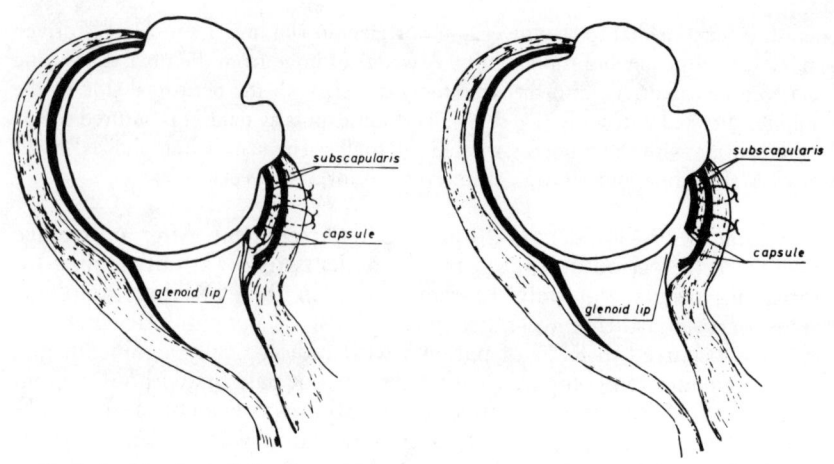

Fig 3–5.—The classic *(left)* and simplified *(right)* Putti-Platt procedures. (Courtesy of Symeonides PP: *Clin Orthop* 246:8–15, September 1989.)

Of 83 patients (85 shoulders) who had the modified operation in 1966–1979, 3 had recurrence and 76 patients had a full range of shoulder motion restored. Anatomical study showed that in the classic method, disruption of the inelastic lateral stump of the subscapularis from the labrum was necessary if lateral rotation was to reach neutral.

The difficult suturing can be eliminated without adversely affecting results. Success of the operation involves shortening the stretched subscapularis; creating, in front of the joint, a double layer of capsule and muscle; and bringing a wide part of the subscapularis below and in front of the humeral head.

▶ The results reported are indeed quite good using the modified Putti-Platt procedure. A critical reader might note that no mention is made of recurrent subluxation after the operation. Some patients may indeed have this in the absence of recurrent dislocations. Also, although ranges of movement after surgery were quite good, the actual motion data are not reported; it would be easier for the reader to analyze the data and reach his own conclusions. It seems that both the subscapularis and anterior shoulder capsule are shortened during this procedure, so attributing shoulder instability only to lengthening of the subscapularis would not seem justifiable on the basis of this material.—R.H. Cofield, M.D.

An Approach to the Repair of Avulsion of the Glenohumeral Ligaments in the Management of Traumatic Anterior Glenohumeral Instability

Thomas SC, Matsen FA III (Univ of Washington)
J Bone Joint Surg [Am] 71-A:506–513, April 1989   3–9

Many patients with recurrent anterior glenohumeral instability have a history of definite trauma that initiated the unidirectional instability. The

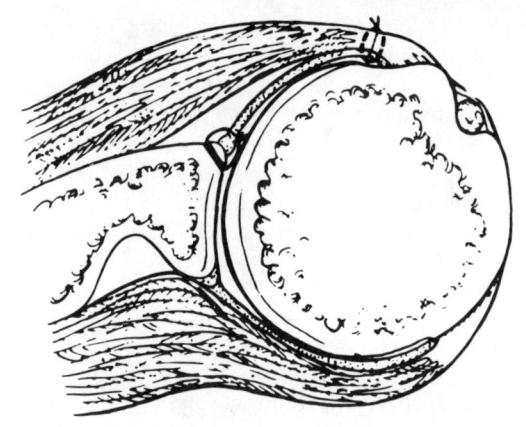

Fig 3-6.—Transverse plane section showing completed repair of the Bankart lesion and anatomical repair of the incision through the subscapularis and capsule. (Courtesy of Thomas SC, Matsen FA III: *J Bone Joint Surg [Am]* 71-A:506-513, April 1989.)

shoulders in these patients usually have ruptures of their glenohumeral ligaments at the point of glenoid attachment, called Bankart lesions. Several surgical procedures are available for stabilizing this type of lesion, but many complications have been reported with the use of screws and staples around glenohumeral joints. A new approach to the surgical repair of recurrent traumatic anterior glenohumeral instability was developed.

During a 9-year period, 49 men and 12 women with an average age of 26.4 years underwent operation for recurrent traumatic anterior glenohumeral instability. Patients with atraumatic anterior instability or multidirectional instability were excluded from the study. Operation involved the direct repair of the structural defect of the capsular ligament using a drilling and suturing technique similar to that described by Rowe in 1978 (Fig 3-6). Although the technique causes some minimal limitation of motion, it eliminates the need for any tendon transfer, bone transfer, or the use of hardware. After an average follow-up of 5.5 years, 39 shoulders in 37 patients were available for evaluation.

Based on the Rowe rating scale, excellent results were obtained in 34 of the 39 shoulders; good results, in 4 shoulders; and poor results, in 1 shoulder. On the basis of the patients' own evaluations, the results were excellent in 33 shoulders, good in 1 shoulder, fair in 3 shoulders, and poor in 2 shoulders. Thus, excellent or good results by the Rowe criteria were obtained in 97%, and by the patients' own evaluations, in 87%. One patient had a redislocation 4 years after operation while doing karate. None of the patients have needed reoperation. The average ranges of motion were 171 degrees of forward elevation and 84 degress of external rotation in abduction. The direct repair of an avulsed glenohumeral ligament as used in this group of patients leaves the healthy tissues intact, minimizes unnecessary dissection, and yields a high success rate.

▶ This modification of the Bankart type of repair may indeed be a significant advance. The dissection is lessened, and the procedure will lead to less scar formation. The modification has both benefits and detriments in the repair of instability problems. The authors are very skilled in patient selection. Some of us may find it difficult to recognize pure traumatic instability and may exclude those with an underlying tendency for capsular laxity: patients who might benefit from a combined Bankart repair and capsular tightening. It would seem that traumatic lesions tend to occur in such people more often than they do in patients without underlying capsular looseness. The results reported are very good though, so from a practical standpoint patient selection apparently can be done effectively.— R.H. Cofield, M.D.

Posterior Subluxation of the Glenohumeral Joint
Fronek J, Warren RF, Bowen M (Hosp for Special Surgery, New York)
J Bone Joint Surg 71-A:205–216, February 1989   3–10

Recurrent posterior subluxation of the glenohumeral joint is more common than was previously thought. The best treatment for this condition is controversial. Physical therapy is agreed upon as the initial therapy, but various surgical procedures have been recommended for cases not responding to conservative treatment. The clinical signs and symptoms of posterior subluxation of the glenohumeral joint were examined in 24 patients and the results of surgical and nonsurgical treatment were evaluated.

The average age was 20 years, and the average follow-up, 5 years. All patients thought that their shoulder joint was loose or unstable or experienced pain during specific activities. Many heard crepitation or clicking in the shoulder. Onset of symptoms often followed trauma or stressful exertion. Anteroposterior radiographs, made with the shoulder in internal rotation, were normal in all but the oldest patient.

Patients were divided into 2 groups according to the severity of their symptoms. Those in group 1 had only moderate disability during strenuous activities and were prescribed a program of physical therapy. Group 2, 11 patients, included 3 who were not helped by the physical therapy program; all had substantial disability during activities of daily life. Patients in group 2 underwent a posterior capsulorrhaphy, with or without a bone block. A splint was worn for 6 weeks to immobilize the arm in neutral rotation and slight extension. After the splint is removed, the patient follows an exercise program designed to strengthen the external rotator muscles.

Physical therapy brought improvement to 10 (63%) of the patients in group 1; 6 could again actively participate in strenuous activities. In group 2, 6 were completely free of pain; 10 had no further episodes of instability. Group 2 patients had more improvement at follow-up than patients in group 1. All, however, were less competitive at their sports. Posterior subluxation or instability appears related to the severity of the initial trauma and the presence of generalized ligamentous laxity.

▶ This very helpful paper describes in some detail the patient characteristics and outlines a quite reasonable surgical procedure. One would like to have slightly more detail about the operative findings and physical examination parameters at the time of follow-up evaluation. About one half of the operative patients had bone grafts supplementing capsular repair. From the information presented, it does not seem that the addition of the bone block added anything to the success of the surgical procedure. Perhaps it is never necessary, or perhaps the capsule, as the authors state, was so thin and weak that the bone block seemed mandatory and success would not have occurred without it. It is difficult to know which view to take given the material presented. The authors appropriately caution us to exclude patients with substantial emotional contributions to their instability, remind us that voluntary instability may occur in the absence of emotional problems, and direct us to consider conservative care as the first line of treatment; however, should operative treatment seem essential, the technique described seems to be safe and effective.—R.H. Cofield, M.D.

Spontaneous Atraumatic Anterior Subluxation of the Sternoclavicular Joint
Rockwood CA Jr, Odor JM (Univ of Texas, San Antonio)
J Bone Joint Surg [Am] 71-A:1280–1288, October 1989   3–11

Little research has been done on atraumatic spontaneous anterior subluxation or dislocation of the sternoclavicular joint. Untreated spontaneous atraumatic anterior subluxation of the sternoclavicular joint may have a benign course. To test this impression, 37 such patients aged 10–36 years were examined. Twenty-nine patients had conservative management with observation and rehabilitation. Eight patients were treated initially at another center. In these patients, operative reconstruction of the sternoclavicular joint or resection arthroplasty was attempted. At an average of 8 years later, the conservatively treated patients had excellent results, with no limitations in activity. The patients treated surgically had several problems, including scars, persistent instability, pain, or limitation of activity resulting in a change in lifestyle.

Spontaneous atraumatic anterior subluxation of the sternoclavicular joint, a rare problem occurring mostly in teenagers and young adults with general ligamentous laxity, has a benign natural course. It should not be treated surgically. Therapy should include education and reassurance.

▶ This is a helpful report. The condition is uncommon but not rare. It is useful to understand that almost without exception patients first seen with atraumatic anterior sternoclavicular joint subluxation do well with time alone. In the small operative group, it is safe to say that reconstruction of the ligaments and capsule to achieve stability was not effective, and resection arthroplasty of the medial end of the clavicle did not seem to improve the patient's situation. The message is clear.—R.H. Cofield, M.D.

Operation for Old Sternoclavicular Dislocation: Results in 12 Cases
Eskola A, Vainionpää S, Vastamäki M, Slätis P, Rokkanen P (Orthopaedic Hosp of the Invalid Foundation: Helsinki Univ Central Hosp, Helsinki)
J Bone Joint Surg [Br] 71-B:63–65, January 1989   3–12

Fresh dislocation of a sternoclavicular joint usually is treated nonsurgically with an arm sling or a figure-of-8 bandage. However, redislocation is common because only half of the medial end of the clavicle has articular contact with the manubrium. Several techniques are available for stabilizing old sternoclavicular dislocations. The effect of late operative treatment in patients with complete sternoclavicular dislocations was evaluated.

Of 8 women and 4 men with an average age of 29 years who underwent operation for painful, old dislocation of the sternoclavicular joint, the average time between trauma and operation was 1.5 years. Eleven patients had had primary treatment with an arm sling for 21 days, and 1 patient had been allowed to mobilize the shoulder immediately. The clavicles of 5 patients were fixed with tendon graft to both the first rib and the manubrium, using the palmaris longus tendon in 4 patients and the plantaris tendon in 1 case (Fig 3–7). Four other patients underwent subperiosteal resection of the medial 2.5 cm of the clavicle without stabilization. In the remaining 3 patients, a graft of fascia lata was used to attach the medial end of the clavicle to the first rib. After a mean follow-up of 4.7 years, only 4 patients had good results: 3 had had tendon grafts and 1 had had a fascia lata graft. Four other patients had fair results. However, all 4 patients having resection of the medial end of the clavicle had poor results, with pain and weakness of the upper extremity. All 4 patients had to give up work and were receiving full disability pensions.

Although resection of the medial end of the clavicle still is recommended by some authors as a treatment for old painful sternoclavicular dislocations, the findings for this group of patients indicate that resection of the sternal end of the clavicle no longer should be used.

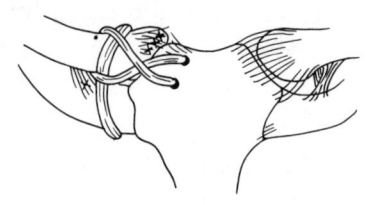

Fig 3–7.—Diagram showing reconstruction with a tendon graft (Courtesy of Eskola A, Vainionpää S, Vastamäki M, et al: *J Bone Joint Surg [Br]* 71-B:63–65, January 1989.)

▶ In old sternoclavicular dislocations, the results are better if it is possible to reduce the clavicle and repair and reinforce the capsule and ligaments. If a resectional arthroplasty must be combined with soft tissue repair because of the presence of arthritic changes, the results will be compromised, and, indeed in these patients, the results were quite poor.—R.H. Cofield, M.D.

Rotator Cuff and Related Syndromes

Ultrasonography in Lesions of the Rotator Cuff and Biceps Tendon
Ahovuo J, Paavolainen P, Björkenheim J-M (Helsinki Univ)
Acta Radiol 30:253–255, May–June 1989   3–13

Tears of the tendons of the rotator cuff traditionally have been diagnosed reliably with arthrography. However, ultrasonography (US) has rapidly become the preferred diagnostic modality for studying rotator cuff tears because it is noninvasive and has a diagnostic reliability approaching that of arthrography. The diagnostic accuracy of US was compared with that of arthrography in identifying rotator cuff tears in 50 men and 38 women with a mean age of 47.3 years who had treatment for chronic pain and shoulder dysfunction resulting from lesions of the shoulder tendons. All patients underwent both US and arthrographic studies that were interpreted independently. Fifteen patients subsequently underwent shoulder operations.

Five of the 15 operated patients had full-thickness tears of the rotator cuff, 1 of whom also had a dislocated biceps tendon. The other 10 patients had no tears, but had degeneration of the rotator cuff tendons. The arthrographic findings of the rotator cuff tendons were verified at operation for the 15 surgically treated patients. However, US revealed a rupture of more than 2 cm in diameter in 3 of the 5 patients with rotator cuff tears, but missed the rotator cuff tears in the other 2 patients. Both patients had rotator cuff tears of less than 2 cm in diameter.

When compared with arthrographic findings, there were 21 true positive, 3 false positive, 57 true negative, and 7 false negative sonograms for full-thickness rotator cuff tears. Thus, US failed to reveal full-thickness rotator cuff tears in 7 patients but did detect tears in 3 other patients whose arthrography studies were negative.

Small rotator cuff tears less than 2 cm in diameter may be difficult to assess with US. Arthrography therefore should be used together with US for patients in whom rotator cuff tears are suspected.

▶ The message is clear. Ultrasonography cannot be relied upon to detect smaller tears of the rotator cuff.—R.H. Cofield, M.D.

Rotator Cuff Sonography: A Reassessment
Brandt TD, Cardone BW, Grant TH, Post M, Weiss CA (Michael Reese Hosp and Med Ctr, Chicago)
Radiology 173:323–327, November 1989

Sonography has been suggested as an alternative to double-contrast arthrography for evaluating shoulder diseases, but lack of agreement on

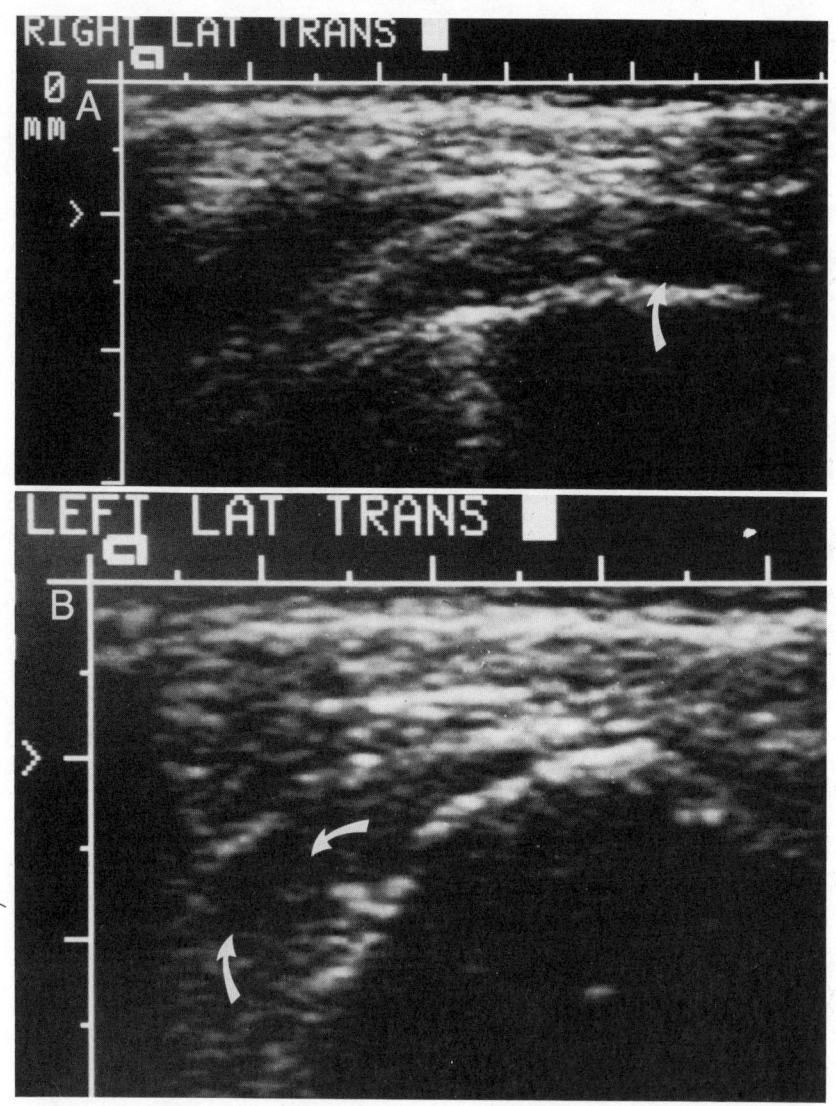

Fig 3–8.—A, focal hypoechoic lesion *(arrow)* within the anterior portion of the symptomatic rotator cuff. A 5-cm tear of the supraspinatus muscle was found during surgery. **B,** a similar lesion within the middle of the asymptomatic rotator cuff *(arrows).* (Courtesy of Brandt TD, Cardone BW, Grant TH, et al: *Radiology* 173:323–327, November 1989.)

what constitutes reliable sonographic signs hinders its acceptance. The usefulness of this method for detecting rotator cuff injury was examined in 62 patients undergoing sonography and double-contrast arthrography and 38 patients undergoing operation after sonography.

When 7 published criteria for defining rotator cuff injury were used, sonography had a sensitivity of 75% and a specificity of 43% compared with arthrography. When the central echogenic band and echogenic foci in the rotator cuff were eliminated as criteria because of their unreliability, the sensitivity was 68% and the specificity was 90%. Assessment of sonography with the reduced number of criteria versus surgery revealed a sensitivity of 57% and a specificity of 76%.

Focal discontinuity of the rotator cuff is considered a reliable sonographic sign, yet false positive examinations were encountered (Fig 3–8). Also, various anatomical features such as the presence of the acromion above the supraspinatus, can preclude a complete examination and cause a false negative diagnosis.

Shoulder sonography has low sensitivity and is hindered by technical and methodologic difficulties. Sonographic examination cannot be recommended yet for evaluating rotator cuff injuries.

▶ This article reinforces the preceding one. In some practices, ultrasonography of the rotator cuff has been quite helpful, but in others, including the experience reported here, ultrasonography has not been as useful as one might wish.—R.H. Cofield, M.D.

Rotator Cuff Tears: Diagnostic Performance of MR Imaging
Zlatkin MB, Iannotti JP, Roberts MC, Esterhai JL, Dalinka MK, Kressel HY, Schwartz JS, Lenkinski RE (Univ of Pennsylvania)
Radiology 172:223–229, July 1989

Magnetic resonance (MR) imaging is a promising technique for evaluating disorders of the rotator cuff. Magnetic resonance imaging studies were compared with arthrograms of the shoulder in patients with suspected rotator cuff injuries who subsequently underwent shoulder surgery.

Thirty-two patients with rotator cuff tendonopathy were evaluated preoperatively by orthopedic history, clinical examination, and MR imaging of the affected shoulder. All patients had positive impingement tests, and all had failed conservative treatment. Eight asymptomatic controls also underwent MR imaging. A scoring system was developed for the imaging studies. Twenty-four of the 32 patients had arthrography within a short interval after MR imaging. Arthrographic studies and MR imaging were reviewed without knowledge of surgical results.

For all rotator cuff tears, MR imaging had a sensitivity of 0.91 and a specificity of 0.88, whereas arthrography had both sensitivity and specificity of 0.71. When the scoring system was used, the sensitivity of MR improved to 1.0 and the specificity to 0.92. There was excellent correla-

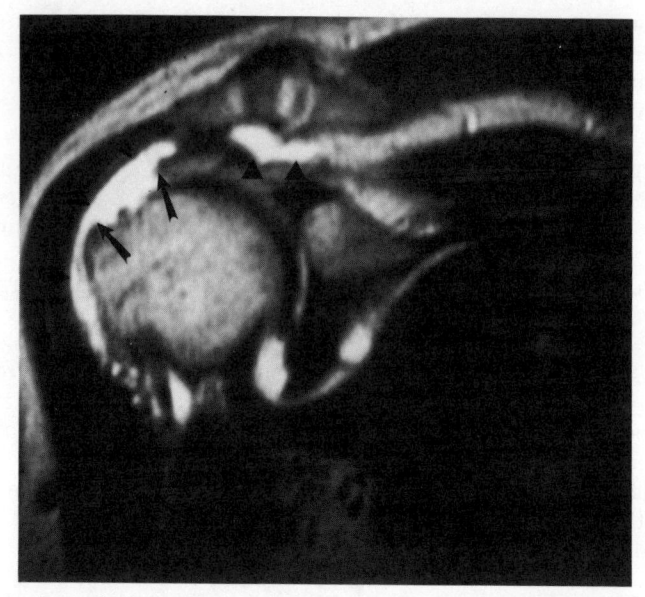

Fig 3-9.—T$_2$-weighted (2,500/80) coronal oblique image at the level of the acromioclavicular joint shows the disruption of the supraspinatus tendon as it is outlined by high-signal-intensity fluid *(arrows)*. A large amount of fluid is also seen in the subacromial and subdeltoid bursae *(arrowheads)*. Increased signal intensity is noted in the proximal retracted tendon edges. (Courtesy of Zlatkin MB, Iannotti JP, Roberts MC, et al: *Radiology* 172:223-229, July 1989.)

tion between the preoperative assessment of the size of the rotator cuff tears and the actual measurement of the tears at surgery.

Magnetic resonance imaging had excellent sensitivity and specificity in detecting rotator cuff injuries. In this study, MR imaging was superior to arthrography, and it provided useful information regarding the size and site of tears and the quality of torn tendon edges (Fig 3-9). When used in conjunction with plain radiography and clinical evaluation, MR imaging should obviate the need for other invasive or noninvasive studies.

Rotator Cuff Tears: Prospective Comparison of MR Imaging With Arthrography, Sonography, and Surgery
Burk DL Jr, Karasick D, Kurtz AB, Mitchell DG, Rifkin MD, Miller CL, Levy DW, Fenlin JM, Bartolozzi AR (Thomas Jefferson Univ Hosp, Philadelphia)
AJR 153:87-92, July 1989
3-16

Arthrography is a highly accurate method of detecting rotator cuff tears. However, the procedure is invasive and relies on indirect visualization of the cuff. To assess the relative accuracy and role of magnetic resonance (MR) imaging in the diagnostic evaluation of rotator cuff tears, the MR findings in 38 patients with suspected rotator cuff tears were compared prospectively in a blind fashion with the results of double-con-

Chapter 3—Shoulder, Elbow and Forearm / **117**

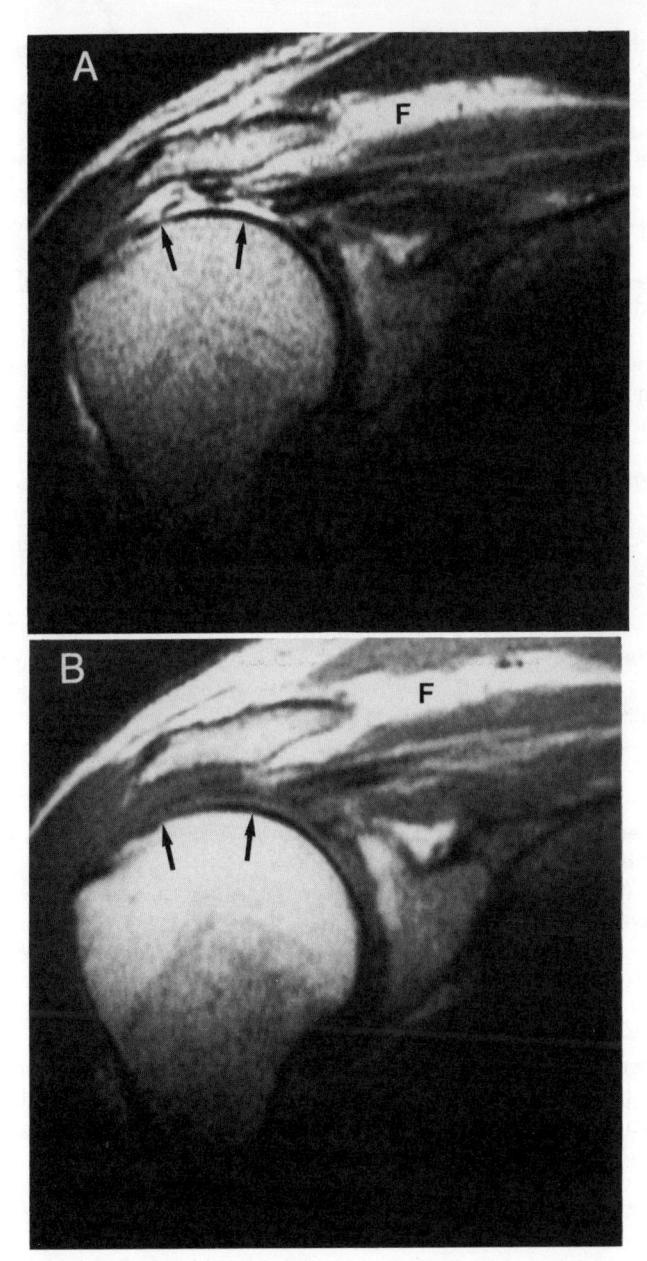

Fig 3–10.—Magnetic resonance images of large rotator cuff tear measuring 6 cm^2 at surgery. **A,** spin-echo 2,000/80 coronal oblique image shows large tear filled with high-signal-intensity fluid and fragments of supraspinatus tendon *(arrows)*. Surrounding fat *(F)* has artifactually high signal intensity because of proximity to surface coil. **B,** spin-echo 600/25 coronal oblique image does not show tear as well as **A** because of low signal intensity of fluid *(arrows)*. Surrounding fat maintains high signal intensity. (Courtesy of Burk DL Jr, Karasick D, Kurtz AB, et al: *AJR* 153:87–92, July 1989.)

trast arthrography in all 38 patients, high-resolution sonography in 23 patients, and surgery in 16 patients.

In the total group of 38 patients, MR showed 22 of 22 rotator cuff tears and 14 of 16 intact cuffs as determined with arthrography (Fig 3–10). The 1 tear missed by both studies measured less than 1 cm^2 at surgery. In the 16 surgically proved cases, both MR and arthrography correctly showed 11 of 12 cuff tears and 4 of 4 intact tears, for a sensitivity of 92% and specificity of 100% for both procedures. In a subgroup of 23 patients, sonography detected 9 of 15 tears and 7 of 8 intact cuffs as determined by arthrography. In the 10 surgically proved cases that included sonography in the evaluation of the rotator cuff, the sensitivity was 63% for sonography, 88% for MR, and 88% for arthrography and the specificity was 60%, 90%, and 90%, respectively.

Magnetic resonance imaging is as accurate as arthrography in the diagnosis of rotator cuff tears. Large rotator cuff tears can be detected reliably with MR, but small tears may be missed. Sonography is not as accurate as MR and arthrography in the diagnosis of rotator cuff tears. Magnetic resonance imaging should be the noninvasive test of choice for the evaluation of rotator cuff disease.

▶ Magnetic resonance imaging is improving dramatically. The above 2 reports mirror what many are experiencing: that MR is as accurate as arthrography for evaluating the rotator cuff. Each test has its advantages and disadvantages, and in difficult patient problems the two may, in fact, complement one another.—R.H. Cofield, M.D.

Comparison of Conventional and Computed Arthrotomography With MR Imaging in the Evaluation of the Shoulder

Habibian A, Stauffer A, Resnick D, Reicher MA, Rafii M, Kellerhouse L, Zlatkin MB, Newman C, Sartoris DJ (Univ of California, San Diego; Mission Community Hosp, Mission Viejo, Calif; Mercy Hosp and Med Ctr, San Diego; New York Univ; Hosp of the Univ of Pennsylvania; et al)
J Comput Assist Tomogr 13:968–975, November–December 1989   3–17

Magnetic resonance (MR), unlike most methods for diagnosing shoulder problems, is a noninvasive procedure without ionizing radiation or bone artifacts. To compare MR with conventional arthrography and computed arthrotomography in assessing the cause of shoulder pain, 18 patients were examined with all 3 methods. Each image was independently reviewed by 2 or 3 experienced examiners with a special evaluation form.

For assessment of rotator cuff tears MR was comparable to conventional arthrography, but examiners were able to diagnose cuff tendinitis with MR. Magnetic resonance allowed staging of the impingement syndrome because of its high-quality soft tissue imaging. Both computed arthrotomography and MR were equally capable of assessing labral lesions and capsular structures and in evaluating instability, but these structures could be evaluated better with MR than with computed arthrotomography if the rotator cuff was completely torn.

Magnetic resonance is a useful method for imaging the glenohumeral joint. The images yielded are equal to or better than those from conventional arthrography or computed arthrotomography. Magnetic resonance has the further advantages of not requiring contrast material and of being noninvasive and easier to perform.

Clinical Presentation of Complete Tears of the Rotator Cuff
Norwood LA, Barrack R, Jacobson KE (Hughston Orthopaedic Clinic, Columbus, Ga)
J Bone Joint Surg [Am] 71-A:499–505, April 1989
3–18

The diagnosis of tears of the rotator cuff, one of the most serious pathologic conditions of the shoulder requiring surgery, often is missed or delayed. Some physicians believe that acute trauma plays an important role in most tears of the rotator cuff, whereas others think a specific traumatic episode occurs in a minority of such patients. The belief that a decrease in the active range of motion of the shoulder is correlated with the extent of tears of the rotator cuff is disputed. Radiographs may or may not be helpful.

Data on 103 patients were analyzed to determine what factors in the patient's history, clinical features, physical examination, and radiographs are most useful in diagnosing the presence and extent of a complete tear of the rotator cuff of the shoulder. An age-matched control group of 51 patients with similar symptoms but normal arthrograms were used for comparison. Two groups of patients with tears of the rotator cuff were identified. Twenty-eight patients (27%) had tears of a single tendon. The histories and physical and radiographic findings for these patients were consistent with a symptomatic local mechanical impingement process in the shoulder.

Sixty patients (80%) of the 75 patients comprising the second group had a history of acute trauma. The patients in group 2 were older and not athletic and had not had previous symptoms severe enough to require treatment. These patients subsequently were found to have a complete tear of more than 1 tendon. Multiple radiographic findings in the shoulder and other co-existing orthopedic conditions were more common in the second group. In the second group, acute trauma in a shoulder that had chronic degenerative changes, instead of localized mechanical impingement, probably caused the tendons to rupture.

Two discrete groups of patients with tears of the rotator cuff were identified. Tendon ruptures in the 2 groups probably were caused by different mechanisms.

▶ You may or may not agree with the conclusions reached by the authors, but these investigators have made many observations that ring true. They offer a detailed description of the differences in the presentation and evaluation of patients with smaller rotator cuff tears versus those with a large extent of tearing.—R.H. Cofield, M.D.

The Influence of Distal Clavicle Resection and Rotator Cuff Repair on the Effectiveness of Anterior Acromioplasty
Daluga DJ, Dobozi W (Loyola Univ Med Ctr, Maywood, Ill; Hines VA Hosp, Hines, Ill)
Clin Orthop 247:117–123, October 1989 3–19

Neer anterior acromioplasty generally is the procedure of choice for symptomatic subacromial impingement. To assess the long-term results of acromioplasty in terms of length of postoperative rehabilitation, residual strength deficits, and effect of the addition of distal clavicle resection or rotator cuff repair, or both, 50 patients with late Neer stage II and III impingement lesions having anterior acromioplasty were evaluated. In addition to the acromioplasty, 13 shoulders had distal clavicle resection, 9 had rotator cuff repair, and 10 had distal clavicle resection and rotator cuff repair.

Based on pain relief, strength, range of motion, and ability to resume full activity, 92% of patients were rated good or excellent. Additional clavicle resection or rotator cuff repair, or both, did not result in an increase in morbidity in overall results. Prolonged rehabilitation, averaging 8.5 months, was seen in all groups, but patients who had additional distal clavicle resection and rotator cuff repair required a 25% longer rehabilitation. Residual strength deficits were evident in 58% of patients, the highest incidence occurring in patients requiring rotator cuff repair and distal clavicle resection (90%). Pain relief was similar in all groups.

Anterior acromioplasty with rotator cuff repair, when a tear is present, yields predictably good to excellent results in patients with shoulder impingement. Rehabilitation is prolonged and improvement can be expected up to about 1 year after surgery.

▶ The more extensive the pathology, the more treatment is necessary, the more prolonged the rehabilitation. Fortunately, the outcome is quite good in most patients, but motion deficits and weakness may occur when tearing becomes extensive.—R.H. Cofield, M.D.

Tenodesis of the Long Head of the Biceps Brachii for Chronic Bicipital Tendinitis: Long-Term Results
Becker DA, Cofield RH (Mayo Clinic, Mayo Found, Rochester, Minn)
J Bone Joint Surg [Am] 71-A:376–381, March 1989 3–20

Surgical tenodesis of the long head of the biceps has been a recommended treatment for chronic bicipital tendinitis for about 50 years. Reports based upon short-term results were quite favorable, although the long-term effectiveness of this procedure has not been analyzed. Of 51

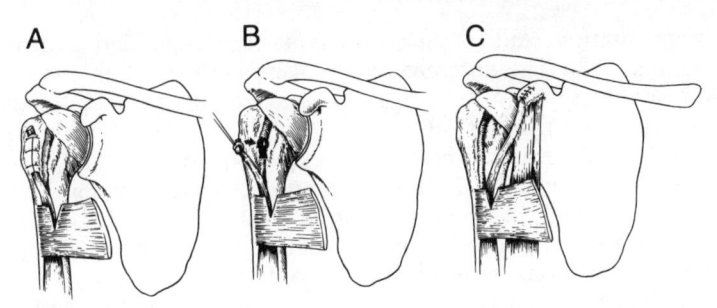

Fig 3–11.—Surgical techniques for fixation of the tendon. A, tenodesis of Hitchcock and Bechtol, performed in 30 shoulders (56%). B, tenodesis of Froimson and Oh, performed in 14 shoulders (26%). C, tenodesis of DePalma and Callery, performed in 10 shoulders (19%). (Courtesy of Becker DA, Cofield RH: *J Bone Joint Surg [Am]* 71-A:376–381, March 1989.)

patients (54 shoulders) followed for an average of 13 years, only 50% had long-lasting satisfactory outcome.

Of the group, 30 were men; the median patient age at the time of surgery was 51 years. In 19 patients, symptoms were traced to a notable injury. Most of the patients had reported severe pain for an average of 2.6 years. Various conservative measures brought only short-term relief. Preoperative radiographs were normal in 43 shoulders. The tendon was tenodesed by 1 of these methods (Fig 3–11). Intraoperative findings were recorded for 38 shoulders. The biceps tendon was described as grossly abnormal in 32, inflamed in 15, having adhesions in 12, and degenerated in 5. Complications occurred in 6 patients; 29 needed additional treatment such as injections or a later operation. At early follow-up averaging 6 months, all but 3 patients had no pain or only slight pain, but at the latest follow-up, 16 shoulders were moderately painful and 10 continued to be severely painful. Physical findings, however, were normal or nearly normal. Active abduction of the shoulder measured more than 150 degrees in all but 1 patient.

Tenodesis of the long head of the biceps achieved a satisfactory result in only 28 of the 54 shoulders in this series. Thus the procedure is not recommended as the primary component in surgical treatment of a painful shoulder.

Biomechanical Evaluation of Rotator Cuff Fixation Methods
France EP, Paulos LE, Harner CD, Straight CB (LDS Hosp, Salt Lake City)
Am J Sports Med 17:176–181, March–April 1989   3–21

The most common techniques for tendon reattachment to the humeral head include suturing the tendon into a bony trough through the cortical surface of the greater tuberosity. Initial fixation strength and failure mode for various rotator cuff reattachment methods (variations of the McLaughlin technique) were assessed.

Repair techniques included standard suture (control), reinforced suture with expanded polytetrafluoroethylene (PTFE) patch and polydioxanone tape augmentation, and stapling with nonarthroscopic and arthroscopic soft-tissue staples. The different repairs were performed on fresh-frozen cadaver shoulder pairs. Repairs were tested to failure in pure tension with the shoulder fixed at 60 degrees of abduction. Load and displacement results were normalized to controls, grouped according to failure modes, and analyzed. The 2 basic failure modes were bone failure, or suture tearing through the bone (indicating weak bone stock), and tendon failure, or suture tearing of the rotator cuff. Gross comparisons of intact and repaired tendons showed that the intact tendon was 2–3 times stronger than the repaired tendon. Based on mode of failure and lack of increased strength after the repair, the use of staples for cuff attachment was discouraged. Polydioxanone tape suture reinforcement did not raise fixation strength; PTFE patch suture augmentation, however, showed significantly higher initial failure loads than did the control and was of specific benefit in shoulders with weak bone stock.

Any difference between the initial strength of staple repairs and that of suture repairs was not significant. Patch augmentation with PTFE of the trough-in-bone procedure showed significantly higher initial failure loads than the trough-in-bone repair alone. In vivo testing of patch augmentation is needed to determine its effects on postoperative strength and tissue healing.

▶ Studies such as this are overdue. This study defines the different failure modes. These authors, as have almost all other investigators, discourage the use of staples. A number of their specimens had failure through the bone of the proximal humerus. This implies that we must be quite careful in preparing the bone for suturing the rotator cuff. If the rotator cuff tendon material is indeed frail, perhaps "augmenting" the repair might be reasonable; however, it is important to recognize, as the authors relate, that in vivo experience will be necessary before a strong recommendation can be made.—R.H. Cofield, M.D.

Frozen Shoulder: Part II. Treatment by Manipulation Under Anesthesia
Parker RD, Froimson AI, Winsberg DD, Arsham NZ (Mt Sinai Med Ctr, Cleveland; Therapy Specialists, Inc, Beachwood, Ohio)
Orthopedics 12:989–990, July 1989   3–22

Frozen shoulder requires early diagnosis and specific treatment. Manipulation with anesthesia followed by vigorous physiotherapy was evaluated in 32 patients with 40 frozen shoulders treated in a 17-year period. Shoulders were manipulated while patients were under general anesthesia to restore normal passive range of motion. Steroid injection was followed by a few days of hospitalization and a few weeks of outpatient physiotherapy. Patients were followed for 2–17 years. Twenty-two patients were interviewed or reexamined. Fifteen had excellent results, and 5 had good results. In 2 patients the outcome was fair. None had poor results. Three patients had recurrences, 2 of whom were diabetic. One patient's course was complicated by transient posterior deltoid paralysis.

Manipulation under general anesthesia is an effective therapy for frozen shoulder in patients who have not regained more than 90 degrees of passive range of motion in physiotherapy.

Good to excellent results can be achieved in more than 90% of patients, with a reduction in the period of morbidity. If surgeons give attention to the details of proper manipulation, the complication rate will be low.

▶ It is important to recognize that only about 2 patients a year had treatment over this 17-year period with the method described. Thus, the authors do not manipulate frozen shoulders frequently; however, their overall approach seems sound. When a person with this diagnosis—and other diagnoses excluded—has significant stiffness and cannot regain movement with therapy, manipulation may be a reasonable treatment alternative. It seemed to be safe for these patients, and the long-term effectiveness was reasonable.—R.H. Cofield, M.D.

Frozen Shoulder and Other Shoulder Disturbances in Parkinson's Disease
Riley D, Lang AE, Blair RDG, Birnbaum A, Reid B (Toronto Western Hosp)
J Neurol Neurosurg Psychiatry 52:63–66, January 1989   3–23

Frozen shoulder, a condition characterized by painful and progressively severe restriction of shoulder joint mobility, has a spontaneous onset and gradual resolution. This condition was noticed in a number of patients who later had Parkinson's disease. The frequency of frozen shoulder and its relationship to the onset of Parkinson's disease were investigated.

A group of 150 patients with Parkinson's disease contributed information on shoulder symptoms and on known predisposing factors for frozen shoulder. These patients were compared with a matched group of 60 persons who had no history of Parkinson's disease.

Of the patients, 65 reported some past or current shoulder disturbance. Of these, 19 satisfied the study's diagnostic criteria for frozen shoulder. The peak time for the occurrence of frozen shoulder was 2 years before the onset of Parkinson's disease. Akinesia in the upper limb ipsilateral to the frozen shoulder was a common first symptom of the disease.

Although none of the controls had had previous diagnoses of frozen shoulder, 1 man appeared to have had symptoms of the condition 7 to 8 months before the study and showed early signs of Parkinson's disease. Frozen shoulder is a known complication of Parkinson's disease, but its appearance before the onset of symptoms has not been recognized previously. Frozen shoulder is predictive not only of the disease but of the site of onset. And those having Parkinson's disease after an episode of frozen shoulder are more likely to be seen first with akinesia than with tremor.

Prosthetic Arthroplasty and Arthrodesis

Nonconstrained Total Shoulder Arthroplasty in Patients With Polyarticular Rheumatoid Arthritis
Barrett WP, Thornhill TS, Thomas WH, Gebhart EM, Sledge CB (Valley Orthopedic Associates, Renton, Wash; Brigham and Women's Hosp, Boston)
J Arthroplasty 4:91–96, March 1989
3–24

The records of 114 patients with polyarticular rheumatoid arthritis who had 140 total shoulder arthroplasties were reviewed retrospectively to assess the degree of pain relief, improvement in range of motion, and durability of the glenoid component fixation. The average follow-up period was 5 years (range, 2–11 years).

Excellent pain relief was achieved in 93% of patients, but improvement in active forward elevation averaged only 34 degrees. External rotation improved from 20 degrees to 40 degrees after operation. In 45% of patients, significant rotator cuff tears were found. Of the humeral components, 75% were secured with a press-fit application, and only 5% showed subsidence ranging from 4 to 7 mm. No humeral components were revised. Radiolucent lines appeared in the glenoid component in 82% of 129 evaluable shoulders, but 94% were nonprogressive. One percent definitely were loose, and 8% probably were loose. Complications occurred in 7% of shoulders, but no deep or superficial wound infections were noted.

Excellent pain relief can be expected for patients with polyarticular rheumatoid arthritis who have had a nonconstrained total shoulder arthroplasty. Because of the compromised status of the rotator cuff, surrounding tissue, and bone stock, the improvement in the range of motion is inferior to that observed in patients with osteoarthritis or monoarticular inflammatory arthritis. Press-fit application of the humeral component is recommended for most patients, whereas cementing is advocated for shoulders with a poor initial press-fit or with inadequate bone stock.

▶ This report reflects quite nicely the current experience on total shoulder arthroplasty in patients with rheumatoid arthritis. Pain relief is typically quite good; return of movement and strength is less than is usually accomplished in osteoarthritis, for instance. Can the results in these categories be improved in patients with rheumatoid arthritis, or has the reconstruction been limited entirely by the soft tissue changes occurring in this disease category? It is difficult to know. For instance, the methods of treating soft tissue contractures at the time of surgery are not described in detail nor is the postoperative rehabilitation regimen explained in depth. Perhaps we need to direct more attention to these 2 things in particular if we wish to improve the motion and strength results after surgery. This suggestion is only a speculation through, for, as these authors imply, improvement in function above the level reported may not be possible because of the nature of the disease.

The radiographic changes occurring after total shoulder arthroplasty never have been studied in depth. These authors mention radiolucent zones around the entire glenoid component in 77 of 129 shoulders. This area certainly deserves our attention. We need more consistent and improved radiographic techniques. Surgeons undertaking this procedure should consider fluoroscopically positioned views of the glenoid bone-cement interface. I am fearful that with consistent use of improved radiographic techniques we will see even more lucent zones than we now recognize. Fortunately, these interface changes have been well tolerated by patients, and the need for revision surgery has been uncommon.—R.H. Cofield, M.D.

Total Shoulder Arthroplasty
Hawkins RJ, Bell RH, Jallay B (St Joseph's Hosp; Univ of Western Ontario, London, Ont)
Clin Orthop 242:188–194, May 1989   3–25

Nonconstrained systems of joint arthroplasties have proved to be effective. Seventy Neer series I or II total shoulder arthroplasties were performed in 65 patients with an average age of 67 years. Thirty-four shoulders had rheumatoid arthritis, and 29 had osteoarthritis. Eighteen patients had rotator cuff tears. Average follow-up period was 48 months.

Satisfactory pain relief was achieved in 91.4% of shoulders, regardless of the disease process. The resultant average increase in range of motion was 60 degrees for forward elevation and 18 degrees for external rotation, and these ranges were significantly greater among patients with osteoarthritis and those with intact rotator cuffs. Radiolucent lines of less than 2 mm were present in 17 humeral components, but none were symptomatic or progressed in thickness. Five glenoid components showed progression of radiolucency. In 2 patients, glenoid loosening needed revision; both patients had rheumatoid arthritis. Complications included 2 glenoid fractures and 2 humeral shaft fractures intraoperatively, symptomatic loosening of the glenoid in 2 patients, and rotator cuff tears in another 2. No infections, neurologic injuries, or vascular injuries occurred.

Total shoulder arthroplasty represents a viable alternate treatment for severe arthritis of the glenohumeral joint. It should be performed only by professionals familiar with surgery of the shoulder, especially with difficult rotator-cuff reconstructions. The eventual outcome of total shoulder arthroplasty can be affected by the etiology of the disease process and the status of the rotator cuff.

Survivorship of Unconstrained Total Shoulder Arthroplasty
Brenner BC, Ferlic DC, Clayton ML, Dennis DA (Denver Orthopaedic Clinic; Univ of Colorado)
J Bone Joint Surg [Am] 71-A:1289–1296, October 1989   3–26

The results of 53 unconstrained total shoulder arthroplasties in 48 patients were reviewed using survivorship analysis. This method takes into consideration a discrete beginning point (the time of arthroplasty), the time intervals, patients present at the start of each interval, the number of failures during that time period, and the number of patients with successful results at that time interval and their most recent follow-up. Failure was defined as the need for revision or the onset of patient's dissatisfaction. The results were also reported, using the American Shoulder and Elbow Surgeons' rating form.

A total of 51 shoulders were followed up for a minimum of 2 years (average, 67 months). After 11 years, the survivorship was 75% for all 51 prostheses, 74% for the 37 Neer prosthesis, and 92% for all prostheses in 25 patients with rheumatoid arthritis. Gristina prostheses were implanted in 14 shoulders, and survivorship was 100% at 4 years. Active forward flexion increased an average of 36 degrees, and external rotation increased 23 degrees. Relief of pain was good or excellent in 82%, improved in 6%, and poor in 12% of shoulders. Radiographic analysis revealed a complete or incomplete radiolucent line around the margin of the glenoid component in 58% of all prostheses. A similar proportion of complete or incomplete radiolucent lines occurred in prostheses that were implanted with pressurization of the cement into the keel-hole in the glenoid fossa as in those that were implanted without the same pressurization.

Survivorship analysis shows that 75% of all unconstrained total shoulder arthroplasties survive after 11 years. The relief of pain, which is the primary goal of total shoulder arthroplasty, is good or excellent in 82% of shoulders. However, radiographic analysis shows a far greater incidence of loosening than is suspected clinically.

▶ Analysis of the failures is quite interesting because the failures are somewhat different from those in other reported series. One patient had instability shortly after surgery; in a second, a subacromial spacer was used that became displaced; 3 others had falls with rotator cuff tearing in all 3 and a fracture in 1; and 1 patient had late glenoid loosening. Five of the 6 arthroplasties that failed did so seemingly because of problems with reconstruction of the soft tissues and not because of component or component-bone interface problems. Based on this experience, we might rightly believe that the technical details of reconstructive surgery in the shoulder will need to focus more fully in the future on soft tissue repair or reconstructive techniques, if failures are to be avoided.— R.H. Cofield, M.D.

Heterotopic Bone Formation Following Total Shoulder Arthroplasty
Kjærsgaard-Andersen P, Frich LH, Søjbjerg JO, Sneppen O (Univ of Aarhus, Denmark)
J Arthroplasty 4:99–104, June 1989

The incidence of heterotopic bone formation (HBF) after hip joint operations has been well described, but the incidence of HBF after shoulder operations never has been assessed. A study was conducted to determine the incidence of HBF after total shoulder arthroplasty.

During a 3-year study period, 53 patients aged 31–78 years underwent 63 Neer Mark-II total shoulder arthroplasties; 10 patients underwent bilateral procedures. Indications included rheumatoid arthritis in 41 shoulders, osteoarthritis in 8 shoulders, traumatic arthritis in 8 shoulders, and miscellaneous lesions in the remaining 6 shoulders. Two patients died within the first year after operation. Three other patients were unavailable for follow-up. After an average follow-up period of 26 months, 58 shoulders in 48 patients were available for evaluation.

At follow-up, 26 shoulders (45%) had heterotopic ossifications, 6 of which had grade III ossification bridging the glenohumeral or glenoacromial space. One patient had a severe bridging ossification located in both the glenohumeral and the glenoacromial space. Heterotopic bone formation occurred more frequently in men than in women; the difference was statistically significant. Ectopic bone formed most often in patients with osteoarthritis or miscellaneous shoulder lesions. Shoulder pain of any kind was reported in 23 shoulders, but pain and the development of HBF were not statistically correlated. Thirty-three patients were given anti-inflammatory drugs during the first postoperative weeks, but the incidence of HBF was not affected by the drug treatment. Although HBF after total shoulder arthroplasty is common, disabling heterotopic ossifications seem to be rare.

▶ This report is quite different from all other reported series of total shoulder arthroplasty. In the other series, heterotopic bone develops in much less than 1% of all shoulders for which this procedure is performed. This report, though, does make us aware that HBF is possible with this operation, and we all should be careful to avoid surgical maneuvers that might cause this to develop. Also, we might consider preventive or prophylactic measures for certain patients undergoing total shoulder arthroplasty who have demonstrated their propensity to form heterotopic bone after arthroplasty in other locations.—R.H. Cofield, M.D.

Shoulder Arthrodesis by External Fixation
Nagano A, Okinaga S, Ochiai N, Kurokawa T (Univ of Tokyo)
Clin Orthop 247:97–100, October 1989   3–28

The choice of pin sites in shoulder arthrodesis after brachial plexus injury may allow for efficient external fixation. A method of pin positioning for shoulder arthrodesis by external fixation was evaluated.

Technique.—The Fischer's external fixator and 5 titanium pins 4 mm in diameter are used. The pins are inserted into the coracoid process from the anterior aspect and the scapular spine from the acromion (Fig 3–12). After the fixation angle of the shoulder is determined, the joint is temporarily fixed with 2 Kirschner wires. Two more pins are inserted into the shaft of the humerus, and all 4 pins are fixed in position by the external fixator. The joint position may be corrected postoperatively, if necessary.

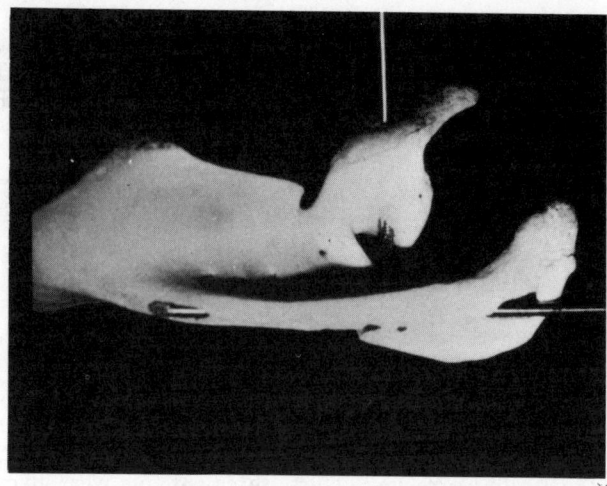

Fig 3-12.—A pin is inserted from the tip of the acromion passing through the scapular spine and viewed from above. (Courtesy of Nagano A, Okinaga S, Ochiai N, et al: *Clin Orthop* 247:97–100, October 1989.)

This operation was performed in 11 cases of brachial plexus injury. All gained solid bone union within 3 months after operation. The external fixator was removed an average of 3 months after surgery. No pin tracts were infected.

One great advantage of this procedure is the postoperative adjustability of the position of the joint, that is, it allows correction of the fixation angle after the operation. In addition, this insertion method holds the scapula more rigid and allows the patient to lie supine.

▶ The placement of pins for external fixation as an adjunct to shoulder fusion is difficult. Many techniques have been suggested, and none is perfect. External fixation as a part of the shoulder arthrodesis procedure may not be the first choice for many surgeons, but it certainly should be considered in selected patients, perhaps those with bone loss, bacterial infection, or severe injury with wound problems.— R.H. Cofield, M.D.

Elbow and Forearm

ELBOW TRAUMA

Transcondylar Fractures of the Distal Humerus
Perry CR, Gibson CT, Kowalski MF (Washington Univ; St Louis Regional Med Ctr)
J Orthop Trauma 3:98–106, June 1989
3–29

Transcondylar fractures of the distal humerus occur in elderly osteopenic patients, and always are caused by low-energy trauma. Transcondylar fractures are characterized by a transverse fracture at the level of the olecranon and coronoid fossae. Stable internal fixation is difficult

Chapter 3—Shoulder, Elbow and Forearm / **129**

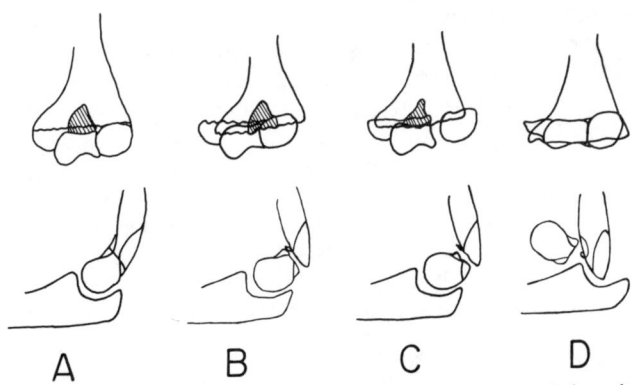

A B C D

Fig 3-13.—All transcondylar fractures have a transverse fracture that extends from the lateral epicondyle through the olecranon and coronoid fossae to the medial epicondyle. This is the only fracture line present in undisplaced (A) and simple displaced (B) fractures. T-type fractures have an additional vertical fracture that separates the capitellum from the trochlea (C). The condyles are dislocated anteriorly from the trochlear notch in fracture dislocations, and the fracture pattern can be either simple or T-type (D). (Courtesy of Perry CR, Gibson CT, Kowalski MF: *J Orthop Trauma* 3:98-106, June 1989.)

to achieve because the distal fragments are small, and most of their surfaces are covered with articular cartilage. A classification system according to displacement into flexion or extension type injuries is proposed.

During a 4-year period, 14 patients had treatment for transcondylar fractures of the humerus. The fractures were grouped into 4 basic patterns: undisplaced, simple displaced, T-type, and fracture dislocation of the humeral condyles from the trochlear notch (Fig 3-13). Treatment of the fractures was based on this classification. Undisplaced fractures were treated in a long arm cast with the elbow flexed to 90 degrees and the forearm in neutral. Displaced fractures were reduced and stabilized with internal fixation.

Adequate follow-up data were available for 7 men and 4 women aged 59-95 years (mean, 70.9 years). All 11 patients had fallen on the outstretched hand. After a follow-up period ranging from 14 to 42 months, all fractures had healed without loss of reduction. None of the patients had postoperative infections. Functional elbow flexion generally was preserved and ranged from 110 degrees to 140 degrees (mean, 123 degrees). However, all patients lost elbow extension. The loss of extension ranged from 5 degrees to 40 degrees (mean, 27 degrees). The results varied according to the type of fracture, with undisplaced fractures having the best prognosis with the least loss of elbow motion.

Because transcondylar fractures in osteopenic patients are difficult to stabilize, the prognosis generally is guarded. The proposed classification system is useful for selecting the optimal treatment for these fractures.

▶ Distal humeral fractures of all types are difficult to treat. The current trend seems to be to further categorize these fractures into their various types and then to develop classification systems within those types that will allow us to understand the fractures more fully and to better select treatment methods. Classifications typically include undisplaced fractures, various types of displacement, and various types of displaced fractures associated with instability. Internal fixation seems to be the accepted treatment for displaced fractures, and rightfully so. Fixation, however, may be tenuous. Surgeons currently consider early movement as part of the treatment regimen. In certain circumstances, early movement will compromise fixation and impair healing. One wonders whether the pendulum will start to swing back toward more ample protection of the fracture to allow healing with certainty and then secondary soft tissue release should that prove to be necessary.—R.H. Cofield, M.D.

Dislocation of the Elbow: An Experimental Study of the Ligamentous Injuries
Søjbjerg JO, Helmig P, Kjærsgaard-Andersen P (Univ of Aarhus, Denmark)
Orthopedics 12:461–463, March 1989

Using human cadaveric elbow specimens, researchers studied the kinesiology of posterior elbow dislocations. An experimental apparatus was designed to determine movement patterns for the joint during the whole range of movement. With a forearm fixed in the neutral position, increasing valgus and external rotary torque was applied at 30 degrees of flexion of the elbow until dislocation occurred. Resulting ligamentous and capsular lesions were recorded and described. Dislocated elbows then were reduced and tested in the apparatus. Researchers plotted movement patterns for a constant torque of 1.5 Nm. In all cases, the force resulting in rupture of the ligaments was greater than 150 Nm.

In 8 specimens, lesions were found on the anterior parts of their ulnar collateral ligaments (AUCL); 5 had lesions on the posterior parts of their medial collateral ligaments. The most common injury on the lateral side of the elbow joint was a tear of the annular ligament.

When the joints were reduced, no specimens could be dislocated in the fully extended position. Application of a combined external rotatory and valgus momentum of 1.5 Nm from about 20 degrees of flexion resulted in posterior dislocation and bilateral ligamentous injury. In cases of persistent valgus instability, restoration of the AUCL is essential.

▶ It is important to remember that although this study nicely describes what supporting structures are torn during dislocation, it does not describe the care that is needed for treatment of elbow dislocation. Reduction of a dislocated elbow and early movement have become the treatment standard. The development of recurrent elbow instability is rare after an acute dislocation; however, if elbow instability persists or recurs, the information in this manuscript will help the surgeon in understanding what structures might need to be repaired or reinforced.—R.H. Cofield, M.D.

Dislocations of the Elbow and Intraarticular Fractures
Josefsson PO, Gentz CF, Johnell O, Wendeberg B (Lund Univ, Malmö, Sweden)
Clin Orthop 246:126–130, September 1989   3–31

Elbow dislocation associated with displaced fracture of the joint articulation carries the risk of osteoarthritis, instability, and dislocation. Data on 23 elbow dislocations in 23 patients, combined with a displaced fracture of the head of the radius, were retrospectively reviewed. Follow-up periods ranged from 3 to 34 years.

All 23 patients underwent surgical treatment, and radial heads were extirpated in 19. Redislocation had occurred in 4 patients, each of whom had an associated fracture of the coronoid process. At follow-up, the most common complaint was reduced range of motion. The most common finding was loss of extension. Severe osteoarthritis with reduced joint space was evident in 12 patients overall, and in two thirds of the patients with resected radial heads.

To help prevent severe instability, a radial head should be preserved and reconstructed when possible. If extirpation is necessary, torn ligaments and muscles should be sutured at the epicondyles. Roentgenographic examination for redislocation should be performed within 1 week after surgery.

▶ This article addresses some of the issues implied by the currently developing classification systems. When fracturing occurs in the presence of a dislocation, treatment may indeed be difficult, and attention must be directed not only to fixation of the fractures but also to maintaining joint stability if success is to be assured.—R.H. Cofield, M.D.

Decompression of the Posterior Interosseous Nerve for Tennis Elbow
Jalovaara P, Lindholm RV (Univ of Oulu, Finland)
Arch Orthop Trauma Surg 108:243–245, 1989   3–32

Pain involving the lateral elbow may have a number of different causes. Tennis elbow usually can be relieved with conservative treatment; however, surgery is necessary for about 10% of patients. The results of decompression of the posterior interosseous nerve (PIN) in 107 patients were reviewed.

Most of the patients were manual workers whose jobs required repetitive tasks using the arms. They experienced local tenderness, pain at rest, and pain during exertion. None had had improvement with conservative treatment or previous operations. During surgery, all sites of compression along the PIN were identified and released. Six patients needed repeated procedures. The overall rate of improvement including all reoperations was 89%. Primary decompression resulted in complete recovery in 30% of patients.

Previous studies reported various rates of success when surgery was directed at entrapment of the PIN. Excellent results ranged from 47% to 71%. The role of PIN in tennis elbow is not fully understood.

▶ Many etiologic factors should be considered when analyzing lateral elbow pain. Posterior interosseous nerve entrapment is one. This article nicely demonstrates that decompression of the PIN alone will not resolve symptoms in the majority of patients.—R.H. Cofield, M.D.

PROSTHETIC ARTHROPLASTY AND OTHER RECONSTRUCTIVE PROCEDURES

Failure of the Wadsworth Elbow: Nineteen Cases of Rheumatoid Arthritis Followed for 5 Years
Ljung P, Lidgren L, Rydholm U (Lund Univ Hosp, Lund, Sweden)
Acta Orthop Scand 60:254–257, June 1989   3–33

During a 4-year period, 19 elbows in 15 patients with rheumatoid arthritis were operated on with insertion of the Wadsworth nonconstrained surface replacement prosthesis (Fig 3–14). The average follow-up period was 5.7 years (range, 4.6–6.9 years).

Six prostheses were revised, for a revision rate of 0.3. Five were revised because of mechanical loosening and 1 because of deep infection. Eight prostheses showed radiographic signs of loosening, which occurred more frequently with the humeral than the ulnar component. Because of progressive loss of bone stock in the distal part of the humerus, spontaneous fractures of 1 of the pillars occurred in 4 elbows.

The Wadsworth elbow prosthesis used in surgical treatment of rheumatoid arthritis was a failure. Better long-term results have been reported with nonconstrained resurfacing elbows with a stemmed humeral component, particularly the capitellocondylar total elbow.

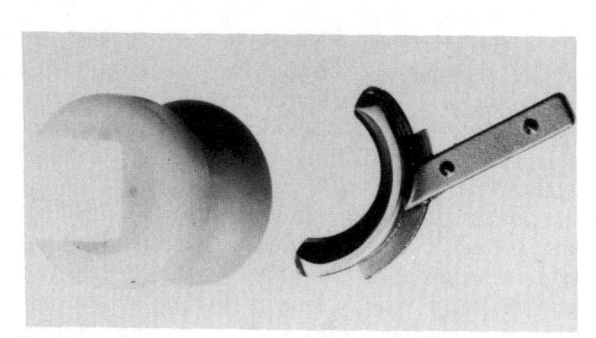

Fig 3–14.—The Wadsworth resurfacing elbow prosthesis. (Courtesy of Ljung P, Lidgren L, Rydholm U: *Acta Orthop Scand* 60:254–257, June 1989.)

▶ It seems that surgeons must avoid using a total elbow arthroplasty wnose humeral component does not include a stem as a part of the prosthetic design.—R.H. Cofield, M.D.

Capitellocondylar Total Elbow Replacement: A Long-Term Follow-Up Study
Weiland AJ, Weiss A-PC, Wills RP, Moore JR (Johns Hopkins Univ)
J Bone Joint Surg [Am] 71-A:217–222, February 1989   3–34

Many operative procedures have been used in attempts to improve function of elbows impaired by injury or disease. An experience with the capitellocondylar unconstrained total elbow prosthesis was reviewed.

Forty total elbow replacements in which a capitellocondylar prosthesis was implanted in 35 patients were examined retrospectively. Follow-up ranged from 4 to 12 years, with a mean of 7.2 years. Pronation, supination, and flexion were improved considerably, although extension was not. In 10 patients (29%) malarticulation or dislocation of the prosthesis occurred. In 2 additional patients, deep infection necessitated prosthesis removal. In 10 patients, 10 prostheses had radiolucent lines on follow-up radiographs; these lines were not associated with pain or loosening. In 7 patients, a transient ulnar-nerve palsy developed in 7 elbows. When the lateral Kocher approach to the elbow was used, the incidence of this complication was decreased from 30% to 15%.

The most important overall factor in determining the clinical success of total elbow arthroplasty is the patient's initial health status. The severity of rheumatoid disease and the postoperative ratings of the elbow were strongly inversely correlated in this series. Although improved postoperative scores do not guarantee improved function, the relief of pain that results from a successful total elbow arthroplasty is a sufficient indication for this procedure.

▶ This report nicely defines the results of patients who had undergone an unconstrained type of total elbow arthroplasty. Loosening of the components was uncommon, but instability and ulnar nerve difficulties were not. Thus, in contemporary care of patients, a surgeon must be quite astute in understanding who to select for this procedure and how to deal with various degrees of instability at the time of surgery. Also, a surgeon must be aware of changes in the operative approach to do total elbow arthroplasty because the current techniques have greatly decreased the frequency of ulnar nerve difficulties. With these 2 types of complications minimized, the unconstrained total elbow replacement becomes a quite satisfactory procedure.—R.H. Cofield, M.D.

The Pritchard Mark II Elbow Prosthesis in Rheumatoid Arthritis
Madsen F, Gudmundson GH, Søjbjerg JO, Sneppen O (The Orthopedic Hosp, Univ of Århus, Denmark)
Acta Orthop Scand 60:249–253, June 1989   3–35

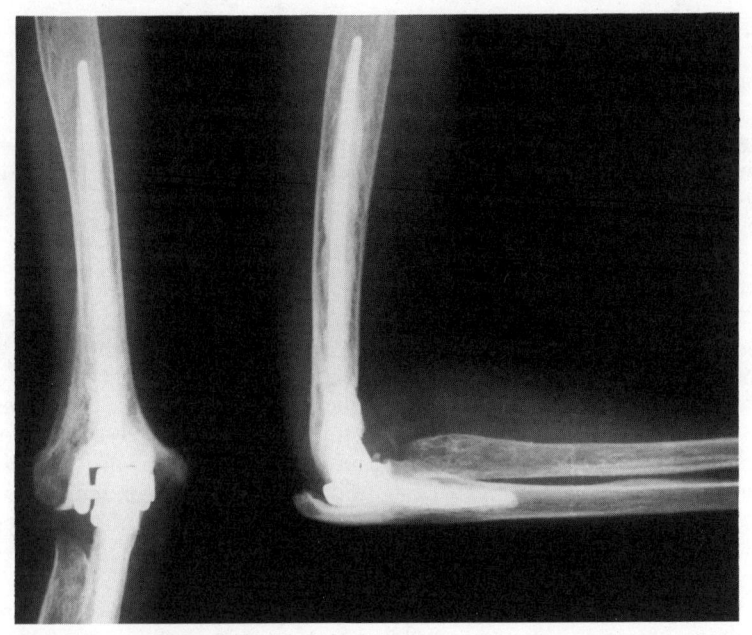

Fig 3–15.—The Pritchard Mark II prosthesis 6 months after arthroplasty. (Courtesy of Madsen F, Gudmundson GH, Søjbjerg JO, et al: *Acta Orthop Scand* 60:249–253, June 1989.)

Some improvements with the Pritchard Mark II elbow prosthesis (Fig 3–15), such as the provision for some rotation and medial–lateral laxity in the hinge, have reduced the incidence of loosening. Twenty-five consecutive rheumatoid elbows treated with the Pritchard Mark II elbow prosthesis were followed prospectively for a mean of 38 months (range, 2–5 years). Fourteen elbows were classified as grade IIIA and 11 as grade IIIB.

Marked pain relief and significantly improved motion were achieved after the operation. Six elbows had radiographic loosening, but only 1 needed revision for pain. Five of the loosenings occurred in grade IIIA elbows. Another elbow required revision because of deep infection. No neuropathies or fractures occurred.

The Pritchard Mark II elbow prosthesis is a good alternate treatment for destroyed rheumatic elbows. Annual radiographic follow-up is warranted to allow revision of a loose prosthesis before large resorption of bone occurs.

▶ If a patient is not a candidate for a less constrained type of total elbow replacement, one of the more constrained designs with some laxity at the hinge seems to be the preferred alternative. The prosthesis described in this article represents one of these types of prosthetic implant. This particular style, however, still has problems with loosening and disassembly at the hinge. For this category of prosthesis, these 2 problems must be minimized.—R.H. Cofield, M.D.

Salvage of Non-Union of Supracondylar Fracture of the Humerus by Total Elbow Arthroplasty
Figgie MP, Inglis AE, Mow CS, Figgie HE III (Cornell Univ, New York)
J Bone Joint Surg [Am] 71-A:1058–1065, August 1989   3–36

Nonunion of supracondylar fractures of the distal end of the humerus are extremely difficult to treat. Nonunions can be treated with open reduction and bone-grafting, provided adequate bone of good quality is available. However, this type of nonunion often occurs in elderly patients with osteopenic bone and poor osteogenic potential. In patients with inadequate bone stock or severe periarticular fibrosis, salvage total elbow arthroplasty may be the only remaining option.

Since 1976, 17 patients underwent 17 total elbow replacements in the treatment of a supracondylar nonunion. Three patients died, leaving 14 evaluable elbows. Of 4 men and 10 women aged 31–77 years, with an average age at operation of 65 years, all had established nonunion. Ten patients underwent 1–4 previous attempts at internal fixation before total elbow replacement was considered. Most of the patients were in pain, had a flail elbow, and were unable to perform activities of daily living. The average preoperative elbow score was 17 points. A semiconstrained elbow prosthesis was used in all patients. Follow-up ranged from 2 to 12 years.

The average postoperative overall score was 84 points. Results were excellent in 6, good in 2, fair in 3, and failed in 3. Seven postoperative complications occurred in 5 elbows. Three elbows needed surgical revision and therefore were considered failures. In 1 of these 3 patients, the implant had to be removed because of infection. The limb was stabilized in an external fixator. Three patients had problems with wound healing, and 1 patient dislocated the elbow. Follow-up radiographs revealed a lucency about the implant in only 2 of the 13 elbows. Heterotopic bone formation was seen in 8 elbows; the epicondyles were present in all 13 elbows.

Total elbow arthroplasty for nonunion of a supracondylar fracture of the humerus is a technically demanding procedure that should be performed only when all other therapeutic options have been exhausted. Satisfactory results in terms of pain relief and functional range of motion often can be achieved if complications can be avoided.

▶ It is clear that the first line of treatment for most nonunions in any location includes internal fixation and bone grafting. In this anatomical setting, that is still true. In certain situations, the first line of treatment might not be possible, and these authors have suggested total elbow arthroplasty as an alternative. They nicely inform us that this treatment choice can be fraught with a number of serious complications, and, although it may be effective treatment for some patients, it is not to be undertaken without due consideration of other less drastic reconstructive options.—R.H. Cofield, M.D.

Total Elbow Arthroplasty for Complete Ankylosis of the Elbow
Figgie MP, Inglis AE, Mow CS, Figgie HE III (Hosp for Special Surgery, New York)
J Bone Joint Surg [Am] 71-A:513–520, April 1989   3–37

Complete ankylosis of the elbow produces severe disability and functional limitations, particularly when other joints in the ipsilateral upper extremity also have limited motion. Complete ankylosis of the elbow usually results in decreased function, but pain is seldom a problem. Because pronation and supination are independent of flexion and extension, pain may be caused by disease of the radial head. Results achieved with conversion of ankylosed elbows to total elbow arthroplasties were reviewed.

Sixteen patients received 19 semiconstrained total elbow replacements for complete ankylosis of the elbow, and were followed-up for 2–12 years. Average elbow scores were 23 points preoperatively and 84 postoperatively. After surgery, the average flexion was 115 degrees; average extension, 35 degrees; and average pronation and supination, 95 degrees. Results were excellent or good in 15 operations. One failure occurred because of a deep infection; after removal of the prosthesis, a satisfactory fascial arthroplasty was achieved. All patients had improved function, and all had relief of pain.

Arthroplasty can succeed only if a patient has a good understanding of the procedure and is willing and able to comply with the postoperative rehabilitation program. Semiconstrained, often custom-fit, implants must be used. The Bryan-Morrey posteromedial approach to the elbow was recommended, as it allows early range-of-motion exercises.

▶ The authors describe the need for the semiconstrained types of total elbow replacement in the care of this problem. Some reconstructive surgeons currently would consider resection arthroplasty with distraction techniques as an alternative to total elbow replacement in patients with ankylosis.—R.H. Cofield, M.D.

Synovectomy of the Elbow in Rheumatoid Arthritis: Long-Term Results
Tulp NJA, Winia WPCA (Slotervaart Hosp, Amsterdam)
J Bone Joint Surg [Br] 71-B:664–666, August 1989   3–38

A study was conducted to assess the short- and long-term results of elbow synovectomy in early and late disease stages in 50 patients with rheumatoid arthritis who had undergone 61 elbow synovectomies. Follow-up ranged from 4 to 10 years (mean follow-up, 6.5 years). Range of motion was measured with a goniometer. Synovectomy of elbows in grades 1 and 2 was defined as early (27 elbows) and in grades 3 and 4 as late synovectomy (34 elbows).

The results were graded as satisfactory in 43 synovectomies and unsatisfactory in 18. Four of the 18 patients with unsatisfactory results later underwent replacement arthroplasty. The average pain score improved from 2.7 before operation to 0.7 after operation. The mean range of flexion improved only slightly, from 89 to 100 degrees. Satisfactory results were achieved in 43 elbows: 20 who had early synovectomy and 23 who had late synovectomy. The difference was not statistically significant.

Analysis of the long-term results in 22 patients who underwent 27 elbow synovectomies before 1980 showed nearly identical success rates after at least 6 years of follow-up. Overall results had had no decline, and results for the long-term group were no different from those of the entire group. These findings support the view that synovectomy performed in destroyed joints is a justifiable operation that can provide at least 10 years of good and painless elbow function before total joint replacement need be considered.

Flexorplasty of the Elbow
Botte MJ, Wood MB (Mayo Med School, Rochester, Minn)
Clin Orthop 245:110–116, August 1989   3–39

Several surgical procedures are available for restoring lost active elbow flexion. Each of these methods has its advocates, and most studies report just a single method for elbow flexor reconstruction. The results of 4 different elbow flexorplasties were compared.

Thirteen men and 3 women aged 17–68 years had treatment for lost or inadequate elbow flexor power. Five patients underwent bipolar pectoralis major transfers, 5 patients had unipolar or bipolar latissimus dorsi transfers, 3 patients underwent free latissimus dorsi transfers, and 3 had triceps-to-biceps transfers. None of the patients were candidates for proximal advancement of the forearm muscles. Each patient was evaluated by physical examination for active and passive ranges of elbow motion, muscle strength of the transfer, and ability to move the hand to the mouth. The mean follow-up period was 31.5 months (range, 4–88 months).

At the follow-up evaluation, the mean antigravity elbow flexion arcs obtained from each procedure were 91 degrees for the pectoralis transfer, 87 degrees for the latissimus dorsi transfer, 11 degrees for the free latissimus dorsi transfer, and 125 degrees for the triceps-to-biceps transfer. Most patients having had pectoralis or latissimus dorsi transfer were able to move their hands to their mouths, most were able to return to work or to school, and most were satisfied with their outcomes. Of the 3 patients having had a triceps-to-biceps transfer, 2 were able to move their hands to their mouths, 2 were able to return to work, and 2 were satisfied with the results. However, none of the 3 patients having had free latissimus dorsi transfer could move their hands to their mouths, 2 were able to return to work, and none were satisfied with their outcomes. Therefore, free muscle transfer for the restoration of elbow flexion cannot be recommended.

▶ The quite poor results of free latissimus dorsi transfer are surprising but should be noted. Unipolar pectoralis major transfer is another consideration not addressed in this article; it may be particularly appropriate in patients who have a concomitant shoulder arthrodesis.—R.H. Cofield, M.D.

FOREARM TRAUMA

Compression-Plate Fixation of Acute Fractures of the Diaphyses of the Radius and Ulna
Chapman MW, Gordon JE, Zissimos AG (Univ of California, Sacramento)
J Bone Joint Surg [Am] 71-A:159–169, February 1989   3–40

In 1975, Anderson and his colleagues reported a 98% union rate for radial fractures and a 96% union rate for ulnar fractures with compression-plate fixation. Modifications of surgical techniques and fixation devices introduced since then were assessed. In addition, the usefulness of routine bone grafting in comminuted fractures, what type of internal fixation influences the rate of refracture, and the desirability of using immediate fixation for open fractures were evaluated in 68 men and 19 women with 129 diaphyseal radial or ulnar fractures. Forty-two patients had both radial and ulnar fractures.

Of the 129 fractures, 68 (53%) were comminuted; 80 (62%) were closed, and 49 (38%) were open fractures. Fourteen of 18 isolated radial fractures were Galeazzi fractures; 10 of 27 isolated ulnar fractures were Monteggia fractures. All nondisplaced closed fractures were treated nonoperatively. Open fractures were internally fixed primarily, using a 3.5-mm or a 4.5-mm AO dynamic-compression plate. Bone grafting was performed routinely in treating comminuted and open fractures.

Union occurred in 125 fractures (97%), and was delayed in 2 (1.5%); 2 fractures (1.5%) did not unite. Only 1 of 68 fractures (1.5%) that needed bone grafting failed to unite. After 12 months follow-up, 79 patients (91%) had excellent or satisfactory functional results, and in 6 (7%), results were unsatisfactory. The operation was rated a failure in the remaining 2 patients. Fractures united in 2 patients with early fixation loss in whom fixation was repeated with 3.5-mm AO plates. Thirty-four plates (26.4%) were removed after fraction union. No refractures occurred in patients who had a 3.5-mm AO plate, but both fractures fixed with a 4.5-mm AO narrow AO plate refractured. The overall fracture union rate was 98.4%.

The use of bone-grafting in treating comminuted and open fractures was supported. Because the 4.5-mm AO plate-and-screw system appears to be too large for most forearm fractures, the 3.5-mm AO system is recommended. Removal of the compression plate is not mandatory, but the long-term effects of retained plates are not yet known.

Post-Traumatic Proximal Radio-Ulnar Synostosis: Results of Surgical Treatment
Failla JM, Amadio PC, Morrey BF (Mayo Clinic and Mayo Found, Rochester, Minn)
J Bone Joint Surg [Am] 71-A:1208–1213, September 1989   3–41

Posttraumatic proximal radioulnar synostosis is rare. It may be caused by a fracture or soft-tissue injury involving the interosseous membrane. Although resection of a posttraumatic proximal radioulnar synostosis can restore useful rotation of the forearm in some patients, it has been suggested that adults who undergo this operation may have a poor prognosis. The incidence of satisfactory outcome after excision of a proximal posttraumatic radioulnar synostosis and which factors might be prognostic of a poor outcome were investigated.

Between 1945 and 1987, 20 skeletally mature patients aged 16–74 years (average, 39 years) underwent excision of a proximal radioulnar synostosis. All patients had difficulty performing activities of daily living because of the loss of forearm rotation. The average time from injury to operation was 18 months. Patients were followed up until the synostosis recurred, or for a minimum of 12 months. The length of postoperative follow-up for all patients averaged 40 months.

Of the 20 patients, 4 had excellent results, 3 had good results, 4 had fair results, and 9 had poor results. At the most recent follow-up, the average total arc of postoperative rotation was 55 degrees, and ranged from 0 to 160 degrees. Thus, about one half of the patients who undergo excision of a proximal posttraumatic radioulnar synostosis can be expected to have satisfactory results. Examination of the 9 patients with poor results suggested that a severe soft tissue injury and a previous unsuccessful attempt at surgical excision may be associated with a poor prognosis.

4 Adult Reconstruction

Introduction

This chapter addresses various aspects of adult reconstructive surgery and a number of areas of general interest such as safer blood replacement practices and the natural history of several orthopedic conditions. The amazing growth in orthopedic surgery, especially the technologic aspects, produces a rich annual literature. We have attempted to select articles of broad interest across this enormous range of subject matter, hoping to capture the essence of what has transpired in the past year. Among the topics covered, several stand out as especially noteworthy: the epidemiology of and multiple factors influencing the incidence of hip fracture, the natural history of osteoarthritis of both the hip and the knee, the results of osteotomy about the hip and knee, and, in a number of papers, the results of meniscal repair of the knee.

Exciting research continues on hip replacement. Among this year's papers are reports of clinical and experimental results using hydroxyapatite coating materials and analyses of titanium alloys as bearing surfaces. The advantages and disadvantages of custom implants are considered, as well as the effect of femoral head size on acetabular failure rates, the variability of cement restriction afforded by different types of intermedullary plugs, the 5-year results of autologous acetabular bone graft for deficiencies, and the incidence, prevention, and treatment of intraoperative fractures in uncemented total hip replacements. A number of papers address infection: its diagnosis, its treatment, and the results of late reimplantation after infected total hip replacement.

Bone stock depletion after total hip replacement is addressed, as well as bone strain many years after total hip replacement, measured in a long-term retrieval study. The natural femur adapted somewhat to an implant, but normal bone strains never were recovered.

Other papers that address the long-term results of total knee arthroplasty confirm the usefulness of the procedure as well as its longevity. One paper points out the frequency of deep venous thrombosis after knee arthroplasty and presents a strong argument for prophylaxis after such surgery. The usefulness of magnetic resonance imaging in diagnostic evaluation of the knee received much attention and is well summarized in the five papers selected. An exciting paper on fresh osteochondral allografting in young patients with cartilage defects of the knee is presented: 78% good results are reported.

"Anterior knee pain" continues to be a confusing diagnostic entity. One paper reports no relationship among the symptoms of anterior knee pain, degree of chondromalacia seen at arthroscopy, and the long-term functional outcome. Another paper suggests that the overwhelming majority of such patients recover with no surgical procedure, emphasizing the need to avoid either open or arthroscopic surgery in these patients if at all possible. Meniscal repair continues to be useful, but it has been pointed out recently that not all tears are amenable to such repair and, indeed, some tears need no repair at all.

Two papers by Dr. Ilizarov outline the scientific principles and results of application of his technique to a variety of problems. Hip arthroscopy, the application of pulsed magnetic fields in disuse osteoporosis, and successful transplantation of rabbit chondrocyte allografts of articular cartilage are exciting avenues of continued research with potential clinical application.

Clement B. Sledge, M.D.
Robert Poss, M.D.

General

Intraoperative Autologous Transfusion in Orthopaedic Patients
Goulet JA, Bray TJ, Timmerman LA, Benson DR, Bargar WL (Univ of California, Davis, Sacramento)
J Bone Joint Surg [Am] 71-A:3–8, January 1989   4–1

Previous reports of autologous transfusion during orthopedic surgery have involved small series of patients. In this study, data on 175 patients having consecutive orthopedic procedures with the use of the autotransfuser in a 2-year period were reviewed. The series included revision hip replacement operations, spinal fusions for scoliosis, elective spinal procedures, surgery for spinal trauma, and reduction of acetabular fractures.

The overall rate of red cells salvaged with use of the autotransfuser was 60%. The mean savings per patient was nearly 2 units, and a mean of 1.7 units of banked blood was transfused, compared with 2.9 units when the autotransfuser was not used. In patients having revision hip arthroplasty or elective spinal surgery, the use of prebanked autologous blood further lowered the mean requirement for homologous blood. There were no complications from air embolism, coagulopathy, or renal failure.

Autologous transfusion is a safe, effective, and economic approach to orthopedic surgery. It substantially lowers the need for banked blood and the risk of associated infectious and immunologic complications. If tumor and infection are absent, intraoperative autologous transfusion may be recommended for all orthopedic operations in which homologous blood may be needed.

Intraoperative Autologous Transfusion in Revision Total Hip Arthroplasty
Wilson WJ (Swedish Hosp Med Ctr, Seattle)
J Bone Joint Surg [Am] 71-A:8–14, January 1989   4–2

The value of intraoperative autologous transfusion in lowering homologous blood requirements was studied in 98 patients who had 100 revision total hip arthroplasties from October 1983 through September 1985. In 50 operations the Haemonetics Cell Saver III was used, and the results were compared with those in the final 50 arthroplasties performed before the cell saver came into use.

With the cell saver a mean of 685 mL of autologous blood, 47% of the estimated loss, was transfused at operation. The mean need for homologous blood transfusion in 39 of these patients over the entire hospital course was 795 mL, compared with 1,160 mL for 46 patients in the control group; the difference was significant.

Four patients in the control group and 11 in the study group were not given homologous blood. The overall saving in homologous blood from the use of autologous transfusion was 42%. No complications were ascribed to use of the cell saver.

Autologous transfusion can save a substantial amount of homologous transfusion in patients who require revision total hip arthroplasty. The actual cost savings are dependent on the cost of homologous blood at a given facility.

Increased Preoperative Collection of Autologous Blood With Recombinant Human Erythropoietin Therapy
Goodnough LT, Rudnick S, Price TH, Ballas SK, Collins ML, Crowley JP, Kosmin M, Kruskall MS, Lenes BA, Menitove JE, Silberstein LE, Smith KJ, Wallas CH, Abels R, Von Tress M (Case Western Reserve Univ, Cleveland; RW Johnson Pharmaceutical Research Inst, Raritan, NJ; Puget Sound Blood Ctr, Seattle; Jefferson Med College, Philadelphia; Univ of North Carolina, Chapel Hill; et al)
N Engl J Med 321:1163–1168, Oct 26, 1989   4–3

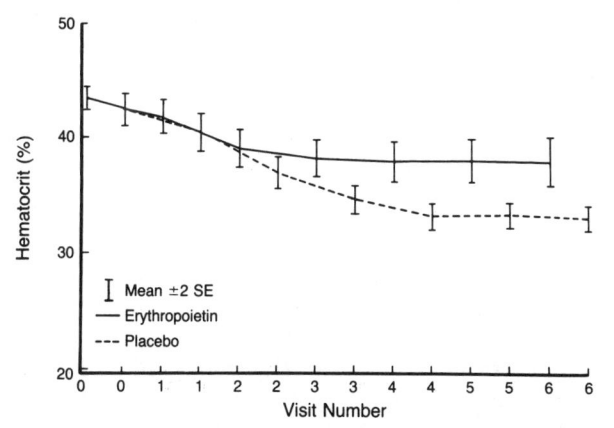

Fig 4–1.—Mean hematocrits for each group before the study and at visits 1 through 6. (Courtesy of Goodnough LT, Rudnick S, Price TH, et al: *N Engl J Med* 321:1163–1168, Oct 26, 1989.)

Can the use of recombinant human erythropoietin increase the amount of autologous blood collected before surgery? In this study 47 adults scheduled for elective orthopedic operations received either 600 units/kg of erythropoietin intravenously or a placebo twice weekly for 3 weeks. About 6 units of blood were collected during this time. The patients also received iron sulfate. Those with hematocrit levels less than 34% were excluded from donation (Fig 4–1).

A mean of 5.4 units was collected for the erythropoietin patients, and 4.1 units, on average, for placebo patients. The mean red blood cell volume donated was 41% greater in the erythropoietin group. All but 1 of 23 erythropoietin recipients were able to donate 4 units or more, compared with 7 of 24 placebo recipients. Adverse effects were comparable between the 2 groups.

Recombinant erythropoietin promotes the ability of elective surgical patients to donate autologous blood, and significant adverse effects are not a problem. Women and children, who have smaller blood volumes, and anemic patients are most likely to benefit from this measure.

▶ Modalities available to reduce the need for homologous blood transfusion include preoperative autologous blood donation and intraoperative autologous transfusion of recovered blood. The first 2 papers (Abstracts 4–1 and 4–2) in this series demonstrate that, in a variety of orthopedic procedures, and in particular in revision total hip replacement, between 50% and 60% of the estimated intraoperative blood loss was recovered and retransfused. When intraoperative losses are replaced with autologous blood, and when a patient has successfully autodonated blood preoperatively, the need for homologous blood transfusion is diminished markedly.

In the third paper (Abstract 4–3), an exciting application of genetic engineering is presented. Recombinant human erythropoietin therapy in preoperative patients allowed the treatment group to donate a volume of red blood cells that was 41% greater than a group given placebo. Thus, it is likely that in the near future patients can donate a greater volume of blood, retain a higher hematocrit, and have returned to them during surgery a greater volume of their own blood loss. These efficacious therapies should diminish further the need for homologous blood transfusion in any elective surgery.— R. Poss, M.D.

Postoperative Blood Salvage Using the Cell Saver After Total Joint Arthroplasty
Semkiw LB, Schurman DJ, Goodman SB, Woolson ST (Stanford Univ)
J Bone Joint Surg [Am] 71-A:823–827, July 1989   4–4

Whether it is feasible and worthwhile to salvage blood from the drainage tubes of patients having total joint arthroplasty was investigated in a prospective study of the Cell Saver. The study group comprised 74 consecutive patients undergoing total hip or total knee replacement. Thirty-five patients received transfusions of blood acquired intraoperatively with the Cell Saver. Fifty patients predeposited autologous blood.

An average of 434 mL of blood was returned to patients having total hip replacement. The average for all hip and knee replacements was 428 mL. Thirteen patients also received nonautologous blood in the perioperative period, but only 4 patients received 3 or more units. The Cell Saver salvaged similar amounts of blood from these patients and from those not needing nonautologous blood. The latter, however, had received more predeposited autologous blood.

The intraoperative use of the Cell Saver is an effective means of salvaging blood and can lower total blood loss by as much as half. If use of the device extends into the immediate postoperative period a significant amount of blood can be retrieved and returned to the patient. Salvaged red blood cells survive as well as autologous cells. Salvage is especially useful when more bleeding is anticipated, as in revision surgery and arthroplasty using noncemented components.

▶ The use of devices to collect, clean, and retransfuse blood lost during orthopedic procedures has been reported widely. This paper describes the use of that technique to retransfuse blood lost during the postoperative period. The Cell Saver was connected to postoperative drains and remained connected throughout a patient's stay in the recovery room. The amount of blood salvaged in the postoperative period was consistently greater than the amount salvaged during the operative procedure (done under tourniquet control), and an average of 434 mL of blood was salvaged that otherwise would have been lost.

As an additional means of diminishing the risk of disease transmission by blood and blood products, this technique deserves further study. Other papers have reported simpler devices for capturing postoperative drainage and returning it to a patient, but questions have been raised about the quality of blood salvaged by these simpler means. The authors of this study have demonstrated that the survival of salvaged red blood cells equals that of autologous cells, suggesting that very little damage to the cells is produced by this method of salvage and reinfusion.— C.B. Sledge, M.D.

Less Pain With Epidural Morphine After Knee Arthroplasty
Nielsen PT, Blom H, Nielsen S-E (Hillerød Hosp, Hillerød, Denmark
Acta Orthop Scand 60:447–448, August 1989   4–5

Inadequate treatment of pain after hip and knee replacement can impede early, active mobilization. The efficacy of epidural morphine in reducing pain after knee arthroplasty was compared with that of systemic opiods in 22 patients. The patients were assigned randomly to receive either epidural morphine, 2–6 mg 3 times daily for 10 days, or intramuscular ketobemidon, 5–7.5 mg for 4 days and then as needed.

Pain scores, as measured with the visual analogue scale, were significantly lower in the epidural treatment group. Knee flexion and range of motion did not differ significantly between groups. Adverse effects to epidural morphine included itching, nausea, and urine retention.

Epidural morphine is superior to systemic opioids in controlling pain after knee arthroplasty. The main disadvantage is respiratory depression, which may occur in up to 5% of patients within 24 hours after epidural morphine administration.

▶ Epidural anesthesia is used widely for orthopedic procedures involving lower extremities. This study points out the usefulness of epidural morphine in the postoperative period for reducing pain after knee arthroplasty and facilitating early functional recovery. Although pain control was excellent in the group given epidural morphine, there was no significant difference between range of motion or maximal knee flexion in the control group and the treatment group. The authors conclude that this is an excellent method of providing pain relief, but they did not demonstrate earlier achievement of functional goals or earlier discharge from the hospital. This has also been our experience.—C.B. Sledge, M.D.

Evaluation of Magnetic Resonance Imaging in the Diagnosis of Osteonecrosis of the Femoral Head: Accuracy Compared With Radiographs, Core Biopsy, and Intraosseous Pressure Measurements
Robinson HJ Jr, Hartleben PD, Lund G, Schreiman J (Univ of Minnesota Hosp and Clinics; VA Hosp, Minneapolis)
J Bone Joint Surg [Am] 71-A:650–662, June 1989   4–6

It generally is believed that an early diagnosis of avascular necrosis of the femoral head would allow prompt intervention in selected patients and would improve the prognosis for the hip. However, available noninvasive techniques for detecting avascular necrosis early are of little diagnostic value, whereas the more accurate invasive examinations require general anesthesia in an operating room. Because preliminary investigations have suggested that magnetic resonance imaging (MRI) may be useful for detecting ischemic necrosis of the femoral head before clinical and radiographic changes are evident, the diagnostic accuracy of MRI was compared with that of other diagnostic techniques in current use.

In phase I of the study, 96 hips in 48 patients who were at high risk for avascular necrosis of the hip were evaluated with MRI and plain radiography. In phase II of the study, 23 hips in 22 patients that were suspected of having early-stage necrosis of the femoral head on MRI but not on plain radiography were further evaluated clinically and with repeated plain radiography, repeated MRI, bone marrow pressure determination, intramedullary venography, and histologic examination of core-biopsy bone specimens.

Of the 23 hips studied in detail for phase II, 18 (78%) had positive changes on MRI, 19 (83%) had positive histologic evidence of avascular necrosis, and 14 (61%) had positive findings by bone-marrow pressure studies and intramedullary venography. Magnetic resonance imaging was particularly useful for the detection of avascular necrosis in hips that were suspected of having Ficat stage 2 or stage 3 changes, with or without radiographic abnormalities. However, the findings in hips that were suspected of having stage 0 or stage 1 changes were at times equivocal.

The sensitivity of MRI as a diagnostic procedure for the detection of Ficat stage 0 or stage 1 changes as indications of very early avascular necrosis is limited, as both false negative and false positive results were observed. However, MRI may be useful in the diagnosis of hips with stage 2 and stage 3 disease.

Correlation of the Findings of Magnetic Resonance Imaging With Those of Bone Biopsy in Patients Who Have Stage-I or II Ischemic Necrosis of the Femoral Head
Seiler JG III, Christie MJ, Homra L (Vanderbilt Univ Med Ctr, Nashville, Tenn)
J Bone Joint Surg [Am] 71-A:28–32, January 1989   4–7

Because of the importance of early diagnosis and treatment in ischemic necrosis of the femoral head, the value of magnetic resonance (MR) imaging was examined prospectively in 15 consecutively treated patients with 16 symptomatic femoral heads. In these cases the MR findings were consistent with a diagnosis of femoral head osteonecrosis, and core decompression was carried out, with biopsy of the contents of the core.

All biopsy specimens were diagnostic of ischemic necrosis. Preoperative MR images consistently showed changes consistent with that diagnosis. Both focal involvement of the superoanterior part of the femoral head and a more diffuse attenuation of the T_1 signal were observed. Signal densities were unchanged on repeat imaging 3 months after core decompression. No fractures and no wound infections occurred. After an average follow-up of 1 year, ischemic necrosis had progressed in 7 of the 16 affected hips.

The MR findings in these cases of stage I and II ischemic necrosis of the femoral head were correlated well with the core biopsy findings. Despite early diagnosis, however, core decompression may not alter the natural course of the diasease. Often a decrease in intraosseous pressure leads to only temporary relief of symptoms.

▶ Two important contemporary questions regarding the diagnosis and treatment of osteonecrosis of the femoral head are: What is the most sensitive method by which early diagnosis can be made? Does early diagnosis and treatment successfully alter the natural history of the disease? When compared with established diagnostic criteria for osteonecrosis (plain radiographs, core biopsies of the femoral head, bone marrow pressure studies, and intramedullary venography), the majority of patients for whom these conventional studies were positive also had positive results of MRI examinations in early-stage osteonecrosis. Results of MRI were falsely negative as well as falsely positive, but the authors conclude that MRI is beneficial in the early diagnosis of osteonecrosis. Patients with grade II or III changes on plain radiographs had uniformly positive MRI findings as well. Despite early diagnosis with MRI and confirmation with core decompression, the authors question whether early diagnosis and treatment with core decompression actually confers long-term improvement or alters the natural history of the disease. It has yet to be demonstrated that the improved diagnostic accuracy in the early stages of osteonecrosis has led to treatment strategies that alter or improve the fate of the hip with osteonecrosis.—R. Poss, M.D.

Core Decompression of the Distal Femur for Avascular Necrosis of the Knee
Jacobs MA, Loeb PE, Hungerford DS (Johns Hopkins Univ)
J Bone Joint Surg [Br] 71-B:583–587, August 1989   4–8

Eighteen patients with avascular necrosis, confirmed pathologically, underwent 28 core decompressions of distal femora between 1974 and 1981. All patients had both rest pain and pain on walking that had failed to improve with nonsteroidal drug therapy and physiotherapy. Follow-up averaged 54 months. Eight-millimeter core biopsy specimens were removed with the Michele instrument.

No orthopedic complications resulted from core decompression. All 7 patients with stage I or II disease had good clinical results, as did 11 of 21 patients with stage III involvement at the time of surgery. Four other patients have experienced progressive pain and probably will need total knee replacement. Six others already have had knee replacement—within an average of 2 years after decompression.

Core decompression at the knee should be considered if severe pain is caused by avascular necrosis and femorotibial alignment is within 5 or 6 degrees of normal. Even patients with stage III involvement have a 50% chance of gaining relief from pain. Tibial and distal femoral osteotomies are preferable in patients with femorotibial malalignment as well as avascular necrosis.

▶ Core decompression of the proximal femur for avascular necrosis is a controversial procedure, with some reports of good results and others of no change. In the current paper, the Hopkins group suggests that core decompression of the distal femur for avascular necrosis is useful. As the criterion for success was pain relief, it can be supposed that decompression may improve pain by relieving intraosseous pressure and stimulating intraosseous nerve endings. Whether this effect is temporary or permanent, and whether it will affect the long-term deterioration of the necrotic area, was not demonstrated.—C.B. Sledge, M.D.

Osteoarthritis of the Knee Joint: An Eight-Year Prospective Study
Massardo L, Watt I, Cushnaghan J, Dieppe P (Bristol Royal Infirmary, Bristol, England)
Ann Rheum Dis 48:893–897, November 1989   4–9

An 8-year follow-up study of the course of osteoarthritis of the knee enrolled 31 patients (mean age, 72 years) who had participated in trials

Change in Clinical Signs and Function Over 8 Years in 31 Patients With Knee Osteoarthritis

	1979	1987
Knee symptoms	31	30
Total knee flexion (mean)	128°	106°
Knee effusion (number with sign)	21	14
Knee crepitus (number with sign)	—	23
Hand symptoms	10	16
Hand signs of osteoarthritis	18	22
Other symptomatic sites	1	3
Other sites with signs of osteoarthritis	5	8
Use of walking aids	5	20
Walking difficulty		
None	9	5
Some	20	13
Severe	0	13
Mean HAQ*	—	1·2 (0–2·8)
Steinbrocker class		
1	—	14
2	—	12
3	—	4
4	—	1
Patient report of change over 8 years:		
Better	—	4
Same	—	7
Worse	—	20

*HAQ, health assessment questionnaire.
(Courtesy of Massardo L, Watt I, Cushnaghan J, et al: *Ann Rheum Dis* 48:893–897, November 1989.)

of intra-articular steroid or a nonsteroidal anti-inflammatory agent. Seventeen patients were obese, and 4 had had unilateral meniscectomy. In most cases the knees or hands were involved at the outset.

All patients remained symptomatic throughout the study (table), although overall pain scores were not changed significantly. Knee flexion deteriorated overall, and 16 patients began using a walking aid during the study period; most patients had a significant loss of walking ability. Only 4 patients believed that their knees were better; 20 claimed that the knees had worsened during the study period. Medical treatment had no obvious role in clinical outcome. Knee radiography showed a predominance of medial compartment disease, which changed the most over time.

It may be that a limited form of "generalized" osteoarthritis involving the knee and hand is frequent. Most of the present patients became significantly disabled during an 8-year follow-up. No factors predicting the clinical outcome could be identified. The radiographic appearances were surprisingly stable compared with the clinical changes.

▶ One of the most embarrassing aspects of orthopedic surgery is that we know so little of the natural history of the diseases we treat in spite of their antiquity. This excellent paper follows the course of 31 patients with osteoarthritis of the knee who were observed carefully over a period of 8 years. Most of us would have predicted an intermittent but steady decline in function and increase in symptoms over the study period, but it is somewhat surprising that the authors found that 4 patients thought that they had had improvement and 20 had worsened to the point at which most became significantly disabled. It is unfortunate that the authors could identify no predictive factors that would allow one to anticipate whether patients will decline, remain unchanged, or improve spontaneously.—C.B. Sledge, M.D.

Epidemiology of Osteoarthritis: Zoetermeer Survey: Comparison of Radiological Osteoarthritis in a Dutch Population With That in 10 Other Populations
van Saase JLCM, van Romunde LKJ, Cats A, Vandenbroucke JP, Valkenburg HA (Erasmus Univ, Rotterdam; Leiden State Univ, Leiden, The Netherlands)
Ann Rheum Dis 48:271–280, April 1989   4–10

Morbidity from osteoarthritis is an important problem in populations with larger proportions of elderly persons. The prevalence of radiologic osteoarthritis was investigated in a random population sample of 6,585 inhabitants of Zoetermeer, The Netherlands. Findings were compared with those in 10 similar population surveys. Overall, 76% of eligible persons participated in the Zoetermeer survey. Previous medical history, rheumatic complaints, life-styles, and other information were gathered by questionnaire. Joints were examined clinically, and blood pressure, height, and weight were recorded. Radiographs also were obtained.

The prevalence of radiologic osteoarthritis was strongly correlated with increasing age and was highest for the cervical spine, lumbar spine, and distal interphalangeal joints of the hands. Prevalence was 10% or less in sacroiliac joints, lateral carpometacarpal joints, and tarsometatarsal joints. Severe radiologic osteoarthritis was rare in persons younger than 45 years. The prevalence of severe radiologic osteoarthritis in elderly persons did not exceed 20% except in the cervical and lumbar spines, distal interphalangeal joints of the hands, and, in women only, metacarpophalangeal joints, first carpometacarpal joints, first metatarsophalangeal joints, and knees. Differences between men and women were slight except for knees and hips. However, women had a higher porportion of severe radiologic osteoarthritis in most of the joints.

The data were comparable with those found in other population surveys. Differences among populations were mostly differences in level. Variations among populations may have been attributable in part to the use of different radiologic criteria as well as to genetic or environmental factors, or both.

▶ One of the factors to be considered in evaluating a patient for joint replacement in osteoarthritis is the natural history of the process in a particular joint: how likely is the process to stabilize, improve spontaneously, or deteriorate? This paper documents the changing frequency of osteoarthritic involvement of all the major joints with age and provides predictive information on the natural history of osteoarthritis. There was no significant difference in the 11 populations studied.—C.B. Sledge, M.D.

Anteversion of the Femur and Idiopathic Osteoarthrosis of the Hip
Wedge JH, Munkacsi I, Loback D (Univ of Saskatchewan, Saskatoon)
J Bone Joint Surg [Am] 71-A:1040–1043, August 1989   4–11

Increased anteversion of the neck of the femur during childhood may lead to osteoarthrosis of the hip during adulthood. Radiographs of the hips of 143 male and 77 female cadavers were studied to establish whether such a cause-and-effect relationship exists. The mean age at the time of death was 71.3 years. Hips were graded as normal or mildly, moderately, or severely osteoarthrotic. Forty-eight femurs of cadavers judged to have idiopathic osteoarthrosis and femurs of 10 normal cadavers were removed and inspected grossly. Final grading—mild, moderate, or severe—was determined by gross findings on dissection. Anteversion of the hip was measured by a reproducible direct method after dissection.

Eighteen cadavers had unilateral and 15 had bilateral osteoarthrosis of the hip, with involvement of the 2 sides being nearly equal. There was no statistically significant difference in the angle of anteversion between the normal hips and each group (mild, moderate, severe) of osteoarthrotic hips, nor was there any significant difference between normal hips and osteoarthrotic hips overall.

In this anatomical investigation, it was not possible to establish a relationship between increased femoral anteversion and idiopathic osteoarthrosis of the hip. Prophylactic derotation osteotomy in patients with increased anteversion of the femur apparently does not alter the risk of later development of osteoarthrosis of the hip; therefore, this procedure cannot be recommended.

▶ Increased femoral neck anteversion historically has been thought to contribute to subsequent development of osteoarthrosis of the hip. This anatomical study failed to demonstrate an association between femoral neck anteversion and osteoarthrosis. The authors properly caution against so-called prophylactic derotation osteotomies in childhood.—R. Poss, M.D.

Primary Osteoarthritis of the Hip Joint in Japan
Nakamura S, Ninomiya S, Nakamura T (Univ of Tokyo)
Clin Orthop 241:190–196, April 1989   4–12

Primary osteoarthritis is rare in Japan; most cases result from congenital hip dislocation and congenital acetabular dysplasia. Data were reviewed concerning 2,000 consecutive patients with osteoarthritis of the hip, excluding rheumatoid disease. Primary osteoarthritis was diagnosed when the center-edge (CE) angle of Wiberg exceeded 10 degrees, the

Sharp angle was less than 45 degrees, and acetabular roof obliquity was less than 15 degrees. In addition, femoral head deformity was absent. Primary osteoarthritis accounted for only 0.65% cases of osteoarthritis. These 13 patients had an average age of 60 years. Follow-up of 9 patients for an average of 39 months showed superolateral progression in some cases and a nonmigratory type of progression in others. In the latter patients the femoral head remained at its original site or shifted somewhat medially. Acetabular roof obliquity was in the high-normal range in those with superolateral progression. The CE and Sharp angles were comparable in the 2 subtypes of primary osteoarthritis.

Primary osteoarthritis of the superolateral type in Japan tends to develop in normal hips with greater acetabular roof obliquity. Biomechanical factors may have a role in the development of this type of osteoarthritis.

▶ Radiographic criteria that define the normal parameters of the Oriental hip were developed. By these criteria, less than 1% of 2,000 hips with osteoarthritis merited a diagnosis of primary osteoarthritis. These findings support the thesis that in Western patients the entity of primary osteoarthritis is exceedingly rare. Even in the small number of Japanese patients with primary osteoarthritis, 1 of the 2 subtypes developed in hips that had a greater degree of acetabular roof obliquity, suggesting a mechanical etiology as well.—R. Poss, M.D.

Roentgenographic Findings in Pigmented Villonodular Synovitis of the Knee
Flandry F, McCann SB, Hughston JC, Kurtz DM (Hughston Orthopaedic Clinic, Columbus, Ga)
Clin Orthop 247:208–219, October 1989   4–13

Because pigmented villonodular synovitis (PVS) is so rare, studies of purely articular lesions are few and those that address roentgenographic findings are fewer still. To determine characteristic roentgenographic findings, data were reviewed on 29 cases of PVS of the knee in 27 patients. All original, serial, and final follow-up roentgenograms were examined jointly by a radiologist and 2 orthopedic surgeons. Films were reviewed for soft tissue, osseous, and degenerative changes, as well as for evidence of extra-articular extension, osteopenia, and loose bodies. Findings were correlated with gross pathology described at surgery.

All cases met the histologic criteria for diagnosis of PVS. Four cases were localized and the remainder were diffuse. Roentgenographic findings were principally in the soft tissues. In some instances there was cystic invasion of bone or degenerative changes, but these findings were rare. When present in diffuse PVS, such changes were most pronounced in the patellofemoral articular surface. In diffuse PVS, large posterior tumefactions usually did not correlate with extra-articular extension. Overall, the clinical behavior of PVS was controlled more by anatomical site and form of disease than by the severity of either histologic or roentgenographic findings.

Although histologically similar, the clinical behavior and response to treatment of localized and diffuse PVS are sufficiently different to warrant their consideration as distinct clinical entities. The clinical behavior of PVS also probably results in large part from the influence of its anatomical site.

▶ Pigmented villonodular synovitis is an unusual condition rarely encountered in any orthopedic surgeon's practice. To understand the clinical behavior of this process it is necessary to review collected series such as the 29 cases reported here. In approximately 20% of these patients recurrence was demonstrated at variable lengths of follow-up, with no demonstrable correlation between either radiographic staging or histologic grade.— C.B. Sledge, M.D.

Cardiac Isoenzyme Values After Total Joint Arthroplasty
Wukich DK, Callaghan JJ, Graeber GM, Martyak T, Savory CG, Lyon JJ (Walter Reed Army Med Ctr and Inst of Research, Washington, DC; Uniformed Services Univ of the Health Sciences, Bethesda, Md)
Clin Orthop 242:232–240, May 1989   4–14

To determine how total joint arthroplasty affects the serum levels of creatine kinase (CO-MB) and lactate dehydrogenase (LD), isoenzyme activity was estimated by automated spectrophotometry and agarose gel electrophoresis in 50 patients in conjunction with hip or knee arthroplasty. Whereas the mean serum level of LD was not significantly increased after hip arthroplasty, that of LD-5 was signficantly elevated on the first postoperative day. The mean serum level of total CK was increased significantly through the third postoperative day, and values of CK-MB were increased on the first 2 days after surgery. After knee arthroplasty, the serum level of LD was increased for the first 2 days, as was the LD-5 fraction, and the total serum CK level was increased up to postoperative day 3.

Three patients had chest pain and ECG changes consistent with myocardial ischemia, which resolved within 24 hours. Each of the 3 had an LD-1:LD-2 ratio greater than 1, but the maximal CK-MB value was only 13 IU/L.

The detection of CK-MB after total joint arthroplasty is not diagnostic of myocardial injury. However, an increase exceeding 50 IU/L, or 5% of total CK, combined with an LD-1:LD-2 ratio of more than 1 should not be ascribed to skeletal muscle injury alone.

▶ Does muscle damage at the time of total joint arthroplasty produce an elevation of cardiac isoenzymes and thereby confuse the diagnosis of myocardial infarction in the postoperative period? The authors of this paper point out that, although the CK-MB levels rose significantly after surgery, it was possible to differentiate that increase from increases caused by myocardial infarction by determining both the serum CK-MB and LD-1:LD-2 levels. If the latter ratio exceeds 1, it is suggestive of myocardial muscle damage.— C.B. Sledge, M.D.

Surgical Management of Advanced Hemophilic Arthropathy: An Overview of 20 Years' Experience
Luck JV Jr, Kasper CK (Univ of Southern California; Orthopaedic Hosp, Los Angeles)
Clin Orthop 242:60-82, May 1989

Advanced hemophilic arthropathy often causes moderate to severe pain and significant incapacity by the third or fourth decade of life. Conservative management with clotting factor concentrate on demand, therapeutic exercises, anti-inflammatory drugs, orthoses, and activity restrictions is effective in most patients. Some, however, may have such severe pain and disability and require so much clotting factor replacement that reconstructive surgery may be a viable alternative.

In a 20-year period, 168 reconstructive procedures were performed for advanced hemophilic arthropathy. Of these, 141 were primary procedures and 27 were reoperations. End-stage arthropathy of the shoulder was treated with either arthroplasty or arthrodesis. Radial head excision with synovectomy and débridement were highly successful for end-stage arthropathy of the elbow. End-stage hip disease proved to be a treatment problem. Experience with various types of hip protheses was rated as fair, with about a 60% revision rate over 20 years. Advanced knee arthropathy was treated with débridement, débridement with patellectomy, osteotomy, fusion, and prosthetic arthroplasty. Knee reoperations usually were necessitated by persisting or recurring symptoms after débridement, patellectomy, or osteotomy. Knee fusions showed good long-term results. Prosthetic arthroplasty of the knee proved stable, with a component failure rate of 2.4% and a reoperation rate for component failure from any cause of 6.8% at 1–14 years. The best treatment for ankle and subtalar joints was athrodesis, rather than prosthetic arthroplasty.

At the latest follow-up examination, all except 1 of the patients who were having recurrent hemarthroses had improvement in terms of frequency of hemarthroses in the involved joint. All had improvement in the level of pain, and all except 2 had improvement in terms of functional capacity. None of the patients who had prosthetic arthroplasty had perioperative infections, but late infections occurred in 10.4% of the 67 athroplasties performed.

Durable functional reconstruction with minimal risk must be the goal in the treatment of end-stage arthropathy.

▶ This paper presents the results of 168 reconstructive procedures in patients with hemophilic arthropathy and represents what certainly must be one of the largest series reported. Excellent control of recurrent hemarthroses and pain was reported and, somewhat surprising, there were no perioperative infections in the patients who had prosthetic arthroplasty, but there was a late infection rate of 10.4%.

The management of advanced hemophilic arthropathy requires a skilled team consisting of an orthopedic surgeon and hematologist. The results can be extremely gratifying as demonstrated in this paper.—C.B. Sledge, M.D.

Reduced Bone Formation in Non-Steroid-Treated Patients With Rheumatoid Arthritis
Compston JE, Vedi S, Mellish RWE, Croucher P, O'Sullivan MM (Univ of Wales; Univ Hosp of Wales, Cardiff)
Ann Rheum Dis 48:483–487, June 1989　　　　　　　　　　　　　4–16

The cellular basis of trabecular bone loss in rheumatoid arthritis was examined by obtaining iliac crest biopsy specimens from 45 patients with definite or classic rheumatoid disease. The patients (mean age, 53 years) had had disease for a median of 4 years. None had ever received systemic steroid therapy. Control values of mean wall thickness, mean interstitial bone thickness, and extent of the trabecular surface covered by osteoid were obtained from 41 healthy controls matched with the patients for age and sex.

Patients and controls did not differ significantly in mean interstitial bone thickness, which is related to resorption depth, or in osteoid surface, which reflects the number of remodeling units. The mean wall thickness, an indicator of the amount of bone formed per remodeling unit, was significantly less in patients than in controls.

Bone loss in rheumatoid arthritis is caused chiefly by reduced bone formation. This suggests that, when treatment is necessary, a drug that stimulates osteoblasts (e.g., sodium fluoride) may be the best choice. The role for routine prophylaxis against bone loss remains unclear.

▶ Patients with rheumatoid arthritis have diminished bone mass regardless of their treatment regimen. This paper demonstrates that the defect is in bone formation, not excessive resorption. It is unfortunate that present methods of managing decreased bone loss involve agents that reduce rates of resorption rather than stimulate bone formation. Although such treatment might be useful in diminishing the bone loss associated with rheumatoid arthritis, it clearly does not attack the primary deficiency in bone formation.—C.B. Sledge, M.D.

Patellar Replacement in Bilateral Total Knee Arthroplasty: A Study of Patients Who Had Rheumatoid Arthritis and No Gross Deformity of the Patella
Shoji H, Yoshino S, Kajino A (Louisiana State Univ; Nippon Med School, Tokyo)
J Bone Joint Surg [Am] 71-A:853–856, July 1989　　　　　　　　　4–17

Indications for using a patellar prosthesis in conjunction with a total knee prosthesis have varied, and whether a patella lacking substantial anatomical deformity should routinely be replaced remains questionable. Thirty-five patients with rheumatoid arthritis of both kenes and no gross patellar deformity underwent bilateral total knee arthroplasty. A total condylar modifier total knee prosthesis was used. One knee of each patient had a patellar replacement. The patients were followed for at least 2 years.

The 2 knees had comparable results with respect to pain relief, arc of motion, functional improvement, and muscle power. No complications were attributed to patellar replacement, and no patient had persistent synovitis that resisted medical care.

Patellar replacement did not improve appreciably the results of total knee arthroplasty in this series. Lateral retinacular release is the key measure for correcting patellar tracking. Acceptable congruence of the patellofemoral articulation can be achieved without replacing the patella as long as its bony anatomy is nearly normal.

▶ A reciprocal relationship between articular cartilage and synovium long has been recognized. In rheumatoid arthritis it generally has been believed that articular cartilage not removed at the time of knee arthroplasty would continue to degenerate and perpetuate an inflammatory process within the joint. This paper reports a small group of patients followed for a little more than 2 years and suggests that the patellar cartilage neither degenerated nor caused a persistent inflammatory response in the knee. Although the results in this study showed similarity between patients with patellar replacement and those without, it stands in stark contrast to most other series that report improved function in patients wtih patellar replacement regardless of whether they have osteoarthritis or rheumatoid arthritis.—C.B. Sledge, M.D.

Arthrodesis of the Cervical Spine in Rheumatoid Arthritis
Clark CR, Goetz DD, Menezes AH (Univ of Iowa)
J Bone Joint Surg [Am] 71-A:381–392, March 1989   4–18

Forty-one patients with rheumatoid arthritis were followed for at least 2 years after cervical arthrodesis. Twenty patients had isolated atlantoaxial subluxation, 5 had isolated cranial settling, and 4 had subaxial subluxation alone. Twenty patients underwent atlantoaxial arthrodesis, and 16 had occipitocervical arthrodesis. Five patients had posterior arthrodesis of the subaxial spine. Two patients also had transoral odontoidectomy, and 1 had an anterior cervical vertebrectomy.

Bony union was present in 16 patients (88%) at last follow-up, and 2 others had stable fibrous union; 3 patients had nonunion. All problems with union occurred in patients having isolated atlantoaxial arthrodesis. Two thirds of the patients had improved clinically, and none was worse. Neurologic status was improved in 11 patients and remained the same in 30. Pain was substantially relieved in all but 2 of 23 patients. Complications included transient hemiparesis, displacement of an anterior graft, and erosion of cement into the occiptal cortex. In 13 patients subluxation developed at a more caudad level, but in only 5 of them did it exceed 3.5 mm.

Impending neurologic deficit is an indication for early cervical spinal arthrodesis in patients wtih rheumatoid disease. The risk of early operative mortality is low. If major instability is evident on x-ray films and neuroradiographic findings are abnormal, posterior arthrodesis should be considered. Postoperative halo immobilization or extension of arthrodesis to the occiput may prevent pseudarthrosis in patients with atlantoaxial instability. Close monitoring is necessary to detect instability at an unoperated-on level of the cervical spine.

▶ This excellent report of 88% bony union in patients undergoing either occiput C2 or C1–C2 arthrodesis demonstrates the usefulness of this surgical procedure. Many previous studies have reported a significant incidence of nonunion and a frightening mortality. Because of their excellent results, the authors suggest arthrodesis in patients with "impending neurological deficit with careful monitoring and precise surgical technique."—C.B. Sledge, M.D.

Deep Vein Thrombosis After Elective Knee Surgery: An Incidence Study in 312 Patients
Stringer MD, Steadman CA, Hedges AR, Thomas EM, Morley TR, Kakkar VV
(King's College Hosp, London)
J Bone Joint Surg [Br] 71-B:492–497, May 1989   4–19

Venous thromboembolism is a major cause of morbidity and mortality after orthopedic surgery, but relatively little is known about the risks after knee surgery. A prospective examination was made of the incidence of deep venous thrombosis (DVT) after a wide variety of elective knee surgeries performed under tourniquet ischemia.

The operated limbs of 312 patients were studied with ipsilateral ascending venography 7 to 10 days after surgery. No patient had any specific prophylaxis against thromboembolism. Patients with symptoms suggestive of pulmonary embolism underwent radioisotope ventilation-perfusion scanning.

Overall, 88 DVTs were diagnosed, for an incidence of 28.2%. The high risk after total knee replacement was confirmed, with an incidence of ipsilateral DVT in 56.4% of patients and symptomatic pulmonary embolism in 1.9%. In contrast, the incidence of DVT with arthroscopy was only 4.2%. Other high-risk procedures were meniscectomy, arthrotomy, patellectomy, synovectomy, and arthrodesis. These procedures were particularly risky in patients aged more than 40 years. The rates of DVT for these procedures ranged from 25% to 67%. In general, the risk of having a postoperative DVT increased from about 10% for patients aged less than 30 years to nearly 50% for patients aged more than 40 years.

Because of the high risk of DVT, prophylaxis against this occurrence is advised for all patients aged more than 40 years who are undergoing elective knee surgery other than arthroscopy. Further research is needed to reach a consensus on a safe and effective prophylactic regimen.

▶ Prophylaxis against venous thromboembolism after hip surgery is now common; prophylaxis after knee surgery is practiced less frequently. This paper documents an incidence of DVT of 28% after elective knee surgery; 56% of patients with total knee replacement had DVT and 1.9% had pulmonary emboli. The evidence presented in this paper argues strongly for routine prophylaxis after total knee arthroplasty in patients aged beyond 40 years.—C.B. Sledge, M.D.

Fat Embolism Associated With Cementing of Femoral Stems Designed for Press-Fit Application
Watson JT, Stulberg BN (Cleveland Clinic Found)
J Arthroplasty 4:133-137, June 1989   4-20

Use of a cemented press-fit femoral component in hip arthroplasty, along with modern cement pressurization, apparently entails a risk of severe fat embolism syndrome. Fat emboli developed in 4 patients after total hip arthroplasty when a cementless, acetabular press-fit component and a cemented, press-fit femoral component were used. No predisposing factors were identified.

Respiratory embarrassment and confusion became apparent as epidural anesthesia resolved. All 4 patients had clinical and radiographic changes of pulmonary edema, as well as severe confusion, tachycardia, and fever. Thrombocytopenia was noted, with an increased sedimentation rate and fat globules in the urine. In addition to supportive care, 1 patient received steroids. There was no functional loss, and all patients had good orthopedic outcomes.

Possible intramedullary debris is generated by the instrumentation used in press-fit implants. The press-fit stem and polymethyl methacrylate cause femoral pressurization, forcing intramedullary fatty debris into the general venous circulation. Epidural anesthesia with an increased venous capacitance allows debris to collect within the proximal femoral veins. When venous return increases after anesthesia, a substantial bolus of fatty debris is present in the pulmonary circulation.

No further embolism has occurred since adoption of thorough cleaning of the proximal femur by pulsatile lavage and use of a vent tube above the medullary plug before cement is introduced. Pressurization is minimized with an undersized implant or by overrasping the proximal femur. Careful titration of anesthesia will minimize fluctuations in venous capacitance and blood pressure.

High-Volume, High-Pressure Pulsatile Lavage During Cemented Arthroplasty
Byrick RJ, Bell RS, Kay JC, Waddell JP, Mullen JB (St Michael's Hosp; Mt Sinai Hosp, Toronto)
J Bone Joint Surg [Am] 71-A:1331-1336, October 1989   4-21

Cardiopulmonary dysfunction at cemented arthroplasty may result from particulate fat and marrow embolism. The value of intramedullary lavage was examined by simulating cemented arthroplasty in dogs. Both low-volume, low-pressure manual lavage and high-volume, high-pressure pulsatile lavage were carried out in dogs with bilateral cemented arthroplasties.

Without lavage the pulmonary artery pressure and pulmonary vascular resistance were increased significantly and arterial oxygen tension was decreased. The intrapulmonary shunt fraction rose. The same changes

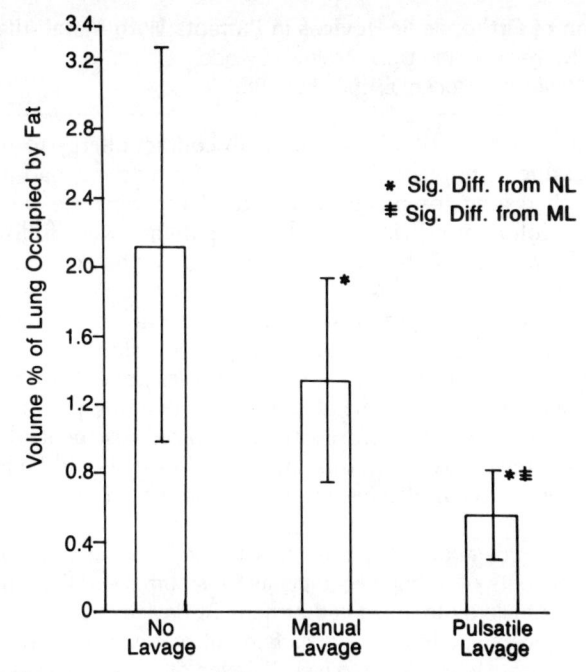

Fig 4-2.—The mean volume percent of lung tissue that was occupied by fat emboli (standard deviation, 1). *Asterisk*, significantly fewer emboli than in the dogs with no lavage. *Triple dagger*, significantly fewer emboli than in dogs undergoing manual lavage. (Courtesy of Byrick RJ, Bell RS, Kay JC, et al: *J Bone Joint Surg [AM]* 71-A:1331–1336, October 1989.)

were seen after low-volume, low-pressure manual lavage, but high-volume, high-pressure pulsatile lavage after reaming limited the circulatory changes. Fat microemboli in the lungs were only 25% as frequent as when no lavage was carried out. Both types of lavage reduced the percentage of lung volume occupied by fat emboli (Fig 4–2).

Apparently, high-volume, high-pressure pulsatile lavage of the reamed intramedullary cavity may reduce pulmonary morbidity from fat embolism after cemented arthroplasty. Lavage may act by evacuating particulate marrow or tissue thromboplastins before pressurization.

▶ Contemporary cementless femoral components are designed to be canal filling so as to achieve stable initial fixation. When used with cement, and with the advances in technique that increase cement pressurization, increased intramedullary pressure can lead to fat emboli. The authors report 4 cases of this syndrome (Abstract 4–20). In the second paper (Abstract 4–21), the merits of high-volume, high-pressure pulsatile lavage are described. In a canine study, high-pressure lavage of the bony surfaces before cement application resulted in a dramatic decrease in fat microemboli to the lungs.

Optimal bone and marrow preparation may decrease some of the adverse effects of the increased intramedullary pressures achieved by contemporary cementing techniques.—R. Poss, M.D.

Implantation of Orthopaedic Devices in Patients With Metal Allergy
Carlsson Å, Möller H (Lund Univ, Malmö, Sweden)
Acta Derm Venereol (Stockh) 69:62–66, 1989   4–22

Follow-up was made of 15 patients wtih contact allergy to nickel who received metallic orthopedic devices. Seven other patients had positive results of patch testing for nickel before total hip replacement and were available for follow-up. The 18 evaluable patients were followed for a mean of 6.5 years. None had any dermatologic or orthopedic complications that could be ascribed to contact allergy.

This is the first long-term follow-up of orthopedic patients in which the outcome was related to the results of preoperative skin testing. Implantation of cemented metal-to-plastic joint prostheses appears to be safe even in patients with preexisting metal allergy. It remains possible that the metal devices used to fix fractures may, if placed just beneath the skin, lead to local eczematous dermatitis. In such cases it should be possible to control the dermatitis until the fracture heals and then remove the device.

▶ As the authors point out, many patients are allergic to one or the other of the metallic components of orthopedic implants. It is surprising, therefore, that so few examples of allergy to implanted orthopedic devices have been reported. In this prospective study the authors carried out preoperative skin testing and identified 15 patients with allergy to nickel. Seven other patients with a positive result of patch testing for nickel also were followed for a significant period of time. No patients manifested any allergy to the implanted device in spite of preoperative tests indicative of sensitivity to nickel. It should be noted that all the devices in this series were cemented, and it is conceivable that the cement barrier around the implanted metallic device prevented extensive contact between the body and the implanted metal.—C.B. Sledge, M.D.

Bone Scintigraphy in Post-Traumatic Reflex Dystrophy
Fanø N, Holm C (Centralsygehuset, Næstved, Denmark)
Scand J Rheumatol 17:455–458, 1988   4–23

Timely treatment of posttraumatic reflex dystrophy (PRD) is critical, but the diagnosis often is difficult to make in the early stages. Bone scintigraphy was carried out with ^{99m}Tc-methylene diphosphonate in 25 patients with pain, tenderness, edema, and vasomotor instability. Five with suspected reflex dystrophy were referred. Ergotherapy had no effect or had exacerbated the symptoms in 8 patients. Multiple sites of increased periarticular activity on 1 side were considered a positive finding.

Scintigraphy was done an average of 11.5 weeks after initial injury. All but 1 study showed multiple periarticular sites of increased activity on 1 side (Fig 4–3). Prednisolone was given subsequently for an average of 12 weeks, and repeat scintigrams showed normalized conditions.

Scintigraphy is a sensitive and specific means of diagnosing PRD. The outlook with prednisolone therapy is dependent chiefly on the degree of

Chapter 4—Adult Reconstruction / **161**

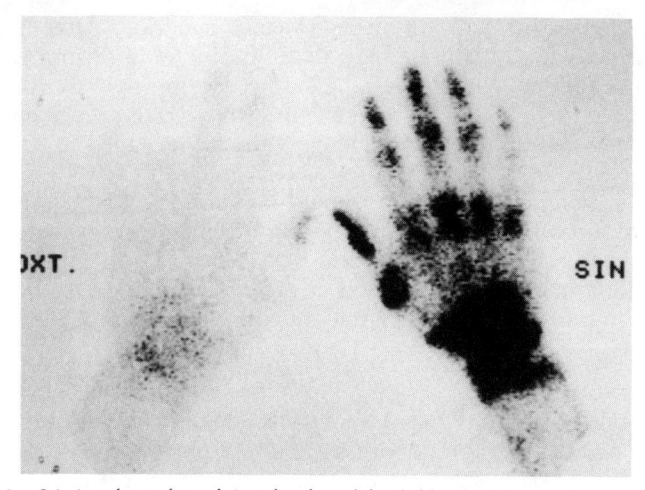

Fig 4–3.—Scintigraphy performed 6 weeks after a left-sided brachial plexus lesion, showing unilateral periarticular uptake in the left hand. (Courtesy of Fano N, Holm C: *Scand J Rheumatol* 17:455–458, 1989.)

functional loss at the time treatment begins. Early treatment can prevent permanent loss of function in patients with PRD.

▶ The diagnosis of reflex sympathetic dystrophy is difficult. The florid case is recognized easily, but many more subtle examples probably are missed. The authors of this paper suggest that bone scintigraphy with technetium can help to establish the diagnosis with sensitivity and specificity of about 96%. The changes seen included increased periarticular uptake around the joints of the involved upper extremity. No patients in this series had involvement of the lower extremity, but the next paper (Abstract 4–24) indicates similar findings in the lower extremity.—C.B. Sledge, M.D.

Reflex Sympathetic Dystrophy of the Knee: Treatment Using Continuous Epidural Anesthesia
Cooper DE, DeLee JC, Ramamurthy S (Univ of Texas, San Antonio)
J Bone Joint Surg [Am] 71-A:365–369, March 1989   4–24

Fourteen patients with confirmed diagnoses of reflex sympathetic dystrophy of the knee were treated in the hospital under epidural block anesthesia; an indwelling catheter was used. The average treatment time was 4 days. Continuous passive motion, manipulation, muscle stimulation, and alternating hot and cold soaks were used during the time of epidural treatment. Previously, 11 patients had chondral shaving for chondromalacia or lateral release procedure for malalignment. Treatment began with 0.5% bupivacaine and continued with morphine, Demerol, or fentanyl.

No complications resulted from treatment. On follow-up averaging 32 months, 10 patients had symmetric ranges of motion. After manipulation, patients who initially had less than 90 degrees of flexion gained 30 degrees on average. Symptoms were resolved completely by the time of the most recent follow-up in 11 patients, whose activity was unlimited. Two patients had intermittent aching, and another failed to gain symptomatic relief.

Reflex sympathetic dystrophy should be considered whenever pain is out of proportion to the degree of injury, or when there is atrophic skin change, decreased skin temperature, hypersensitivity to touch, stiffness and swelling, or some combination of these. Epidural blockade with appropriate mechanical measures can lead to total symptomatic relief in many cases.

▶ Continuous epidural anesthesia has been reported to be successful in treating patients with reflex sympathetic dystrophy of the lower extremity. Eleven of the 14 patients in this series had complete resolution, 1 experienced no relief, and 2 were improved. Technetium bone scan showed increased uptake in 5 of the 7 patients in whom it was done. Of great interest is the fact that 9 of the 11 patients had symptoms of reflex sympathetic dystrophy before their first knee operation. More careful evaluation of enigmatic knee pain, using technetium scintigraphy and diagnostic epidural blocks, might have prevented unnecessary surgery in those patients.— C.B. Sledge, M.D.

Cryopreserved Articular Chondrocytes Grow in Culture, Maintain Cartilage Phenotype, and Synthesize Matrix Components
Schachar N, Nagao M, Matsuyama T, McAllister D, Ishii S (Univ of Calgary, Alta; Sapporo Med College, Hokkaido, Japan)
J Orthop Res 7:344–351, May 1989   4–25

Fresh graft tissue, a desirable alternative to artificial materials in surgery to replace injured or diseased joints, is in limited supply. One method of preserving transplant tissues for long periods is cryopreservation, freezing to ultralow temperatures. For these grafts to be successful, chondrocytes must survive freezing and remain able to produce normal matrix components: proteoglycans and type II collagen. With samples of articular cartilage (AC) from rabbits, attempts were made to discover whether cryopreserved AC chondrocytes were able to proliferate in tissue culture while maintaining their phenotype.

Chondrocytes were isolated from AC samples and divided into 3 groups: fresh control cells (C), cells frozen for 1 day (F1), and cells frozen for 7 days (F7). Cultures of the 3 groups were maintained for 14 days. Similar growth rates were observed for C, F1, and F7. An initial lag phase, extending from day 1 to day 4, was followed by an exponential growth phase reaching confluence on the sixth or seventh day. Morphology was comparable for the control and frozen-thawed cells. Because no spindle-shaped cells were seen, there was apparently no change to a fibroblast cell type. All 3 groups showed signs of proteoglycans production by day 3, and this grew more intense throughout the experiment.

Though results of this animal study cannot be applied directly to adult AC in a clinical setting, its successful outcome does suggest that cryopreservation of cartilage-bearing allografts for transplantation is a promising method of storage.

Total Hip Reconstruction

Shape the Implant to the Patient: A Rationale for the Use of Custom-Fit Cementless Total Hip Implants
Bargar WL (Univ of California, Davis)
Clin Orthop 249:73-78, December 1989   4-26

The closer an implant fits the endosteal canal, the less reaming and reshaping are necessary. Excessive reaming can weaken supporting bone and create stress concentrations. For an optimal result it is not enough to routinely use the largest size possible. In 156 cases the implant was customized with a CT-generated computer-assisted design (CAD) and computer-assisted manufacturing (CAM) prosthesis. The use of data from a CT scan in implant design lessens distortion, compared with roentgenographic methods, and avoids magnification errors. Modern CAD-CAM technology shortens the design and manufacture time and provides better dimensional accuracy.

The 81 primary total hip arthroplasties and 75 revision arthroplasties have been followed up for an average of 22 months; 48 hips were followed up for 2 years or longer. In primary cases patients given a customized implant had less pain at all follow-up intervals, compared with the pain of earlier patients when the same surgeon used off-the-shelf prostheses. Less than 20% of patients who had revision arthroplasties had more than slight pain. The use of custom components decreased the need for structural bone grafting, and stability was achieved in situations where this would not have been possible if off-the-shelf components were used.

Two operations failed because of aseptic loosening. Subsidence of more than 3 mm of the collarless custom design occurred in 8% of patients, mainly in early revision cases; this complication now has been nearly eliminated.

Although custom-designed devices cannot yet be recommended in all cases of cementless total hip arthroplasty, surgeons should critically assess the fit of off-the-shelf devices before operation. If an optimal fit is not possible, the use of a T-generated CAD-CAM custom prosthesis should be considered.

Fit the Patient to the Prosthesis: An Argument Against the Routine Use of Custom Hip Implants
Capello WN (Indiana Univ, Indianapolis)
Clin Orthop 249:56-59, December 1989   4-27

Although custom-designed implants have a role in the occasional instance of massive loss of femoral bone, there is a question of whether routine use of a custom or individualized femoral prosthesis is preferable to using an off-the-shelf implant in cementless hip arthroplasty. There are many arguments against this routine practice apart from cost. If custom or individualized implants are to be used routinely there must be an accurate and reproducible means of determining the internal configuration of the femoral canal. However, all methods including CT carry a risk of error. Errors probably are inevitable, and they are recognized only when the device is delivered to the surgeon.

Even if it were possible to determine routinely and accurately the internal configuration of the femur, whether implants are truly customized is questionable. Any compromises necessary will be made relative to the implant; for instance, metal will be removed to make it implantable. Trimming is necessary proximally, so the potential exists for distal fixation and this could lead to significant proximal stress shielding.

The clinical results in both primary and revision arthroplasties are quite encouraging, and recent modifications may improve the results even further. Undersizing is one of the prominent reasons why current implants fail.

▶ The arguments for and against the use of custom-made cementless femoral components are presented. There is general agreement that the primary requirement for successful cementless total hip arthroplasty is an initial stable fit. Many contemporary femoral stems have been designed so that this stable fit is achieved by maximal fit and fill of the femoral canal. Previous work has demonstrated that the geometry of the femoral canal in a human population is widely variable. There are 2 questions then: What is adequate fit, that is, can sufficient implant stability be achieved by fitting an off-the-shelf prosthesis of optimal design to the so-called average femur? Second, by custom design, is the fit and fill actually improved when compared with off-the-shelf prosthesis? The issue is complicated when one recognizes that to achieve excellent fit, one must combine not only a well-designed prosthesis but expert instrumentation and surgical technique.

Further issues are the cost of 1 method vs. the other and the issue of quality control. To what extent should the surgeon be responsible for the design and material adequacy of the implant that he uses? The reader should find these 2 arguments for and against the routine use of custom implants to be helpful in considering the appropriate role of this technology in contemporary total hip replacement.—R. Poss, M.D.

Size of the Femoral Head and Acetabular Revision in Total Hip-Replacement Arthroplasty
Morrey BF, Ilstrup D (Mayo Clinic and Mayo Found, Rochester, Minn)
J Bone Joint Surg [Am] 71-A:50–55, January 1989

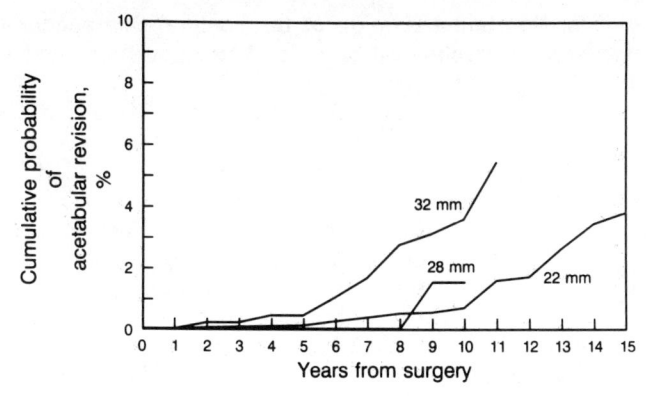

Fig 4–4.—Kaplan-Meier survival curves for the 32-, 28-, and 22-mm femoral components. The probability of revision is cumulative with each successive year of follow-up. (Courtesy of Morrey BF, Ilstrup D: *J Bone Joint Surg [Am]* 71-A:50–55, January 1989.)

There is some evidence that acetabular loosening after hip replacement arthroplasty is more frequent when the 32-mm femoral head is used than the 22-mm component. Fifty-nine revisions done for aseptic acetabular loosening—after more than 6,000 total hip arthroplasties for degenerative arthritis or traumatic arthritis—were reviewed.

Revisions were necessary in about 1% of hips given a 22-mm femoral head component and in about 2.5% of those given a 32-mm component. Two of 520 hips given a 28-mm femoral head component required revision. Cumulative-probability survival curves are shown in Figure 4–4. The dimensions of the acetabular wall were smaller in hips with a 32-mm component than in those given the 22-mm femoral head. Loosening was more likely to occur in men and in patients aged less than 60 years.

Because the larger femoral head component came into use some years after the smaller one did, better results should have been achieved, but this is not the case.

▶ The first principle of Charnley was to achieve low-friction arthroplasty, and the means by which that was accomplished was to utilize a small-diameter femoral head. The theoretic advantage of a large-diameter femoral head is that greater stability is conferred and the unit load on the polyethylene is diminished. These advantages are achieved at a cost of higher frictional forces at the bearing surface (and a thinner polyethylene component).

A very large literature on dislocation of total hip replacement has failed to confirm that a larger-diameter femoral head component does confer increased stability. In this paper, the consequences of increased frictional forces, that is, an increased incidence of acetabular component loosening, are seen in the group of patients who had 32-mm femoral head components.—R. Poss, M.D.

Examination of Rotational Fixation of the Femoral Component in Total Hip Arthroplasty: A Mechanical Study of Micromovement and Acoustic Emission
Sugiyama H, Whiteside LA, Kaiser AD (DePaul Biomechanical Lab, Bridgeton, Mo; Jikei Univ, Tokyo)
Clin Orthop 249:122–128, December 1989   4–29

Rotational loosening is an important cause of failure of the femoral component of total hip arthroplasties. The role of torsional loading in loosening of cementless femoral components was examined in preserved human femora. A cemented Ortholoc implant with a microtextured proximal surface also was studied. Cement was manually mixed with and without canal irrigation or vacuum-mixed with canal irrigation. All components were implanted by the same person.

Analysis of the micromovement data showed that both torque to 50-μ subsidence and torque to failure were quite low with cementless fixation and with poor cement technique, but were markedly improved by pulsed irrigation. Pressure injection and vacuum mixing of cement further improved the results. Acoustic emission was, however, detected even in the most carefully implanted cement specimens under conditions of torsional loading that commonly occur in daily activities.

Deeply penetrated cement appears to fail by microfracture of the cement mantle. Cementless fixation of the intramedullary stem provides inadequate fixation against torsional loading. Even with the best cement technique, torsional failure can occur in the course of normal daily use. Improved torsional fixation is needed badly.

▶ The role of torsional loading of femoral components is receiving attention, and properly so. The largest forces across the hip are in the sagittal plane and are generated by stair climbing and rising from low chairs. Therefore, it is important that a criterion of stable femoral fixation be that an implant resists not only bending and axial forces, but torsional ones as well. In this laboratory study, the authors demonstrate that optimal surgical and cement technique are required to resist deleterious torsional forces. Even with optimal cement technique, torsional failure can occur as a result of daily activities over a long period. Design of femoral components should address the need for torsional stability.— R. Poss, M.D.

Torsional Stability of the Femoral Component of Hip Arthroplasty: Response to an Anteriorly Applied Load
Nunn D, Freeman MAR, Tanner KE, Bonfield W (London Hosp Med College; Queen Mary College, London)
J Bone Joint Surg [Br] 71-B:452–455, May 1989   4–30

Torsional loading on the proximal part of the stem of a femoral hip prosthesis is responsible for causing femoral fracture. Rotational instability of femoral components has not been well studied because it is nearly impossible to assess rotational movement on plain radiographs. A stereophotogrammetric study has estimated the magnitude of the rotational force acting on the anterior aspect of the femoral head of an uncemented prosthesis to be about 4 degrees. A study was done to measure the movement resulting from an anteriorly applied load on hip prostheses inserted into cadaveric femora, and to assess the effect of the movement on rotational femoral head stability.

Rotation within the bone was measured with a strain-gauged cantilever screwed to the greater trochanter. Rotation within the bone was measured with and without preservation of the femoral neck, with and without the use of cement, and with a prosthesis that had longitudinal ridges on the stem and was implanted without cement. Each bone was loaded to 400 newtons, and the deflection was recorded. The bone was then loaded to 800 newtons, simulating an average full body weight, and the process was repeated.

The displacement of a ridged cementless prosthesis with the femoral neck intact did not differ statistically from that of a cemented prosthesis with the neck excised under loads of 400 or 800 newtons. However, the displacement of the smooth cementless prosthesis with the neck intact was significantly greater than that of the cemented prosthesis with the neck intact. The displacement of the smooth prosthesis with the neck intact also was greater than that of the ridged implant with the neck intact and that of the cemented prosthesis with the neck excised, but the difference did not reach statistical significance. Bones with uncemented smooth prostheses were fractured at loads only a little greater than 400 newtons with the neck intact, and often were fractured at loads of approximately 200 newtons with the neck excised. All bones with ridged implants were fractured at loads between 400 and 800 newtons with the neck resected, but none were fractured with the neck intact. Bones with cemented prostheses were capable of withstanding loads of up to 1,800 newtons without fracture.

Torsional instability may be a problem in uncemented hip prostheses. Preservation of the femoral neck and the addition of ridges to the metaphyseal region of the prosthesis increases resistance to rotation.

▶ The authors demonstrate that changes in femoral design can effect greater torsional stability. Cemented prostheses were more stable than cementless prostheses. Retention of the femoral neck and longitudinal ridges in the femoral component conferred greater rotational stability to the prosthesis. Whether these or other design features prove to be the best means by which rotational stability is conferred, it is important that we recognize the importance of achieving rotational stability in design of femoral components.—R. Poss, M.D.

Air Inclusion in Bone Cement: Importance of the Mixing Technique
Lindén U, Gillquist J (Univ of Linköping, Sweden)
Clin Orthop 247:148–151, October 1989

The mechanical properties of bone cement are largely dependent on the porosity created during mixing. Manual mixing produces a cement of unpredictable porosity. Manual mixing was compared with mechanical mixing of Simplex P bone cement, with or without centrifugation or vacuum.

The percent porosity was reduced in mechanically mixed cement specimens compared with manually mixed specimens. Even with centrifugation, manually mixed cements had higher porosity. An uneven distribution of pores was evident in centrifuged specimens. Mechanical mixing in a vacuum was associated with the lowest porosity. Mechanical mixing produced a more dense cement than manual mixing. Mixing in a vacuum improved all cement specimens, regardless of the mixing method used.

Mechanical mixing of bone cement in a vacuum produces a product of optimal quality. In this way it is possible to lessen the amount of cement needed to join the implant to bone. Shrinkage and exposure of bone to monomer consequently are minimized.

▶ Reduction of porosity in cement can only enhance its strength and reduce crack initiation and propagation of cracks. Therefore, there is good reason to prepare cement using some method that reduces its porosity. This study demonstrates once again that manual mixing of cement is the least optimal method by which cement should be prepared. Centrifugation or vacuum mixing confers more predictable porosity reduction. In this study vacuum mixing was found to be superior to centrifugation. The conclusion to be drawn from most published studies is that either centrifugation or vacuum mixing are desirable adjuncts to contemporary cementing technique.—R. Poss, M.D.

Subsidence of the Femoral Component Related to Long-Term Outcome of Hip Replacement
Loudon JR, Older MWJ (Victoria Infirmary, Glasgow, Scotland; King Edward VII Hosp, Midhurst, England)
J Bone Joint Surg [Br] 71-B:624–628, August 1989   4–32

Some cemented prostheses are designed to slip or subside within the cement mantle if a more optimal position for load transmission is needed. Reportedly, small amounts of prosthetic subsidence occur in the first year after implantation. Increased amounts of subsidence are associated with the development of radiologic signs in the proximal femur and at the bone-cement interface.

The relationship among subsidence, radiologic signs, and long-term clinical outcome was assessed in 102 patients who had undergone primary low-friction arthroplasty between 1969 and 1972 and had survived for 9–13 years. Clinical outcome was evaluated by grading for pain, function, and range of motion. Radiographs were obtained to assess the presence or absence of 6 defined radiologic signs. Clinical outcome was rated satisfactory when the patient had minimal or no pain and satisfactory function with the prosthesis in situ. Clinical outcome was rated unsatisfactory if the prosthesis had been revised or removed, or was still in situ because the patient was not medically fit to undergo revision, but the prosthesis caused severe pain or functioned unsatisfactorily.

At 1 year after arthroplasty, all 102 prostheses functioned satisfactorily. At 9–13 years after arthroplasty, 10 prostheses had become unsatisfactory, 7 of which had been revised. Three were radiologically loose and unacceptably painful. Review of the radiographs showed that fracture of the cement at the prosthesis tip had appeared within 1 year in 29 prostheses and thereafter in an additional 13. Of 42 prostheses with fractured cement tips, 6 had undergone revision and 2 were symptomatically loose. The remaining 34 prostheses with cement tip fractures had satisfactory long-term clinical results. Of the 60 prostheses without cement tip fracture, only 1 hip had been revised for breakage and 1 prosthesis was symptomatically loose. The remaining 58 prostheses were functioning well.

Subsidence of more than 5 mm was seen in 14 of the 92 prostheses with clinically satisfactory outcomes and in 8 of the 10 with unsatisfactory outcomes. The difference was highly significant. Every prosthesis had 1 or more radiologic signs at long-term follow-up, regardless of clinical outcome. An unsatisfactory outcome was associated wtih 3.4 radiologic signs per film, and a satisfactory outcome, with 2.3 radiologic signs per film.

Fracture of the cement tip in low-friction arthroplasty is associated with increased femoral subsidence and radiographic changes that adversely affect long-term clinical outcome of hip replacement.

▶ Progressive subsidence of a femoral component over time and fracture of the cement at the tip of the prosthesis are associated with a higher incidence of failure of total hip replacement. The degree to which optimal surgical and cement techniques can be used should diminish the incidence of mechanical failure of femoral fixation 10 years after total hip arthroplasty.—R. Poss, M.D.

Intramedullary Plugs in Cemented Hip Arthroplasty
Beim GM, Lavernia C, Convery FR (Univ of California, San Diego; VA Med Ctr, La Jolla)
J Arthroplasty 4:139–141, June 1989   4–33

The intramedullary plugs used in cemented hip arthroplasty to reduce the loosening rate are made of 3 different materials, but there are little data on behavior under standard conditions of use. Bone, polymethyl methacrylate, and polymeric plugs from 2 different manufacturers were inserted in intramedullary canals 9–14 mm in diameter and were compared for migration, leakage of cement, and time that different pressure ranges could be maintained (Fig 4–5).

The polymethyl methacrylate plugs showed the least migration and leakage. Cement pressure greater than 100 psi could be maintained for longer than 6 minutes. Bone plugs usually began to migrate with the in-

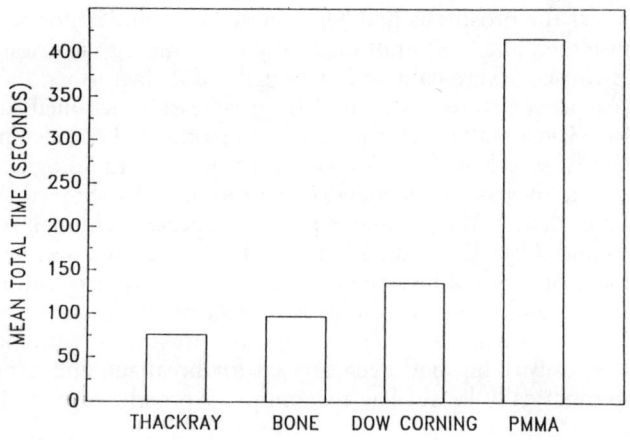

Fig 4–5.—Relative ability to withstand more than 50 psi. (Courtesy of Beim GM, Lavernia C, Convery FR: *J Arthroplasty* 4:139–141, June 1989.)

troduction of pressure and continued to do so; they also had extensive cement leakage. High intramedullary pressures were not maintained. Thackray and Dow polymeric plugs showed extensive or complete cement leakage. Migration was common unless prevented by cement that had leaked. High pressures were not maintained. The Thackray plugs seemed too large for the canals and often broke off when inserted.

Selection of intramedullary plugs is important in cemented joint arthroplasty. The various plugs have different holding characteristics. Thackray plugs are not suitable if the intramedullary canal diameter is less than 13 mm.

▶ There is now a consensus among investigators that the use of intramedullary plugs in cemented total hip arthroplasty contribute to the pressurization of cement and to the achievement of a uniform cement mantel. This study points out that all plugs are not equal and that the goal of increased intramedullary pressure and, therefore, enhanced microinterlock is achieved more predictably when a cement plug is used. Surgeons should not assume that plugging the canal with any device confers the optimal or desired result.—R. Poss, M.D.

A Long-Term Follow-Up Study of Total Hip Replacement With Bone Graft: Correlations Between Roentgenographic Measurement and Hip Mobility
Matsuno T, Masuda T, Hasegawa I, Kanno T, Ichioka Y, Matsuno S, Hirai K (Hokkaido Univ; Hokkaido Orthopedic Mem Hosp, Sapporo, Japan)
Arch Orthop Trauma Surg 108:14–21, January 1989   4–34

Congenital hip dislocation and secondary osteoarthritis are common in Japan. The deficient acetabulum has presented serious problems in total hip replacement, but good results can be achieved with ideal positioning of the acetabular component in the true acetabulum. Results were reviewed in 50 total hip replacements in which acetabular deficiency was treated by autologous bone grafting from the femoral head. Forty-four patients with congenital hip dislocation were operated on at an average age of 55 years.

On follow-up averaging 5 years, solid union was achieved consistently, and there was no loosening of either the acetabular or femoral component. Satisfactory pain relief occurred, and 25 patients were able to walk without canes after surgery. Thirty-four hips had a range of flexion exceeding 90 degrees. Two patients had recurrent dislocation in the first year after surgery. Three had trochanteric problems from wire fracture. There were no nerve palsies.

In patients with arthritis secondary to congenital hip dislocation, positioning the acetabular component in the true acetabulum through bone grafting on its superolateral aspect provides optimal functional results and minimizes the risk of long-term loosening.

▶ The authors present excellent 5-year results of total hip replacement in which acetabular defects were corrected by placement of the acetabular component in the anatomical position and acetabular bone stock restored laterally by autologous bone grafting from the femoral head. The issue of the long-term fate of the acetabular allograft or autograft is not resolved. Some published studies suggest continued satisfactory results from this approach, whereas others, notably the reports of Harris and associates (1–5) warn of greater rates of impending failure after 6 or more years.

The issue still is unresolved and must await further careful long-term studies.— R. Poss, M.D.

References

1. Harris WH, et al: *J Bone Joint Surg [Am]* 59:752, 1977.
2. Harris WH: *Orthop Rev* 6:67, 1977.
3. Harris WH: *Orthop Rev* 9:107, 1980.
4. Gerber SD, Harris WH: *J Bone Joint Surg [Am]* 68:1241, 1986.
5. Woolson ST, Harris WH: *J Bone Joint Surg [Am]* 65:1099, 1983.

Aseptic Loosening in Total Hip Arthroplasty Secondary to Osteolysis Induced by Wear Debris From Titanium-Alloy Modular Femoral Heads
Lombardi AV Jr, Mallory TH, Vaughn BK, Drouillard P (St Anthony Med Ctr, Columbus, Ohio)
J Bone Joint Surg [Am] 71-A:1337–1342, October 1989   4–35

Since 1984, titanium alloy components have been used in the present facility for total joint arthroplasty. Two recent patients needed revision hip arthroplasty about 3 years after initial surgery because of aseptic loosening. The loosening had resulted from severe osteolysis induced by metallic debris from the modular head of the femoral component. The osteolysis (Fig 4–6) resolved after revision arthroplasty. In both cases black-stained, hypertrophic synovial tissue was found, and the surface of the modular femoral head had a burnished appearance.

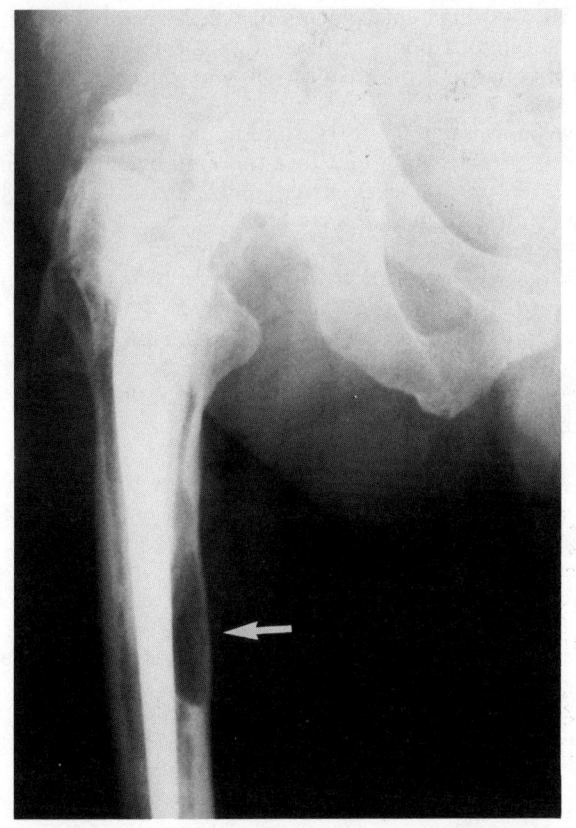

Fig 4-6.—Radiograph made 3 years after the index operation showing osteolysis of the proximal part of the femur. (Courtesy of Lombardi AV Jr, Mallory TH, Vaughn BK, et al: *J Bone Joint Surg [Am]* 71-A:1337-1342, October 1989.)

Wear debris was generated by the titanium alloy modular femoral head in these cases. The process occurred in about 3 years. The prostheses were passivated, but the protective layer obviously failed. Perhaps non-ion-implanted titanium alloy should not be used as a bearing surface in hip or knee arthroplasty. If osteolysis occurs from this cause, revision should be done as soon as possible, with thorough débridement to preserve bone stock by limiting osteolysis and to minimize the long-term effects of exposure to metal ions.

▶ This study demonstrates that titanium alloy, when used as a bearing surface in total hip replacement, produces increased amounts of wear debris. The authors suggest that the process of ion implantation may improve the wear characteristics of titanium, but properly point out that these conclusions are based on in vitro data only. Whether titanium alloy is a satisfactory material as a bearing surface is not yet fully resolved. In a recent study (1) the authors reported quite satisfactory results and minimal deleterious effects from 20 STH titanium prostheses that had been analyzed. They conclude that titanium is an appropriate bearing surface in the absence of acrylic or metallic interposed particles, and in the absence of loosening of the prosthesis. In another convincing study, however, the authors (2) report that titanium is an unsatisfsctory bearing surface even when used in cementless arthroplasty. They noted marked accumulations of metal and polyethylene debris in the tissues and deleterious bone response to these particles. Now the weight of published literature suggests that titanium alloy is not satisfactory as a bearing surface.—R. Poss. M.D.

References

1. McKellop HA, et al: *J Bone Joint Surg [Am]* 72A:512, 1990.
2. Nasser S, et al: *Clin Orthop*, in press, 1990.

An Analysis of the Changes in the Surfaces of Metallic Femoral Components in Hip Prostheses: A Study of 60 Prostheses Removed After 1–20 Years
Pazzaglia UE, Pedrotti L, Ramella R, Zatti G (Policlinico S Matteo, Pavia, Italy)
Ital J Orthop Traumatol 15:223–229, June 1989 4–36

Although only alloys with high resistance to corrosion are used in prostheses, degradation of the metallic surface remains a possibility. The behavior of metallic surfaces in real-life conditions was examined in the femoral components of 60 hip prostheses removed after 1 to 20 years.

Changes were seen only in cemented prostheses. Both corrosion phenomena characteristic of the steel components used and wear phenomena secondary to mobilization were observed. Wear-related changes occurred in both steel components and in Co-Cr alloy. Areas of prosthetic breakage did not coincide with areas of degradation on the metallic surface. Degradation caused by friction was seen at all time intervals, but that related to corrosion was noted only in prostheses removed after 5 years or longer.

Changes in the surfaces of the metallic compounds do not appear to be the result of contact with interstitial fluids alone. Metallic particles can stimulate a macrophagic reaction and thereby contribute to corrosion or to friction-related wear that follows mobilization of the prosthesis.

▶ Long-term changes in the surface characteristics of a variety of alloys used in total hip replacement were analyzed 1 to 20 years after surgery. Alloys of stainless steel and cobalt chromium had changes attributable to both corrosion and abrasion against their cement bed. The long-term fate of metallic components is determined by a variety of factors, including the in vivo microenvironment and the relative motion of the prosthesis and its interface.—R. Poss, M.D.

Biologic Response to Hydroxylapatite-Coated Titanium Hips: A Preliminary Study in Dogs
Thomas KA, Cook SD, Haddad RJ Jr, Kay JF, Jarcho M (Tulane Univ)
J Arthroplasty 4:43–53, March 1989   4–37

Use of a plasma-sprayed hydroxyapatite (HA) coating on an implant surface can shorten the time to adequate fixation strength and increase maximal fixation strength. The amount of bone-implant apposition or bony ingrowth increases as a result. The biologic response was studied in adult dogs bearing HA-coated load-bearing endoprostheses for up to 1 year. A straight Ti-6A1-4V alloy stem was used, with pockets of pure titanium porous coating or a grooved macrotexture on its anterior, posterior, and medial sides. The articulating heads were of the same alloy.

In sections of uncoated grooved implants, no direct bone-implant apposition was seen proximally after up to 10 weeks. In contrast, HA-coated grooved implants had extensive direct bone-coating apposition after 5 weeks. No fibrous tissue interposition was seen in HA-coated implants. There was no evidence that the HA coating deteriorated or separated from the substrate material. Uncoated porous implants had ingrowth at 10 weeks equivalent to that seen with HA-coated devices after 6 weeks.

These findings support previous reports of increased bone deposition and proliferation on HA-coated implants. It seems likely that HA coatings can enhance the fixation of load-bearing implants. Applying HA coating onto a porous surface has no advantage.

▶ In dogs, HA-coating consistently produced extensive and direct bone coating apposition after 5 weeks compared with similar implants that were uncoated. When HA-coated or uncoated porous implants were compared, the HA-coated implants demonstrated an equivalent amount of bone upgrowth but at an earlier period in the post operative course.

A number of clinical and laboratory studies suggest that HA coating confers an early and abundant bone upgrowth to the coating. The important clinical question that remains is, what is the fate of the HA coating with time? Is it stable? Will it degrade with time and produce particulate wear debris? Will its bond to the metallic substrate be maintained? In this study the answers to those questions are reassuring. If HA enjoys a similar fate in clinical application, its use will improve significantly the clinical and radiographic results of cementless total hip arthroplasty. That question, however, is a very large one and can be answered only through further careful clinical and laboratory studies.— R. Poss, M.D.

Experimental and Clinical Experience With Hydroxyapatite-Coated Hip Implants
Geesink RGT (State Univ of Limburg, Maastricht, The Netherlands)
Orthopedics 12:1239–1242, September 1989   4–38

The excellent biologic and mechanical properties and interface characteristics to bone of hydroxyapatite-coated implants were first demonstrated in a plug implant study of dogs. That study provided direct evidence of bonding between hydroxyapatite coating and bone. Periosteal tissue, mature osteocytes, and young osteoblasts were seen in direct contact with the coating without any intervening fibrous tissue. The study also confirmed the biocompatibility between hydroxyapatite and bone.

A subsequent total hip replacement study of dogs further investigated the biologic characteristics of hydroxyapatite coatings under mechanical loading. That study demonstrated that hydroxyapatite-coated prostheses are much better incorporated into bone than any of the other devices presently in use. The coatings acquired such tight bonds with the surrounding bone that, 6 weeks after implantation, powerful extraction forces were required to cause fissuring and fracturing.

Since 1986, nearly 100 patients have received hip replacement systems with hydroxyapatite-coated hip implants at the State University of Limburg. Most patients had diagnoses of osteoarthritis or avascular necrosis of the femoral head. Postoperative complications included 2 hip luxations and 1 femoral fracture involving some shortening of the leg which healed without further complications. Very few patients had significant postoperative pain. The almost complete absence of midthigh pain was particularly striking. The mean Harris hip score after 3 months was 84, approaching 98 after 6 months and longer. Many patients had Harris ratings of 100 within 3 months after operation.

Follow-up in this first series of patients having hydroxyapatite-coated hip prostheses has been less than 2 years. The preliminary results accumulated to date indicate excellent early postoperative clinical and functional results. However, long-term follow-up is still the final test against the current generation of cemented or cementless implants.

▶ This review of the experimental and clinical experience to date with hydroxyapatite-coated implants was made by one of the first clinicians to investigate its use. The short-term benefits are encouraging, but the ultimate application of this technique must await further clinical follow-up.— R. Poss, M.D.

Wear Characteristics of the Canine Acetabulum Against Different Femoral Prostheses
Cook SD, Thomas KA, Kester MA (Tulane Univ)
J Bone Joint Surg [Br] 71-B:189–197, March 1989
4–39

Cartilage degeneration was studied in canine acetabula after the implantation of prostheses having articulating surfaces of low-temperature isotropic (LTI) pyrolytic carbon, cobalt-chromium-molybdenum (Co-Cr-Mo) alloy, and titanium (Ti-6A1-4V) alloy. The prostheses had hemispheric heads with straight stabilizing stems and were in place for 2 weeks to 18 months.

Cartilage that articulated with LTI pyrolytic carbon showed less gross wear, fibrillation, and eburnation than did cartilage articulating with the metallic surfaces. In addition, there was less loss of glycosaminoglycan and less subchondral bone change. The likelihood of cartilage surviving at 18 months was 92% with LTI pyrolytic carbon and 20% with either of the metallic alloys.

Every attempt should be made to preserve the natural femoral head, but if a prosthesis is required, a material such as LTI pyrolytic carbon is best. Degenerative cartilage change is considerably more pronounced when metallic alloys are used.

▶ In this experimental study, low temperature isotropic pyrolytic carbon, cobalt-chromium alloy, and titanium alloy were compared as articulating surfaces in canine acetabula. The carbon femoral heads produced significantly fewer mechanical and biochemical changes in the articular cartilage and subchondral bone than either of the metallic surfaces. In the next few years we will see increased research into newer materials as bearing surfaces in total joint replacement.—R. Poss, M.D.

Aggressive Granulomatous Lesions After Hip Arthroplasty
Tallroth K, Eskola A, Santavirta S, Konttinen YT, Lindholm TS (Orthopaedic Hosp of the Invalid Found, Helsinki)
J Bone Joint Surg [Br] 71-B:571–575, August 1989 4–40

Aggressive bone resorption may be observed around the cemented femoral component of a total hip replacement. Prosthetic loosening is the usual result. Nineteen patients who required revision surgery because of aggressive granulomatosis were among 417 patients having revision arthroplasty in a 5-year period. The diagnosis was made when large focal lytic areas were seen around the prosthesis in the absence of infection.

Usually, initial arthroplasty was for primary osteoarthritis. Cement had been placed digitally without an intramedullary plug. Stress pain commonly was the first clinical sign of granuloma. Most lesions appeared to have begun in the area of the lesser trochanter. Revision arthroplasty was done 9 years on average after primary hip surgery and 14 months after aggressive granulomatosis was diagnosed. In some cases lesion area had doubled within an average of about 2 years. Fourteen stems were loose at the time of revision surgery. Histologic studies showed collagen deposition with histiocytes and giant cells containing cement particles. Bacterial cultures were negative in all cases.

Aggressive granulomatosis is a distinct entity that progresses at varying rates. Because rapid growth of the lesions can lead to spontaneous fracture, revision arthroplasty should be considered shortly after the diagnosis is made. The authors perform revision arthroplasty using uncemented titanium prostheses and bone grafting.

▶ In a subset of patients the biologic response to accumulated wear debris is an accelerated granulomatous reaction that rapidly depletes bone stock and may subject the patient to pathologic fracture. This group of patients should be followed carefully and revision surgery performed early before extensive bone loss occurs.— R. Poss, M.D.

Femoral Fracture During Non-Cemented Total Hip Arthroplasty
Schwartz JT Jr, Mayer JG, Engh CA (Anderson Clinic, Arlington, VA; Univ of Maryland)
J Bone Joint Surg [Am] 71-A:1135–1142, September 1989   4–41

Intraoperative femoral fracture occurs in up to a fourth of uncemented total hip arthroplasties. Data were reviewed on 1,318 consecutive arthroplasties of this type done between 1977 and 1986. There were 39 intraoperative femoral fractures, for an incidence of 3%. Only half of the injuries were diagnosed at the time of surgery. Fractures occurred both proximally (Fig 4–7) and distally near the tip of the prosthesis (Fig 4–8). Most fractures were incomplete and minimally displaced, and did not impair the stability of the femoral prosthetic component.

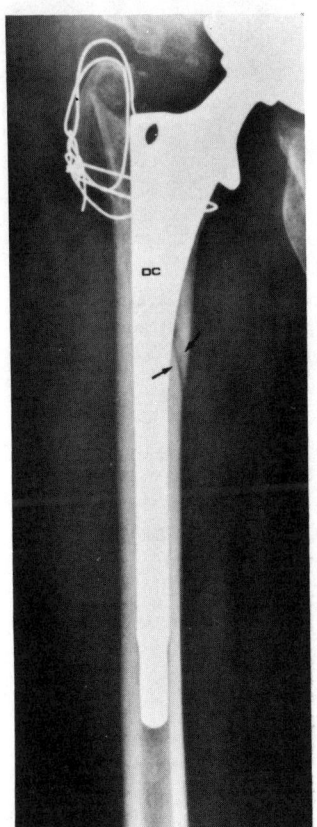

Fig 4–7.—Roentgenogram showing a complete proximal femoral fracture *(arrows)*. (Courtesy of Schwartz JT Jr, Mayer JG, Engh CA: *J Bone Joint Surg [Am]* 71-A:1135–1142, September 1989.)

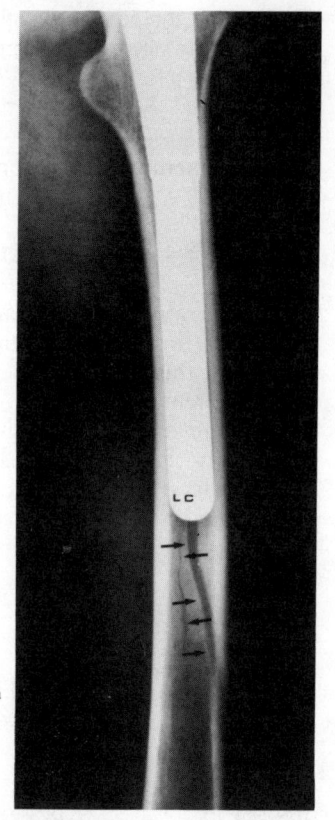

Fig 4–8.—Roentgenogram showing an incomplete displaced femoral fracture *(arrows)* distal to an anatomical medullary locked prosthesis. The posterior part of the cortex remained intact. (Courtesy of Schwartz JT Jr, Mayer JG, Engh CA: *J Bone Joint Surg [Am]* 71-A:1135–1142, September 1989.)

Complete proximal fractures were stabilized with a partially or fully coated prosthesis to assure distal fixation. Those found at surgery were fixed by cerclage wiring. If an incomplete distal fracture was detected postoperatively and the posterior femoral cortex was intact, a spica cast was applied. The patients with fracture did not differ from those without fracture with regard to residual pain, walking ability, or implant stability. Only 1 patient with fracture lacked stable fixation 2 years postoperatively.

The incidence of fracture has lessened since a template was introduced in preoperative planning to determine the proper site of the pilot hole and the proper size of implant. Enlarged broaches and fully fluted rigid reamers were used, and the pilot hole was enlarged to prevent eccentric reaming. In addition, stems that totally fill the femoral canal have been used more frequently.

▶ Intraoperative femoral fracture is a not uncommon complication of cementless total hip arthroplasty, and its incidence is increased compared with cemented total hip arthroplasty because of the goal of maximal initial stabilization. Most authors report a decreasing incidence of this complication as further experience is gained with a particular prosthesis and its instrumentation. The authors report that only half of the fractures were diagnosed at the time of surgery, thus the surgeon must maintain a high index of suspicion for this complication. Proximal fractures, when recognized, are easily treated, but distal fractures present a more formidable treatment challenge. When the fractures are recognized and appropriately treated, this group of patients enjoys a favorable prognosis similar to that of their counterparts who have not sustained fractures.— R. Poss, M.D.

Biomechanical and Histologic Invstigation of Cemented Total Hip Arthroplasties: A Study of Autopsy-Retrieved Femurs After In Vivo Cycling
Maloney WJ, Jasty M, Burke DW, O'Connor DO, Zalenski EB, Bragdon C, Harris WH (Massachusetts Gen Hosp, Boston; Harvard Med School)
Clin Orthop 249:129–140, December 1989   4–42

To mechanically assess successfully cemented femoral components of total hip arthroplasty after years of excellent in vivo service, 11 femurs with cemented femoral components were taken at autopsy from 8 patients who died 2 weeks to 17 years after arthroplasty. Five intact femurs also were obtained. The implants had been stable clinically and roentgenographically. In the biomechanical analysis bone strain and stability of the implant were examined in the single-extremity stance and stair-climbing positions by using a 100-pound spinal load.

Remarkable stability was observed; the maximal axial micromotion was 40 μ. Strain gauge studies showed marked stress shielding in the proximal medial femoral cortex (Figs 4–9 through 4–11). Strain in the calcar region remained abnormal even 17 years after surgery. All the prostheses had remarkable axial stability in both single-extremity stance and simulated stair-climbing loading.

Marked stress shielding of the proximal medial femoral cortex is noted after placement of a cemented femoral component. Stress-related disuse osteoporosis is a serious concern. The present findings demonstrate inti-

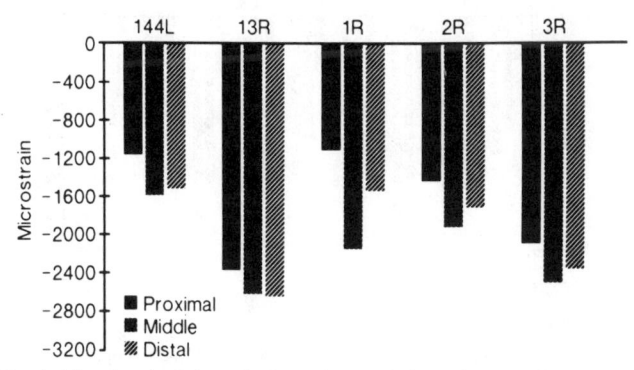

Fig 4–9.—Axial strains along the media femoral cortex in intact femurs. (Courtesy of Maloney WJ, Jasty M, Burke DW, et al: *Clin Orthop* 249:129–140, December 1989.)

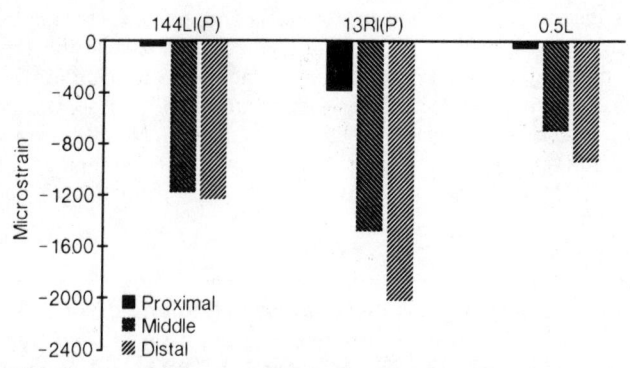

Fig 4–10.—Axial strains along the medial femoral cortex immediately after THA. (Courtesy of Maloney WJ, Jasty M, Burke DW, et al: *Clin Orthop* 249:129–140, December 1989.)

mate osseointegration at the bone-cement interface. In the absence of cement fragmentation the interface is well maintained for many years after arthroplasty.

▶ As the longevity of total hip arthroplasty has increased, an important question becomes whether bone adaptation to the altered strain distribution imposed by metallic femoral stems will result in deleterious stress shielding or catastrophic depletion of bone stock. In this autopsy study of hips recovered as long as 210 months after initial implantation, the authors establish some important findings. First, acute implantation of a prosthesis drastically alters the normal strain distribution patterns of the femur, the most important of which is proximal strain bypass. When strain gauge studies were performed on femurs in which the implant had been present for as long as 17 years, proximal strain bypass to some degree was still evident. This analysis was performed on femurs in which implants, relatively small by today's standards, were cemented. An issue of current concern is whether the very large and stiff metallic prosthe-

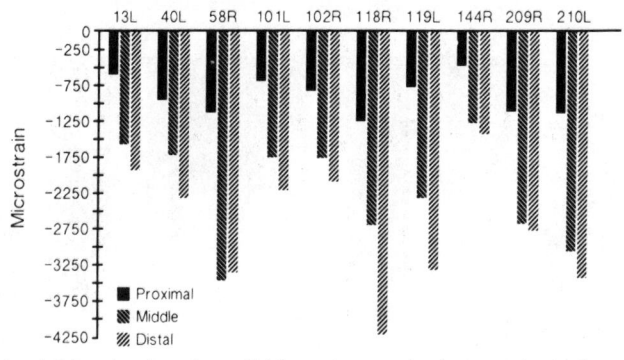

Fig 4–11.—Axial strains along the medial femoral cortex after long-term in vivo bone remodeling. (Courtesy of Maloney WJ, Jasty M, Burke DW, et al: *Clin Orthop* 249:129–140, December 1989.)

sis currently being used will impose tolerable levels of strain bypass over the long term.—R. Poss, M.D.

Plain Radiographs Inadequate for Evaluation of the Cement-Bone Interface in the Hip Prosthesis: A Cadaver Study of Femoral Stems
Jacobs ME, Koeweiden EMJ, Slooff TJJH, Huiskes R, van Horn JR (Univ of Nijmegen, The Netherlands)
Acta Orthop Scand 60:541–543, October 1989   4–43

To determine if plain radiographs accurately represent the true cement-bone interlock, a comparison was made of radiographs and macroscopic morphology on cross sections of 11 human femurs into which an endoprosthesis had been inserted. Four femurs were obtained postmortem from patients with a hip arthroplasty, and 7 cadaver femurs were cemented under various conditions. Radiographs were taken of all the femurs, which then were cut for macroscopic inspection of the cement-bone interface with respect to gross interpretation, depth of cement penetration, integrity of the bone bed, and lamellation of the cement.

In cadavers, radiographs did not distinguish between broken trabeculae within the cement and good penetration of cement into intrabecular spaces. Radiolucencies in both cadaver and autopsy specimens were not necessarily indicative of blood, air, or soft tissue interposed between cement and bone; they sometimes resulted from a particular arrangement of trabeculae in the wall of the femur. In autopsy specimens seen years after surgery, plain films did not show sheets of new cortical bone that anchored the implant.

Plain radiographs are unreliable indicators of the true nature of the cement-bone interface. Previously reported results indicating that radiolucent lines on these films demonstrate radiolucent material interposed between bone and cement were not supported by these data.

Roentgenographic Changes in Proximal Femoral Dimensions Due to Hip Rotation
Bell AL, Brand RA (Univ of Iowa Hosps)
Clin Orthop 240:194–199, March 1989   4–44

Radiographic evaluation and follow-up of total hip arthroplasties (THA) is difficult because standard anteroposterior (AP) hip radiographs are often inconsistent in terms of patient orientation and distance between the patient and the x-ray source. However, inconsistency can distort the width of a radiolucent line or hide it at the cement-bone interface.

How relatively small amounts of femoral rotation may affect the measurement of proximal femoral dimensions on supine anteroposterior (AP) hip radiographs was studied in 3 human adult right femurs that were radiographed in anatomical position at 15 degrees, 30 degrees, and 45 degrees of both internal and external rotation (Fig 4–12).

All 3 femurs had a similar pattern of increases and decreases in dimensions with rotation, but the pattern varied from level to level. As little as 15 degrees or less of internal or external femoral rotation caused significant changes in proximal femoral dimensions on the supine AP hip radiograph, and the magnitude of the changes increased with increasing rotation. These changes are comparable to the medullary canal expansion of a normal adult femur over 5–10 years.

To obtain accurate measurements of proximal femoral dimensions over time, the rotations used in each examination should be matched precisely to those in previous examinations. Radiographic techniques for consistent visualization of total hip arthroplasties already have been described. One is the use of a chariot, or rotating transparent plastic support by which the standing patient is held in position and consistently oriented with respect to the x-ray source and film cassette. Time and cost constraints probably will prevent widespread acceptance of this technique.

Fig 4–12.—A, lateral view, and B, anteroposterior view of a femur oriented in anatomical position as defined by Ruff and Hayes. The femur was subsequently rotated (internally or externally) about the indicated longitudinal axis. The labeled proximal femoral levels (levels A, B, C, and D) in the anteroposterior view correspond to the levels of measurement: (1) level A, the distal margin of the lesser trochanter (DLT); (2) level B, 25 mm distal to the DLT; (3) level C, 50 mm distal to the DLT; and (4) level D, 100 mm distal to the DLT. (Courtesy of Bell AL, Brand RA: *Clin Orthop* 240:194–199, March 1989.)

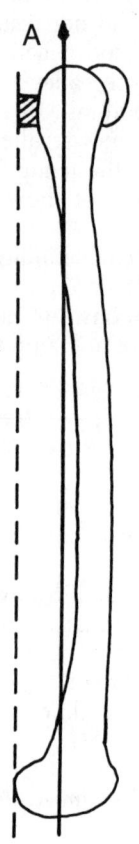

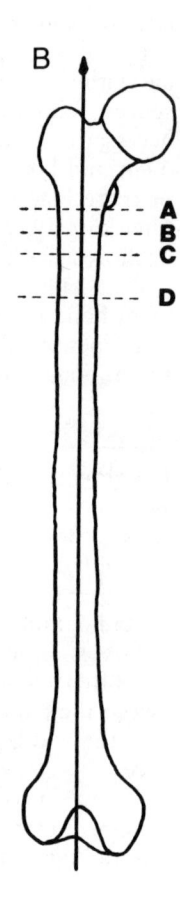

▶ Documentation of the adequacy of fixation of hip prosthesis is dependent on interpretation of plain radiographs. These 2 studies (Abstracts 4-43 and 4-44) alert us to some of the inadequacies of these methods, and so call for a more cautious interpretation of radiographic results. Serial radiographic measurements must be performed in a consistent and reproducible protocol if meaningful interpretations are to be extracted.— R. Poss, M.D.

Arthroscopic Surgery for Synovial Chondromatosis of the Hip
Okada Y, Awaya G, Ikeda T, Tada H, Kamisato S, Futami T (Kokura Mem Hosp, Kitakyusyu, Japan)
J Bone Joint Surg [Br] 71-B:198–199, March 1989   4-45

Although arthroscopy is being used increasingly, it has not often been used for the hip. One girl had a successful arthroscopic operation for synovial chondromatosis.

Girl, 16 years, had intermittent left hip pain when skipping and had some reduction of abduction and medial and lateral rotation. Arthroscopy under general anesthesia showed many tiny cartilaginous bodies, some loose in the joint and others firmly attached to the synovium of the acetabular fossa. Synovial biopsy and examination of the fragments showed synovial chondromatosis. When the patient declined open surgery, the chondroid fragments were removed arthroscopically via the same lateral approach. Hundreds of the bodies were removed; a few were left embedded in the synovium about the ligamentum teres. A check arthroscopy 4 months later showed new cartilaginous bodies and no deformation of the articular surfaces. The patient was free of pain and had normal motion 1 year after operation.

Arthroscopy now has been carried out successfully in conditions such as osteoarthritis, torn acetabular labrum, aseptic necrosis of the femoral head, and Perthes' disease. When the anterior and lateral approaches are used, it is possible to examine practically the entire hip. A 6.5-mm arthroscope makes it possible to remove small fragments from a joint or take a biopsy through a single puncture.

▶ Reports of the application of arthroscopic examination and treatment to problems about the hip will become more frequent. Arthroscopic biopsy, lavage and removal of loose bodies, examination of the articular surfaces, and examination of the acetabular labrum are early applications of this technique to the hip. Further experience and improvements in arthroscopic technique will define further the role of arthroscopic surgery in the hip joint.— R. Poss, M.D.

Ligaments and Meniscal Injuries

Open Meniscus Repair: Technique and Two to Nine Year Results
DeHaven KE, Black KP, Griffiths HJ (Univ of Rochester Med Ctr, Rochester, NY)
Am J Sports Med 17:788–795, November–December 1989

The preliminary results of open repair of peripheral meniscus tears were published earlier. The intermediate results after open repair of acute and chronic peripheral meniscus tears were reviewed in 92 patients aged 12–40 years who underwent repair of peripheral meniscus tears in 104 knees between 1976 and 1983. Follow-up data were available for 80 repairs in 74 patients; 18 patients were lost to follow-up.

Of the 80 repairs, 39 were done in the acute stage and 41 were done in the chronic stage. Thirty-three of the 34 patients who underwent repair of an acute meniscus tear and 21 of the 41 patients who underwent repair in the chronic stage had associated acute ruptures of the anterior cruciate ligament (ACL). Forty-four patients with 49 repairs were evaluated by a return clinic visit that comprised a detailed questionnaire, physical examination including knee arthrometer measurements with the KT-1000, and radiographic examination consisting of standing anteroposterior views of both knees in extension and 45 degrees of flexion. The other 30 patients responded to a detailed questionnaire alone.

During an average follow-up of 4.6 years, 9 (11%) of the 80 repaired menisci tore again. The interval between repair and retear ranged from 6 to 34 months. Seven retears occurred in chronic tears, and 2 occurred in acute tears. Three of the 9 retears occurred through the repair zone and required meniscectomy because of extensive damage to the body of the meniscus. Retear in the other 6 cases occurred at different sites; the original repair sites were found to be well healed at reoperation. Retears occurred in 1 of 26 isolated repairs, 2 of 38 repairs done with ACL stabilization, and 6 of 16 repairs done in ACL deficient knees that were not stabilized. Standing radiographs showed normal compartments in 40 of the 41 repairs.

In view of the well-reported significant incidence of degenerative changes after meniscectomy in the treatment of a torn meniscus, and the satisfactory results obtained to date with open repair, retention and repair of the meniscus is highly recommended.

▶ This paper carefully documents the results of repair of meniscal repairs in 104 knees. These results of open repair of peripheral tears of the menisci demonstrate an excellent intermediate-term result. The authors point out that their indication for arthroscopic repair is limited to tears within the vascular zone far enough away from the peripheral rim to make open repair difficult. In addition, they advise carrying out ACL stabilization in young persons with high physical demands. The authors strike a good balance between open and arthroscopic repair, repair of the ACL, or conservative management.—C.B. Sledge, M.D.

Non-Operative Treatment of Meniscal Tears
Weiss CB, Lundberg M, Hamberg P, DeHaven KE, Gillquist J (Univ of Rochester, NY; Univ Hosp, Linköping, Sweden)
J Bone Joint Surg [Am] 71-A:811–822, July 1989   4–47

A selective approach in the treatment of meniscal tears preserves as much meniscal tissue as possible. To identify a subset of clinically stable meniscal tears that can be managed conservatively, the results of 3,612 arthroscopic procedures performed for the treatment of acute or chronic meniscal lesions, with or without an associated ligamentous lesion, were reviewed retrospectively. Eighty meniscal tears in 75 patients were assumed to be stable based on clinical judgment. Of 70 longitudinal tears, 52 were lateral and 18 were medial meniscal lesions. Ten were vertical radial lesions, and all involved the lateral meniscus.

Fifty-two patients were followed for 2 to 10 years. Only 6 required additional intervention, because of symptoms that were unrelated to meniscal tear. Thirty-two patients underwent repeat arthroscopy at an average of 26 months (range, 3 to 100 months) after the initial arthroscopy. Twenty-six patients had longitudinal tears, and 6 had radial tears. Seventeen longitudinal tears healed completely, whereas 5 radial tears showed no evidence of healing and 1 had extended. Neither chronic ligamentous laxity nor a meniscal tear precluded healing of the stable longitudinal tears. No localized degenerative changes were found in the adjacent articular cartilage in any of the stable vertical longitudinal or radial meniscal lesions. Except for the 6 patients who had additional surgery, none of the 52 patients who completed a questionnaire reported symptoms of a meniscal lesion, and none of the 42 patients who were reexamined 2 or more years after the operation had signs of a meniscal lesion.

Stable vertical longitudinal tears, especially in the vascular outer area of the meniscus, have great potential for healing. The tear should be left alone unless no other lesions are present and it causes sufficient disability to warrant treatment. Stable radial tears have little potential for healing, but their optimal management could not be established in this study.

▶ Eighty meniscal tears identified in 3,612 arthroscopic procedures were judged to be stable and managed nonoperatively. Stable longitudinal tears did very well, and healing was demonstrated at repeat arthroscopy in 17 of 26 such tears. Radial tears did not heal and produced late symptoms. If a longitudinal meniscal tear, either of partial thickness or full thickness, is deemed to be stable at initial evaluation, nonoperative treatment appears to be effective and is clearly preferable to operative treatment.—C.B. Sledge, M.D.

Anterior Cruciate Ligament: Its Normal Response and Replacement
Butler DL (Univ of Cincinnati)
J Orthop Res 7:910–921, October 1989   4–48

The knee is one of the most frequently injured joints in the human body. When it is injured, the anterior cruciate ligament (ACL) often is disrupted. The human ACL is a primary restraint to anterior tibial displacement at both 90 degrees and 30 degrees of flexion. The ligament has a complex macrostructure composed of bundles of different lengths, curvatures, and orientations. Subunits from the human anterior and posterior cruciate and lateral collateral ligaments have similar material properties; however, the linear modulus, maximal stress, and strain energy density to maximal stress of the ACL are significantly less than similar properties of the patellar tendons. Axial stress of the tissue subunits is nonuniform during tensile loading. This finding may be partially attributable to differences in bundle crimp period and crimp angle.

When stiffness, strength, energies, and elongation to maximal force and failure were compared in 9 commonly used human ACL substitutes, only the bone-patellar tendon-bone unit had stiffness and maximal force greater than the ACL.

▶ This award-winning paper reviews a long series of research projects on the ACL. The mechanical properties, geometric arrangement, and healing potential are examined and compared with the mechanical properties of 9 commonly used ACL substitutes. The patellar tendon substitute showed significant loss in structural and material properties in both the dog and primate, and it was not improved by maintaining a vascular supply or by using intermittent passive motion.— C.B. Sledge, M.D.

Surgical or Non-Surgical Treatment of Acute Rupture of the Anterior Cruciate Ligament: A Randomized Study With Long-Term Follow-Up
Andersson C, Odensten M, Good L, Gillquist J (Univ of Linköping, Sweden)
J Bone Joint Surg [Am] 71-A:965–974, August 1989   4–49

Some studies have reported unsatisfactory long-term results after acute repair of ruptured anterior cruciate ligaments (ACLs). To determine whether repair with augmentation of the ACL using part of the patellar tendon might improve results, 111 patients with injuries that included acute rupture of the ACL were randomized to 3 treatment groups. One group received simple repair of all injured structures; another group underwent repair of all injured structures and augmentation of the ACL with a strip of the iliotibial band; and the third group underwent repair of all injured structures except the ACL. At 45 or more months after surgery 107 patients were available for reexamination.

At the most recent follow-up patients who had repair and augmentation of the ACL had significantly more stability and significantly fewer subsequent meniscal tears. Patients who received augmentation also needed fewer reconstructions for symptoms of instability. Patients with augmented repair had better knee function and higher levels of activity than patients in either of the other treatment groups. Researchers also found that 64% of the patients with ruptures of the ACL also had meniscal tears. More than half of these tears needed primary treatment.

In patients with rupture of the ACL, repair and augmentation of the ACL results in better function of the knee and a higher level of activity than simple repair, or repair of only peripheral lesions. Because patients with this injury frequently have associated injuries needing primary treatment, arthroscopy is recommended for all patients with acute ruptures of the ACL.

▶ The optimal treatment for acute rupture of the ACL remains unsolved. Some studies report good results without operative intervention, others report excellent results with reconstruction, and still others show good initial results but late deterioration. This paper analyzes the results of 3 different approaches: simple repair of the injured structures; augmentation of the ACL with the iliotibial band; and repair of all injured structures except for the ACL. The authors conclude that patients having repair of the torn structures and augmentation of the ACL with a strip of iliotibial band did significantly better than the other 2 groups. Only 30% of the patients who did not have repair of the ACL returned to participation in competitive sports, as did a similar proportion of patients wtih repair of all structures except the ACL, in strong contrast to the 71% of patients who had augmentation and were able to return to competitive sports.

The strength of this paper lies in that it is a randomized, prospective study with a follow-up averaging almost 5 years.—C.B. Sledge, M.D.

Four- to Ten-Year Followup of Unreconstructed Anterior Cruciate Ligament Tears
Pattee GA, Fox JM, Del Pizzo W, Friedman MJ (Southern California Orthopedics and Sports Med Group, Van Nuys, Calif)
Am J Sports Med 17:430–435, May–June 1989   4–50

The optimal management of anterior cruciate ligament (ACL) tears remains controversial. The long-term objective and functional results and patient satisfaction after nonoperative treatment of ACL tears were evaluated retrospectively 4–10 years after ACl tears were documented by arthroscopy and mild to moderate pivot shifts under anesthesia.

Forty-nine patients average age 27 years had complete tears initially managed nonoperatively. Two thirds of the knees had tears of 1 or both menisci, requiring partial meniscectomies. Because of persisting symptoms of disabling instabilty, 9 patients (18%) underwent reconstruction of the ACL at an average 26 months after initial injury. The remaining 40 patients were evaluated at an average 5.6 years (range, 4–10) after documentation of the tear.

Of the 40 patients treated nonoperatively, 25 (62%) had satisfactory subjective results. Eight (20%) had returned to their preinjury level of athletic activity without restrictions, 10 (25%) functioned at the same levels but with symptoms and with some patients requiring bracing, 17 (43%) had reduced their level of sports participation, and 5 (12%) no longer engaged in sports. Only 2 patients (5%) required subsequent meniscectomies.

Physical examination showed pivot shifts in 27 patients (87%). Instrumented laxity testing showed a difference between injured knee and normal knee of 3.1 mm with a 20-lb force. Radiographic studies were normal in 7 (35%) of 20 knees, whereas 13 (65%) showed mild degenerative changes. Overall, objective results were satisfactory in only 7 (23%) of 31 patients, but functional results were satisfactory in 19 (61%).

Apparently, many patients have adapted well to their ultimate functional disability through modification of activities. Few patients, however, return unrestricted to their preinjury level of function after nonoperative management of ACL tears.

▶ Few areas in orthopedics are more controversial than the torn ACL. In this paper, 49 patients with complete tears had nonoperative management. Eighteen percent eventually underwent reconstruction. Sixty-two percent of those treated nonoperatively had satisfactory subjective results, but only 20% returned to their preinjury levels of athletic activity. This study would appear to confirm the suggestion that the ACL should be repaired in persons who wish to participate in functionally demanding running and cutting activities.—C.B. Sledge, M.D.

Non-operative Management of Acute Grade III Medial Collateral Ligament Injury of the Knee: A Prospective Study
Mok DWH, Good C (St George's Hosp, London)
Injury 20:277–280, September 1989   4–51

Complete rupture of the medial collateral ligament of the knee traditionally has been managed by immediate surgical repair. The value of protected motion was assessed in 25 patients seen from 1985 to 1987 with acute complete ruptures and associated anterior cruciate ligament (ACL) injury. The average age was 28 years. Five patients had tears in the sheath of the ACL. Nine had partial cruciate ligament tears and 11 had complete ruptures. Patients were mobilized in a cast brace and underwent physiotherapy.

The patients were hospitalized for 1 week on average and lost 4 weeks from work. All returned to their preinjury level of sports activity. Four of 16 knees assessed 18 months after injury had moderate medial laxity. Further follow-up showed no tendency toward greater ligamentous laxity of the medial collateral ligament. Slight anterior laxity persisted in anterior cruciate-deficient knees but caused no functional problems.

Conservative treatment is an appropriate initial approach to acute rupture of the medial collateral ligament, even if the ACL also is injured.

▶ The management of complete tears of the medial collateral ligament has evolved over the past several years from routine surgical repair and prolonged postoperative immobilization to more conservative treatment with nonoperative management coupled with early guided motion. The authors of this paper clearly demonstrate that conservative management produces excellent results, even if the ACL also is injured.—C.B. Sledge, M.D.

Knee Pain

Arthroscopy in Patients Wtih Recalcitrant Retropatellar Pain Syndrome
Osgood JC, Kneisl JS, Barrack RL, Alexander AH (Naval Hosp, Oakland, Calif)
Othop Rev 18:1177–1183, November 1989   4–52

Patients with recalcitrant retropatellar pain syndrome (RPPS) have pain localized to the peripatellar region after stair-climbing, prolonged sitting, or repeated kneeling. The arthroscopic findings in patients with RPPS were correlated with the long-term clinical course. Patients were excluded if they had histories consistent with meniscal or cruciate injuries, or if they had previous knee surgery.

Forty-one of 81 patients were followed for 24 to 73 months. The mean length of follow-up was 51 months. Investigators recorded arthroscopic findings, graded the status of chondral surfaces, and correlated these with clinical findings using a modified Insall rating system. Cartilage irregularities were routinely débrided.

At follow-up, nearly equal numbers of patients improved, were worse, or stayed the same. There was no correlation between the severity of objective chondromalacia at arthroscopy and the severity of long-term functional impairment. Débridement of lesions did not improve the outcome. Missed intra-articular pathology was found in only 4% of patients at arthroscopy. These findings suggest that nonoperative treatment is the procedure of choice in patients with RPPS. Arthroscopy should be reserved for very selected cases.

▶ Anterior knee pain, referred to as retropatellar pain syndrome in this paper, is an illusive diagnosis describing a symptom complex caused by a number of different pathologic entities. This paper evaluates the role of arthroscopy in evaluating patients with enigmatic knee pain. The authors report no correlation between the severity of observed chondromalacia and the severity of long-term functional impairment. Treatment did not appear to affect the outcome. The authors state that arthroscopy should be reserved for very selective cases.—C.B. Sledge, M.D.

A Conservative Approach to Anterior Knee Pain
Whitelaw GP Jr, Rullo DJ, Markowitz HD, Marandola MS, DeWaele MJ (Boston City Hosp; Waltham Physical Therapy Associates, Waltham, Mass)
Clin Orthop 246:234–237, September 1989   4–53

Pain in the anterior knee area can represent a number of disorders. Data were reviewed on 85 consecutive outpatients aged 11 to 62 years who had pain beneath or adjacent to the patella that was aggravated by increased activity, stair-climbing, or prolonged sitting. There was tenderness beneath the facets on patellofemoral compression or forced excursion. Crepitus, effusion, or a reduced range of motion was noted in 60% of the 114 affected knees.

Nearly 90% of the patients reported improvement in their knee symptoms after a disciplined physical therapy program, which included stretching exercises, electrical quadriceps stimulation, progressive straight-leg raising, isometric and short-arc quadriceps sets, and ice application. Standard doses of nonsteroidal anti-inflammatory drugs were advised. Two thirds of patients considered themselves improved after a mean follow-up of 16 months. More than half of the patients reported an increased level of activity compared with that at presentation.

Patients with anterior knee pain who lack obvious bony, ligament, or meniscal injury should receive physical therapy and nonsteroidal anti-inflammatory drugs. Activities that produce pain should be limited, but patients should participate in a home exercise program.

▶ Anterior knee pain describes a constellation of symptoms arising from any of a number of different conditions. This paper demonstrates that 90% of patients will have improvement with time, physical therapy, and nonsteroidal anti-inflammatory drugs. A program of this type should be followed before patients are subjected to surgery, either arthroscopic or open.—C.B. Sledge, M.D.

Cartilage Damage

Contact Pressures in the Patellofemoral Joint During Impact Loading on the Human Flexed Knee
Haut RC (Gen Motors Research Labs, Warren, Mich)
J Orthop Res 7:272–280, March 1989

Bone fracture is a criterion used by the automotive industry in assessing the potential for lower extremity injury caused by impact on the flexed knee, but studies with animal models indicate that irreversible cartilage damage may result from overpressures within the patellofemoral joint without fracture. Progressive degenerative disease may result from such an injury.

Contact pressures were measured in 9 cadaver specimens during impact loading of the isolated flexed knee. Loads were delivered with a free-flight inertial mass having either a rigid or foam-padded interface. The patella or femur fractured at impact loads of about 8.5 kilonewtons (kN). The patellofemoral pressure averaged about 25 megapascals (MPa) for 8 kN of impact load on the joint flexed 90 degrees. Pressure distribution was nonuniform, and the contact area varied with both the level of contact load and the degree of joint flexion. At 70% of the fracture load for the knee flexed 90 degrees, nearly 35% of the contact area was exposed to pressures exceeding 25 MPa.

Pressures observed in this study probably can lead to fissures and lacerations of the cartilage. A foam padding system can help distribute loads over the knee and about the patella, lowering patellofemoral contact pressures.

▶ Cartilage is known to be susceptible to damage by direct pressure (1) and to exist in the normal joint within a very carefully controlled range of mechanical pressure. It has been proposed that bone will fracture to dissipate energy and protect the articular cartilage from lethal loads. This paper, however, suggests that loads previously considered lethal to chondrocytes may be encountered during impact of the flexed knee on the dashboard of an automobile and may explain posttraumatic osteoarthritis of the patellofemoral joint after such injuries.—C.B. Sledge, M.D.

Reference

   1. Repo RU, Finlay JB: *J Bone Joint Surg [Am]* 59:1068, December 1977.

A System for Grading Articular Cartilage Lesions at Arthroscopy
Noyes FR, Stabler CL (Cincinnati Sportsmedicine Ctr; Deaconess Hosp Ctr, Cincinnati)
Am J Sports Med 17:505–513, July–August 1989

Several classification systems have been devised to describe and categorize damages to articular cartilage. However, each system has certain limitations and deficiencies that can lead to confusion. A new classification system describes articular cartilage abnormalities in simple terms.

The proposed system is based on 4 separate and distinct variables: the description of the articular surface, the extent (depth) of involvement, the diameter of the lesion, and the location of the lesion. The articular surface is described as smooth and intact, closed lesion (grade 1); damaged, open lesion (grade 2); and bone exposed (grade 3). Each grade is divided into subtypes A or B depending on the depth of involvement. Subtypes A and B in grade 1 are characterized as soft (1A) and loss of resilience (1B); in grade 2 are based on surface damage less than (2A) or equal to or more than (2B) one half the thickness of the cartilage; and in grade 3 depend on whether the subchondral bone has a normal contour (3A) or shows evidence of cavitation with actual loss of bone (3B). The diameter of the lesion is recorded at 5-mm intervals from less than 10 mm to more than 25 mm. The location of the lesion on the femur and tibia as well as on the patella are noted. The degree of knee flexion also is recorded for patellofemoral lesions.

Although somewhat qualitative and subjective, this classification system enables a surgeon to record observed articular cartilage changes during the initial arthroscopy and subsequent follow-up arthroscopies. This proposed system is helpful in comparing treatment results between different studies. In addition, a point scaling system is applicable for research purposes to facilitate computerization and statistical analysis of data.

▶ Arthroscopy has created a unique opportunity to observe the articular cartilage of joints earlier than was generally the case when open surgery was the only resort. To relate the changes in articular cartilage to the subsequent course of the patient, it is necessary to have some objective system of classifying cartilage damage. The system proposed in this paper is an improvement over previous systems and has the advantage of being fairly intuitive: the surface is described in 3 categories and the depth of the lesion described by a suffix A or B. In addition, the diameter and location of the lesion are specified. If this system becomes widely accepted, it may be possible to relate cartilage damage to the subsequent course and predict which lesions are more worrisome, which lesions are less worrisome, and, for example, what type of lesion in the lateral compartment of a knee would prejudice against successful outcome from tibial osteotomy.—C.B. Sledge, M.D.

Osteochondritis Dissecans and Other Lesions of the Femoral Condyles
Bradley J, Dandy DJ (Newmarket Gen Hosp; Addenbrooke's Hosp, Cambridge, England)
J Bone Joint Surg [Br] 71-B:518–522, May 1989

Femoral condylar lesions seen in 5,000 consecutive arthroscopies were reviewed to distinguish and characterize acute and old osteochondral fractures, chondral separations, chondral flaps, and osteochondritis dissecans.

Chondral separation was defined as full-thickness separation of an area of normal articular cartilage, exposing subchondral bone. If only part of the cartilage thickness was involved, a chondral flap was diagnosed. In developing osteochondritis dissecans, a single area of ossification develops separately from the main body of an otherwise normal epiphysis. In late osteochondritis, loose bodies arise from a concave defect on the condyle. If disappearance of subchondral bone left a cavity roofed by a plate of cortical bone, idiopathic osteonecrosis was diagnosed.

Old osteochondral fractures were distinguished readily from late osteochondritis dissecans. Both developing and late osteochondritis were found only on the medial femoral condyle. An expanding concentric lesion typically appeared in the second decade of life and progressed to a concave steep-sided defect in the mature skeleton. Idiopathic osteonecrosis was distinguished from other disorders by bone loss and the absence of cortication.

Osteochondral fractures result from acute trauma, not a "dissecting" pathologic process. Developing osteochondritis dissecans is characterized by an expanding concentric lesion at the margin of an otherwise normal epiphysis. Mobile fragments attached at their periphery by articular cartilage represent separation of an osteochondritic fragment from its bed.

▶ The authors propose a useful method of classification of lesions of the femoral condyles, especially osteochondritis dissecans, and suggest criteria to distinguish between recent lesions and late lesions. As efforts continue to develop systems of nomenclature and evaluation for cartilage lesions to unravel the natural history of such lesions, classification systems such as the one proposed in this paper become especially useful.—C.B. Sledge, M.D.

Effects of Salicylate on Chondrocytes From Osteoarthritic and Contralateral Knees of Dogs With Unilateral Anterior Cruciate Ligament Transection
Slowman-Kovacs SD, Albrecht ME, Brandt KD (Indiana Univ, Indianapolis)
Arthritis Rheum 32:486–490, April 1989 4–57

Salicylates suppress proteoglycan synthesis by normal articular cartilage, and this inhibitory effect is much greater in osteoarthritic (OA) cartilage. To determine whether isolated OA chondrocyte is inherently more susceptible to the effects of salicylate on glycosaminoglycan (GAG) metabolism, isolated chondrocytes from the articular cartilage of dogs with unilateral OA and normal controls were incubated in the presence or absence of sodium salicylate.

Salicylate suppressed GAG synthesis by chondrocytes in the OA knees as much as it inhibited GAG synthesis by normal chondrocytes. In contrast, chondrocytes in the contralateral knees of dogs with unilateral OA were notably resistant to the effects of salicylate.

Salicylate has a direct effect on the OA chondrocyte. The OA chondrocytes, however, are no more vulnerable to the effects of salicylates than are those in normal cartilage.

▶ The role of salicylates in treatment of osteoarthritis and chondromalacia has been controversial for many years. Early reports suggested a beneficial effect in experimental OA, but subsequent studies, such as this, have failed to demonstrate any protective effect. Indeed, this paper reports that salicylates suppress proteoglycans (in both normal and osteoarthritic cartilage) and suggests that salicylates may indeed be detrimental in the treatment of osteoarthritis by preventing synthesis of new matrix.—C.B. Sledge, M.D.

Resurfacing of the Knee With Fresh Osteochondral Allograft
Meyers MH, Akeson W, Convery FR (Univ of California, San Diego; Rancho Los Amigos Hosp, Downey, Calif; Parkland Mem Hosp, Dallas)
J Bone Joint Surg [Am] 71-A:704–713, June 1989 4–58

The promising results of replacing the articular surfaces of various joints with fresh osteochondral allografts prompted a trial of this procedure in 58 patients who had disabling pain after previous attempts had failed. The diagnoses included osteochondritis dissecans of the femoral condyle; patellar chondromalacia; traumatic arthritis of the tibial plateau; and unicompartmental degenerative arthritis. Follow-up averaged 3.5 years. Weight bearing was not allowed until graft incorporation was evident on x-ray film, which usually required 12–20 weeks.

A modification of the hip rating system of d'Aubigné and Postel (table) indicated excellent results in 13 knees, good results in 14, and fair results in 4. Nine failures occurred, for a success rate of 77.5%. All 10 operations for osteochondritis of the femoral condyle succeeded. One infection ultimately necessitated amputation.

A fresh osteochondral shell allograft is recommended for the treatment of posttraumatic arthritis of the patella and chondromalacia of the patellofemoral joint, as well as posttraumatic arthritis and defects of the tibial plateau. The femoral condyle is treated in this way for traumatic defects,

Knee-Rating Scale

No. of Patients Preop.	Points*	Criteria	No. of Patients Postop.
		Pain	
2	1	Severe; not relieved by rest and analgesics	0
15	2	Severe; relieved by rest and analgesics	0
13	3	Moderate; regular analgesics needed	1
1	4	Mild; occasional analgesics needed	2
0	5	Minimum; occasional ache	8
0	6	None	20
		Function	
3	1	Bedridden or household walker with two canes or crutches	0
5	2	Time and distance outside limited; walks with canes or crutches	0
15	3	Walks >0.8 km with external aids; going up and down stairs limited	1
6	4	Walks >0.8 km with or without external aids; going up and down stairs not limited	1
2	5	No canes; limps	16
0	6	Unlimited walking without a limp	13
		Range of motion	
0	1	<60° of flexion	0
1	2	15 to 90° of flexion	0
4	3	0 to 90° of flexion	0
5	4	>90° of flexion; ≤15° extension lag	1
21	5	>90° of flexion without extension lag	8
0	6	≥130° of flexion without extension lag	22

*Excellent, 18 points; good, 15–17 points; fair, 12–15 points; and poor, less than 12 points. (Courtesy of Meyers MH, Akeson W, Convery FR: *J Bone Joint Surg [Am]* 71-A:704–713, June 1989.)

osteochondritis, or avascular necrosis. The procedure is not recommended for unicompartmental degenerative arthritis involving both the femur and tibia.

The allograft must be fresh and should not include more than 1 cm of subchondral bone. Chips of autologous bone are used to lift the graft as needed for maximal contact with host bone; a firm press-fit must be obtained except in the patella, where screws are used. The joint must be stable. Early joint motion is important, but weight bearing is prohibited until the graft is totally incorporated.

▶ The treatment of cartilage defects in young patients has no satisfactory answer; they generally are considered too young for joint replacement, but the presence of a full-thickness cartilage lesion in a weight-bearing joint often produces chronic disabling symptoms. Resurfacing such defects with living articular cartilage is an attractive possibility. The success rate of 78% reported in this series is cause for cautious optimism; infection resulting in amputation tempers one's enthusiasm. The 12- to 20-week period of non-weight bearing after the operation is troublesome, but appears to be warranted. It is unfortunate that the results in this series are reported as excellent, good, fair, or poor on a cumulative basis; with no result is it possible to determine whether the cause of a less than excellent result was incomplete pain control, limited function, or decreased range of motion. Nevertheless, in selected lesions involving 1 surface of the knee, this technique shows promise if the results reported in this paper can be duplicated by other investigators.—C.B. Sledge, M.D.

Repair of Rabbit Articular Surfaces With Allograft Chondrocytes Embedded in Collagen Gel
Wakitani S, Kimura T, Hirooka A, Ocho T, Yoneda M, Yasui N, Owaki H, Ono K
(Osaka Univ, Osaka; Natl Defense Med College, Tokorozawa, Japan)
J Bone Joint Surg [Am] 71-A:74–80, January 1989   4–59

Transplantation of isolated chondrocytes to rabbit articular surfaces has had a low success rate. To overcome the loss of viability in the transplanted cells and help fix the chondrocytes in the defect, chondrocytes were isolated from articular cartilage, preserved at $-196C$, thawed, suspended in solution, gelated, and then transplanted into full-thickness defects in the articular cartilage of rabbits.

The histologic appearance of the repaired tissue 24 weeks later was similar to that of hyaline cartilage in at least 75% of rabbits, as opposed to the fibrocartilage in control defects. Autoradiographs showed that the chondrocytes in repair tissue originated from the transplanted cells. The newly synthesized collagen in the experimental group was mostly type II, unlike the control group, which had type I collagen. Direct and indirect blast formation reactions showed no significant immunologic enhancement by either chondrocytes or collagen in the rabbits that had cell transplantation.

The use of allograft chondrocytes embedded in collagen gel holds promise for treating damaged articular cartilage in human beings. The chondrocytes remain viable during preservation and transplantation. The collagen gel can be molded to fit the defect, fixes the cells, and provides a good environment for matrix macromolecular synthesis.

▶ The authors demonstrate that allograft articular chrondrocytes embedded in a collogen gel can be transplanted successfully into full-thickness defects in rabbit articular cartilage. These results point toward further research, the result of which may provide the basis for biologic resurfacing of articular cartilage defects.—R. Poss, M.D.

The Biologic Concept of Continuous Passive Motion of Synovial Joints: The First 18 Years of Basic Research and Its Clinical Application
Salter RB (Univ of Toronto)
Clin Orthop 242:12–25, May 1989   4–60

The concept of continuous passive motion (CPM) of synovial joints is derived from the limited ability of articular cartilage to heal or regenerate, and from the adverse effects of immobilization on joints. Many studies have confirmed that CPM stimulates pluripotential mesenchymal cells to form articular cartilage and accelerates the healing of articular tissues. Continuous passive motion is superior to both immobilization and intermittent active motion in preventing joint stiffness and stimulating articular healing. Its usefulness is suggested by studies of intra-articular fractures, septic arthritis, patellar tendon lacerations, and periosteal grafts.

Devices of CPM are being produced for the ankle, ankle-knee-hip, finger, elbow, and shoulder. Continuous passive motion has been started immediately after operation and continued for at least 1 week. Clinical devices operate at a rate of 1 complete cycle in 45 seconds. Indications have included open reduction of fractures; arthrolysis for posttraumatic arthritis; release of joint contractures; total arthroplasty; tendon repair; ligament reconstruction; and synovectomy for rheumatoid disease. Patients who have received CPM are relatively free of pain. It is possible that the continuous generation of proprioceptive impulses blocks the transmission of pain impulses to the brain.

▶ Doctor Salter has pursued the concept of CPM for 20 years and has produced an impressive body of evidence to support its usefulness in the treatment of patients with intra-articular fractures, acute septic arthritis, articular grafts, and more recently, total joint replacements. In this paper he reviews the basic research leading up to this important contribution to the management of joint injuries.—C.B. Sledge, M.D.

Magnetic Resonance Imaging

Magnetic Resonance Imaging of Achilles Tendon Ruptures
Keene JS, Lash EG, Fisher DR, DeSmet AA (Univ of Wisconsin, Madison)
Am J Sports Med 17:333–337, May–June 1989   4–61

Reportedly, magnetic resonance imaging (MRI) can demonstrate Achilles tendon rupture. To determine the amount of separation between the ends of the tendon or the condition and orientation of the torn fibers, MRI images of 3 acute Achilles tendon ruptures were correlated with findings during surgical repair. The findings were specifically compared as to the condition of the tendons (e.g., shredded or uniform), and orientation (e.g., anterior or retrograde), of the fibers. Width of the diastasis was noted between the ends of the tendon with and without ankle flexion.

All parameters were assessed accurately with MRI. Tendon tears were best delineated on the sagittal T_2-weighted sequence (Fig 4–13). The T_1-weighted sequence assisted in differentiating fat from hemorrhage and in excluding occult bone trauma.

Magnetic resonance imaging is not needed to establish the diagnosis of Achilles tendon rupture. If further information regarding the condition, separation, or orientation of the ends of the tendon is desired, MRI is an accurate noninvasive means of evaluating these parameters. This tech-

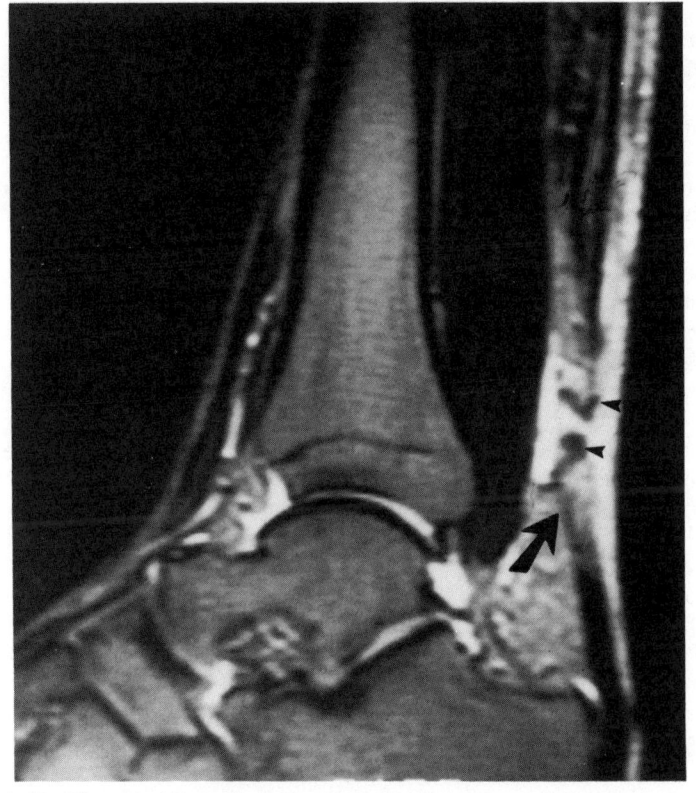

Fig 4–13.—The sagittal T_2-weighted (TR, 2,000; TE, 90) image reveals that the location of the Achilles tendon tear represents a 2-cm gap composed of high signal blood and small fragments *(arrowheads)* of low signal, nonapposed tendon. The distal end of the tendon *(arrow)* has high signal intensity representing intra-tendinous hemorrhage. (Courtesy of Keene JS, Lash EG, Fisher DR, et al: *Am J Sports Med* 17:333–337, May–June 1989.)

nique is suggested: The ankle is plantar-flexed 25 degrees. Axial T_2-weighted images 10 mm thick are obtained to localize the tendon for thin sagittal slices. Axial sections also help delineate additional abnormalities (e.g., anterior hemorrhage). Then 3-mm-thick sagittal T_1- and T_2-weighted images are obtained through the proximal and distal ends of the tendon and the diastasis. Thicker sections are not recommended because some clarity is lost.

▶ As experience with MRI increases, diagnostic capabilities for the musculoskeltal system are being realized. Rupture of the Achilles tendon usually is established easily on physical examination, but the width of the gap and the status of the torn ends cannot be appreciated. In this study, MRI is demonstrated to provide a useful noninvasive method of visualizing the torn ends of the Achilles tendons and demonstrating the width of the gap. It should be a useful adjunct in certain cases to facilitate planning of operative intervention or, perhaps, help with the decision to treat these tears with closed treatment or operative repair.—C.B. Sledge, M.D.

Treatment of Dislocation of the Hip, Detected in Early Childhood, Based on Magnetic Resonance Imaging
Bos CFA, Bloem JL (Univ of Hosp, Leiden, The Netherlands)
J Bone Joint Surg [Am] 71-A:1523–1529, December 1989   4–62

Closed reduction is the preferred treatment for children with congenital dysplasia of the hip that is diagnosed after the child begins to walk; arthrograms are taken to confirm reduction. In 7 children in whom congenital dislocation of the hip was diagnosed after they began to walk, magnetic resonance imaging (MRI) provided important data for treatment.

In 5 children, closed reduction could not be achieved and open reduction was necessary. Preoperative MRI indicated an inverted labrum, capsular adherence to the ilium, and a displaced transverse ligament. In 2 patients, MRI disclosed a stretched capsule; after closed reduction, the capsule appeared to have been detached from the acetabular rim. Subsequent to prolonged immobilization, the capsule had shrunk. These children appeared to have long-standing congenital dislocation of grade I described by Ogden and by Dunn.

In persistent congenital hip dislocation, MRI allows better treatment planning than possible with plain films or arthrograms alone. The images show 2 different developmental patterns. Some hips in Ogden's and Dunn's grade I classification with persistent dislocation treatable by closed reduction with prolonged immobilization constitute a subgroup of this grade not previously described.

▶ Recent literature has recommended ultrasonography as a valuable diagnostic tool in the discovery of clinically inapparent congenital hip dislocation. In this paper, the role of MRI is assessed in the detection and planning of treatment in children in whom congenital dislocation is diagnosed after they begin to walk. These imaging modalities should greatly accelerate improvements in the detection and treatment of this continuing and seemingly preventable problem.—R. Poss, M.D.

Common Pitfalls in Magnetic Resonance Imaging of the Knee
Watanabe AT, Carter BC, Teitelbaum GP, Bradley WG Jr (Huntington Med Research Inst, Pasadena, Calif)
J Bone Joint Surg [Am] 71-A:857–862, July 1989   4–63

How often do normal ligamentous and tendinous structures mimic pathologic changes in the knee? In a review of magnetic resonance (MR) examinations of 200 knees in patients aged 8 to 83 years, most studies were done for suspected internal derangement of the knee.

The course of the transverse geniculate ligament simulated a tear of the anterior horn of the lateral meniscus in 22% of sagittal MR scans, but no tear was found in the patients having arthroscopy. The anterior branch of the meniscofemoral ligament—Humphry's ligament—was seen in one third of the studies. The posterior branch, or Wrisberg's ligament, also was identified in one third of scans. Only 1 of 32 patients having arthroscopy actually had a loose body. In about one fourth of studies the bursa of the popliteus tendon simulated a tear of the posterior horn of the lateral meniscus. Two of 11 patients had a tear at this site on arthroscopy. Increased signal intensity consistently was present at the site of the intraligamentous bursa of the medial collateral ligament and between the lateral collateral and lateral capsular ligaments.

Normal structures of the knee are a common source of potential false-positive diagnoses of internal derangement. A close knowledge of the normal anatomy will help avoid this pitfall.

▶ Magnetic resonance imaging of the knee is still in its infancy, and only a fraction of the information available on these studies is currently understood. This review of 200 knee examinations reveals that normal structures, if not recognized, can give rise to a false positive diagnosis of abnormality, especially meniscal tears. The ligaments of Wrisberg and Humphry can be misinterpreted as osteochondral or meniscal fragments. The bursa of the popliteus tendon can simulate a tear of the lateral meniscus.

As we gain more experience with this powerful method of examination of the knee, it is important to correlate the images with other examinations, including physical examination, until experience and better resolution improve the accuracy and reliability. False positives, rather than false negatives, complicate interpretation; a negative examination can be accepted with more confidence.—C.B. Sledge, M.D.

Double-Blind Assessment of the Value of Magnetic Resonance Imaging in the Diagnosis of Anterior Cruciate and Meniscal Lesions
Glashow JL, Katz R, Schneider M, Scott WN (Lenox Hill Hosp, New York)
J Bone Joint Surg [Am] 71-A:113–119, January 1989   4–64

An accurate noninvasive diagnostic test for internal derangement of the knee is needed. Magnetic resonance (MR) imaging has many advantages, but its objective accuracy for this purpose is not known. The usefulness of MR imaging in the accurate interpretation of pathologic intra-articular changes in the knee was assessed in a prospective double-blind study.

Forty-seven patients scheduled to have arthroscopy and 3 who were to have arthrotomy volunteered to undergo MR imaging before surgery. The radiologists had no clinical or radiographic data on the patients before the assessment of MR images. Radiologists' interpretations were not known to the surgeon before arthroscopy or arthrotomy was performed. Observations were limited to findings in the menisci and anterior cruciate ligament. For pathologic findings in the menisci, MR imaging had a positive predictive value of 75%, a negative predictive value of 90%, sensitivity of 83%, and specificity of 84%. For complete tears of the anterior cruciate ligament, MR imaging had a positive predictive value of 74%, a negative predictive value of 70%, sensitivity of 61%, and specificity of 82%.

When combined with clinical and radiographic examination, MR imaging provides the most accurate noninvasive source of information for pathologic findings in the menisci and anterior cruciate ligament.

▶ Fifty patients who were to undergo either arthroscopy or arthrotomy had evaluation of their knees with MR imaging before surgery. Assuming that observation of the anterior cruciate ligament and menisci at the time of surgery is infallible, MR imaging was found to have a positive predictive value of 75% for meniscal injuries, a negative predictive value of 90%, and somewhat lower predictive value for anterior cruciate ligament injuries. The authors appropriately stress the necessity for both clinical and routine radiographic examination of the knee, in addition to MRI, to establish the appropriate pathologic diagnosis as no single technique is entirely reliable.—C.B. Sledge, M.D.

Chronic Complicated Osteomyelitis of the Lower Extremity: Evaluation With MR Imaging
Mason MD, Zlatkin MB, Esterhai JL, Dalinka MK, Velchik MG, Kressel HY (Hosp of the Univ of Pennsylvania, Philadelphia)
Radiology 173:355–359, November 1989   4–65

Recent studies have shown that magnetic resonance (MR) imaging is useful in diagnosing bone and soft tissue infection and in defining the limits of infection. The diagnostic performance of MR imaging in determining the presence or absence and extent of active infection in patients with extensive acute and chronic bone and soft tissue deformity from previous trauma and surgical procedures was reported.

Fourteen patients underwent preoperative MR imaging with a 1.5-tesla superconducting magnet. Magnetic resonance imaging findings were confirmed by reviewing the clinical, surgical, histologic, and microbiologic records of the patients. Eleven of 14 examinations were true-positive, 2 were true-negative, 1 was false-positive, and none was false-negative. Five indium scans were true-positive; 3 were true-negative; none was false-positive; and 3 were false-negative. In 2 amputated extremities, there was a close correlation between the extent of disease on surgical and pathologic assessment and that on MR imaging, which delineated the course of sinus tracts.

Magnetic resonance imaging appears promising in the detection of osteomyelitis superimposed on chronic tissue changes from old infection, trauma, and surgery. It was helpful in the surgical planning for the patients in this series.

▶ It is difficult to determine the extent of involvement in osteomyelitis with conventional clinical or radiographic techniques. This study suggests that MR imaging is more sensitive than indium scanning and gives a better estimate of extent of involvement.—C.B. Sledge, M.D.

Vascular Damage Trauma

The Use of Quantitative Bacterial Counts in Open Fractures
Moore TJ, Mauney C, Barron J (Charlotte Mem Hosp, Charlotte, NC)
Clin Orthop 248:227–230, November 1989   4–66

Late infection remains a problem in treating open fractures. Once sepsis develops, significant morbidity may be expected. The recent trend toward early soft tissue coverage of open fracture wounds prompted a prospective study of quantitative bacterial counts in 50 patients with 52 such fractures. The average age was 31 years. Thirty-five patients had multiple injuries. Thirty-eight patients had lower limb fractures, and 14 had upper extremity fractures.

Forty-one fractures were associated with positive quantitative bacterial counts. Late sepsis developed in 4 of 8 patients having counts exceeding 10^5 and in 2 of 44 having lower counts. Bacterial counts were not correlated with the time of débridement. A significant porportion of patients had gram-negative isolates.

There is evidence that a quantitative bacterial count after débridement of an open fracture is more predictive of infection than are quantitative counts made before débridement. If the count exceeds 10^5 at any time, further medical treatment should be considered before definitive fracture care and soft tissue coverage.

▶ Much controversy has surrounded the question of whether quantitative bacterial counts in open fractures are useful. The authors of this paper demonstrate the usefulness of quantitative bacterial counts *after* débridement and cleansing of open fractures and suggest that this is much more predictive of outcome than counts done before débridement.—C.B. Sledge, M.D.

Arterial Injury Complicating Knee Disruption
Varnell RM, Coldwell DM, Sangeorzan BJ, Johansen KH (Univ of Washington; Harborview Med Ctr, Seattle)
Am Surg 55:699–704, December 1989   4–67

Dislocation of the knee (DK) is accompanied by a substantial risk of popliteal artery injury, and the use of arteriography in ruling out occult arterial injury in DK is well accepted. Because DK may occur and then reduce spontaneously, an occult arterial disruption may still be present despite absence of an obvious dislocation. Hence, arteriograms have been performed routinely in all trauma patients who have sustained extensive knee ligamentous disruptions (LD) without DK. The validity of this policy was tested in 30 patients, 19 with DK, and 11 with severe LD.

The incidence of major (22% vs. 18%) or minor (38% vs. 36%) vascular abnormalities did not differ significantly between patients with DK and those with LD. Doppler arterial pressure measurements were highly predictive of major arterial injury. No clinically significant arterial injury was discovered among the 17 patients who underwent formal arteriographic examination in the angiography suite. In contrast, 4 of 12 patients (33%) who had "1-shot arteriograms" in the operating room had major vascular injuries.

Arterial injury should be ruled out in all trauma patients with severe knee LD, whether or not DK is present. Doppler pressure measurements in screening injured extremities for occult arterial injury prove promising. The "1-shot arteriogram" provides rapid localization of the level of injury in a patient highly suspected clinically to have vascular injury. A combined digital angiographic-surgical suite may be optimal in the management of potential vascular injuries, including knee disruption.

▶ Dislocation of the knee is a serious injury, frequently resulting in amputation. As the frequency of this injury is increased with increased numbers of pedestrian–automobile collisions, improved management becomes mandatory. Because of the high rate of amputation accompanying unrecognized injury to the popliteal artery, the authors recommend arteriography in all patients first seen with grossly unstable knees. They point out that Doppler pressure measurements are highly predictive of major arterial trauma and may be used to select appropriate patients for arteriography. Avoiding an unnecessary trip to the angio suite will significantly expedite getting these patients to the operating room for wound care.—C.B. Sledge, M.D.

Vascular Injury About the Knee: Improved Outcome
Thomas DD, Wilson RF, Wiencek RG (Wayne State Univ, Detroit)
Am Surg 55:370–377, June 1989   4–68

Forty-one patients seen within 8 years with 43 vascular injuries about the knee were reviewed. Injuries included 34 to popliteal arteries, 5 to tibial-peroneal trunks, 3 to isolated popliteal veins, and 1 to the proximal anterior tibial artery. Gunshot injuries predominated in this series. Two thirds of patients had fractures. The popliteal vein was injured in more than half the patients, and one third had nerve injuries. Nine patients were in shock when first seen.

Primary arterial repair was carried out in 19 extremities. A lateral repair was used for a tibial-peroneal trunk injury. Saphenous vein grafts were used in 13 limbs, and a vein patch in 1. Expanded polytetrafluoroethylene grafts were used in 5 extremities. Nine popliteal vein injuries were repaired primarily, and 1 was treated with a saphenous vein patch. Fasciotomy was done initially on 27 lower extremities.

Four patients needed major limb amputations. Significant wound infection or local tissue necrosis developed in 9 patients, necessitating multiple débridements. Three of these patients went on to amputation. Osteomyelitis developed in 4 patients. Local tissue complications occurred only in limbs with ligated veins. One patient died in renal failure caused by prolonged shock and myoglobinuria.

Amputation rates for popliteal artery injury have decreased markedly. Factors influencing the prognosis include the severity of injury; associated vein, nerve, bone, and soft tissue injuries; and the warm ischemia time. Delay in operating for longer than 6–8 hours increases the amputation rate. Angiography is useful, especially in patients with knee dislocation. Early fasciotomy promotes limb salvage.

▶ Severe vascular injuries associated with trauma to the knee are limb-threatening unless properly managed. This paper emphasizes that every effort must be made to reduce warm ischemia time and carry out early vascular repair and fasciotomy in most cases. One technique that can diminish the delay between arrival in the emergency room and definitive establishment of perfusion is to carry out arteriographic studies in the operating room rather than accept a significant delay for formal arteriographic studies before proceeding to the operating room. In spite of the excellent care described in this paper, 4 patients needed amputation, emphasizing the severe nature of these vascular injuries that often are accompanied by severe disruption of muscle, nerve, and bone.—C.B. Sledge, M.D.

Compartment Syndrome

Evaluation of Injection Techniques in Recording of Intramuscular Pressure
Styf J (Univ of Göteborg, Sweden)
J Orthop Res 7:812–816, October 1989   4–69

Needle manometry is a valuable complement to clinical signs in diagnosing acute and chronic compartment syndromes. However, the accuracy of pressure reading by the injection technique has not been evaluated.

Intramuscular pressure was recorded with a 1.2-mm needle and a 1.05-mm Myopress catheter connected to an electromagnetic transducer. The catheter had 4 side holes in the tip. Three different studies were performed: in the first study, intramuscular pressure was recorded unilaterally in the anterior tibial muscle of 12 healthy subjects. The second study evaluated different ways of recording pressure with the needle injection technique in 12 patients with bilateral medial tibial syndrome. In the third study, the accuracy of pressure reading on the manometer gauge using the naked eye was compared with pressure monitoring on a chart recorder. Subjects were the same as those in the second study.

After an injection of 0.07 mL, intramuscular pressure was significantly higher when it was recorded with the injection needle. Pressure recorded with an injection needle using the "meniscus method" was significantly closer to preinjection pressure compared with the injection technique described by Whitesides and others.

Pressure readings either using the meniscus method after injection or using a catheter or needle with multiple side holes improve the accuracy of the injection technique. The needle manometer technique is easily available and simple to perform. Use of the recommended methods will eliminate its drawbacks.

▶ Evaluation of intracompartmental pressures is performed frequently in patients with trauma to the lower extremities. A number of techniques are available to measure these pressures with varying ease and accuracy. This paper discusses the techniques of needle manometry and demonstrates excellent accuracy when following the precise techniques described by the authors. A needle or catheter with multiple side holes is recommended, and the "meniscus method" of determining the end point improves the accuracy.—C.B. Sledge, M.D.

The Significance of Intracompartmental Pressures in the Diagnosis of Chronic Exertional Compartment Syndrome
Mannarino F, Sexson S (Wright State Univ; St Elizabeth Hosp, Dayton, Ohio)
Orthopedics 12:1415–1418, November 1989   4–70

Chronic exertional compartment syndrome is a prevalent cause of lower limb pain in athletes, but the value of intracompartmental pressure estimates in making this diagnosis is uncertain. The results of compartment pressure testing were reviewed for 15 patients—6 with bilateral chronic lower leg pain—who underwent fasciotomy because of resistance to conservative treatment. Twenty regular recreational athletes served as a control group. Compartment pressures were measured with the wick catheter technique.

Resting compartment pressures in symptomatic patients averaged 14 mm Hg, and exercise pressures averaged 81.5 mm Hg. There was no particular intracompartmental pressure level above which symptoms consistently developed. The controls had average resting and exercise compartment pressures of 10 and 63 mm Hg, respectively. Nineteen of the 21 operations gave excellent or good results, and 2 were failures. No complications developed.

Resting and exercise compartment pressure measurements suggest chronic exertional compartment syndrome but are not conclusive. Pressures greater than 100 mm Hg are more predictive. The clinical presentation and the reproduction of symptoms on pressure testing are most useful in making the diagnosis.

▶ Exertional compartment syndrome is now a well-recognized clinical entity, but the authors of this paper point out that the manometric determination of exercise compartment pressure is not conclusive. They suggest that the clinical presentation and the reproduction of symptoms with exercise are the critical factors in making a diagnosis. Pressure readings greater than 100 mm Hg strongly support the diagnosis.—C.B. Sledge, M.D.

Osteotomy

Function After Tibial Osteotomy for Medial Gonarthrosis Below Aged 50 Years
Odenbring S, Tjörnstrand B, Egund N, Hagstedt B, Hovelius L, Lindstrand A, Luxhöj T, Svanström A (Lund, Skövde, Eksjö, and Gävle, Sweden)
Acta Orthop Scand 60:527–531, October 1989   4–71

Can sports and other activities be resumed after osteotomies in young and active middle-aged patients with early gonarthrosis? Twenty-nine patients aged 50 years and younger underwent 30 tibial osteotomies for stage I medial gonarthrosis. The median age was 42 years. Earlier knee injury had been reported for 20 extremities, and 17 knees had had meniscectomy. Closing wedge osteotomies were done.

Twenty-four patients believed they had had improvement after a median follow-up of 11 years. Twenty were able to walk 2 km or more without pain, and 12 could walk without limit. Three patients had no pain when running. Nine patients maintained high levels of activity through work or jogging. Lysholm scores for the corrected and undercorrected knees were comparable. Disease progressed in 3 patients, 2 of whom were undercorrected. Two knees, 1 of them excessively overcorrected, had lateral arthrosis at follow-up.

The degree of correction was not correlated with the Lysholm score in these cases. Recurrent varus deformity is not always associated with an unsatisfactory outcome. High tibial osteotomy is beneficial to young patients with gonarthrosis who wish to maintain active life-styles. Previous meniscectomy does not dispose to progressive gonarthrosis after tibial osteotomy.

▶ Medial compartment osteoarthritis can be treated with either tibial osteotomy or unicompartmental replacement. In the young patients reported in this series, tibial osteotomy, if effective, would be preferred to implantation of an artificial device. In this series of 29 patients with a median age of 42 years, 24 patients had improvement at follow-up averaging 11 years. This optimistic report suggests that tibial osteotomy certainly should not be abandoned, especially in patients for whom implants are not appropriate. The longevity of the good results in this series also is noteworthy.—C.B. Sledge, M.D.

Upper Tibial Osteotomy for Secondary Osteoarthritis of the Knee
Morrey BF (Mayo Clinic, Rochester, Minn)
J Bone Joint Surg [Br] 71-B:554–559, August 1989   4–72

Thirty-four consecutively seen patients aged less than 40 years underwent proximal tibial osteotomy for secondary degenerative arthritis; 33 were followed up 3 years or longer after surgery. The mean follow-up was 7.5 years. Primary abnormalities were medial meniscectomy and fracture in 11 cases each, medial plus lateral meniscectomy and osteochondritis with medial meniscectomy in 4 cases each; and osteochondritis dissecans in 3 cases.

Twenty-four operations (73%) gave satisfactory results (Table 1). Knee motion was unchanged postoperatively; no patient lost more than 5 degrees of flexion–extension. Patients with a fracture or medial meniscectomy had comparable results. All knees with both medial and lateral meniscectomies had poor outcomes (Table 2). Radiographs showed little loss of correction at last follow-up; loss of correction did not explain surgical failures. Complications included a superficial infection and a nonfatal pulmonary embolism. Eight patients needed further surgery.

Osteotomy is as effective in younger patients with secondary osteoarthritis as in older patients with primary arthritis. The prognosis is related

TABLE 1.—Pain and Activity Level Before and After Tibial Osteotomy in 33 Knees at Latest Follow-Up or Before a Revision Operation

	Pain				Activity level		
	None	Mild	Moderate	Severe	Normal	Minimal limitation	Moderate limitation
Before	0	4	22	7	0	9	24
After	13	7	6*	7	20	9*	4

*Not all these results were recorded as unsatisfactory; some had improved by 1 grade as a result of the osteotomy.
(Courtesy of Morrey BF: J Bone Joint Surg [Br] 71-B:554–559, August 1989.)

TABLE 2.—Result Related to Diagnosis

Diagnosis	Result Satisfactory	Unsatisfactory	Follow-up in years Mean (range)
Medial meniscectomy	8	3	7.1 (2 to 12)
Fracture	9	2	7.5 (1 to 12)
Medial and lateral meniscectomy	0	4	7.0 (6 to 8)
Osteochondritis dissecans	3	0	8.3 (6 to 11)
Osteochondritis dissecans and medial meniscectomy	4	0	7.3 (3 to 12)
Total	24	9	7.5 (1 to 12)

(Courtesy of Morrey BF: *J Bone Joint Surg [Br]* 71-B:554–559, August 1989.)

to the underlying cause of arthritis; osteotomy should be avoided after a lateral meniscectomy. Failures tend to occur relatively early after osteotomy.

▶ This is another paper reporting the medium-term follow-up of young patients undergoing tibial medial compartment osteoarthritis. Seventy-three percent of results were satisfactory; loss of correction was mild and did not explain the failures, and complications were infrequent. This paper provides yet another confirmation of the usefulness and safety of tibial osteotomy in selected patients.—C.B. Sledge, M.D.

Effect of High Tibial Osteotomy on Upper Tibial Venous Drainage: Study by Intraosseous Phlebography in Primary Osteoarthritis of Knee Joint
Day A, Sarma UC, Dave PK (All India Inst of Med Sciences, New Delhi)
Ann Rheum Dis 48:188–193, March 1989   4–73

An altered intraosseous vascular pattern leads to increased intraosseous pressure in osteoarthritis. The effects of high tibial osteotomy on vascular patterns in the upper tibia were studied with intraosseous phlebography in 5 patients with predominantly medial compartment osteoarthritis and genu varum and in 5 controls with normal knees. Studies were repeated 3–6 months postoperatively. Conray-280 was injected into cancellous bone in the upper tibias of patients and controls under anesthesia.

Preoperative studies of the patients with arthritis showed engorged, tortuous medullary sinusoids and slow dye clearance compared with the findings for controls. In no case was dye totally cleared within 30 minutes. The osteotomies united in all patients, and rest pain was totally relieved.

Postoperative phlebograms showed the almost total disappearance of sinusoidal outlines. Dye clearance times were markedly improved, though still abnormal, ranging from 6 to 15 minutes. Control clearance times were 3–6 minutes.

Relief of venous congestion is associated with relief of venous pain after high tibial osteotomy in patients with osteoarthritis of the knee. The relief obtained with a fenestration operation supports this conclusion, as does the lack of relationship between correction of deformity and immediate relief of pain.

▶ Why does tibial osteotomy relieve the pain of medial compartment osteoarthritis? A number of studies have shown that symptomatic relief does not relate closely to angular correction, so some other mechanism must be involved. In this paper, the authors suggest that intraosseous hypertension produces the symptoms with distention of nerve endings around engorged vessels in the osteoarthritic joint. After osteotomy, relief of venous congestion was associated with pain relief.—C.B. Sledge, M.D.

Results of Chiari Pelvic Osteotomy for Established Osteoarthritis of the Hip: A Five- to Ten-Year Follow-Up Study
Sterkers Y, Goutallier D (Hôpital Henri Mondor, Créteil, France)
Fr J Orthop Surg 3:26–32, March 1989   4-74

No ideal treatment is available for established osteoarthritis of the hip in young and middle-aged persons. Total hip replacement has a potential for medium-term loosening, particularly in young and active persons. Conservative procedures therefore are recommended for younger patients, provided the operation stabilizes the hip for a reasonable period. Since 1977, Chiari osteotomy has been used to treat established osteoarthritis in young adults and later was combined with intertrochanteric osteotomy.

Within 5 years, 32 Chiari osteotomies were performed in 31 patients (mean age, 42 years) who had established osteoarthritis of the hip. Twelve hips were classified as stage III and 20 as stage IV with the De Mourgues and Patte classification. Acetabular dysplasia without subluxation or deformtiy of the femoral head was found in 7 hips. Two hips were subluxated but had spherical femoral heads. Twenty hips had flattened femoral heads; 18 were subluxated and 2 were not. Primary osteoarthritis was observed in 3 hips. Seventeen Chiari osteotomies were isolated acetabular procedures. In 10 hips intertrochanteric valgus osteotomy preceded Chiari osteotomy at the same operation. Nine of these 10 combination procedures were done in subluxated hips with flattened femoral heads. In the remaining 5 hips pelvic osteotomy was performed as a salvage operation to delay deterioration after previous intertrochanteric osteotomy.

No infections, injuries to major vessels, or involvement of major nerves occurred except for an episode of transitory paralysis of the common peroneal nerve in 1 patient. All Chiari and intertrochanteric osteotomies united with simple bed rest for 45 days without internal fixation or plaster casting. One acetabular roof became necrotic, requiring prosthetic replacement 1 year later.

After 6 years and 4 months of follow-up, 25 hips had no clinical deterioration. Twenty-four hips either had increased or unchanged joint space and in 20 hips, improved congruity was seen. Functional results were good or excellent in 22 hips. Seven hips had clinical deterioration, 5 of which were treated with prosthetic hip replacement. The radiographic results mirrored the clinical results. Except for rapid destructive osteoarthritis, no formal contraindications could be demonstrated.

Chiari osteotomy seems to be the best salvage procedure for treating established osteoarthritis of the hip in younger patients. Older age, primary osteoarthritis, rapid deterioration, necrotic appearance or complete disappearance of the joint space probably should be considered contraindications.

▶ The Chiari pelvic osteotomy is a useful salvage procedure for adults with established osteoarthritis. Thirty-two hips were treated with either Chiari osteotomy alone or in combination with intertrochanteric osteotomy. At a mean follow-up of 6.4 years, 78% of the patients had no clinical deterioration. In younger, active patients who meet the clinical and radiographic criteria for joint preserving osteotomies, the likelihood of achieving satisfactory clinical results for at least 5 years is high. These alternative procedures should be considered when evaluating the appropriate treatment for such patients.— R. Poss, M.D.

Biomechanical Analysis of Hip Function After Chiari Pelvic Osteotomy
Koržinek K, Muftić O (Univ of Zagreb, Yugoslavia)
Arch Orthop Trauma Surg 108:112–115, February 1989   4–75

The Chiari pelvic osteotomy may lead to favorable biomechanical changes in the hip joint through femoral head medialization and shortening of the medial lever-load arm (Fig. 4–14). In contrast, unfavorable changes may occur if the abductor muscles are shortened and the resulting gluteal force is reduced. These changes are more apparent when the pelvic osteotomy is combined with intertrochanteric varus osteotomy. In some cases good radiologic results are not accompanied by a good clinical outcome.

The biomechanical results of Chiari pelvic osteotomy in 34 patients operated on during 1979–1985 were examined. A majority of patients were aged 14–15 years at the time of surgery. The best results were achieved when lateralization and distal displacement of the greater trochanter were carried out. The ratio of gluteal force to weight declined after operation, and the reaction-weight ratio also decreased.

Supplemental lateralization and distal displacement of the greater trochanter substantially improve the functional results of the Chiari pelvic

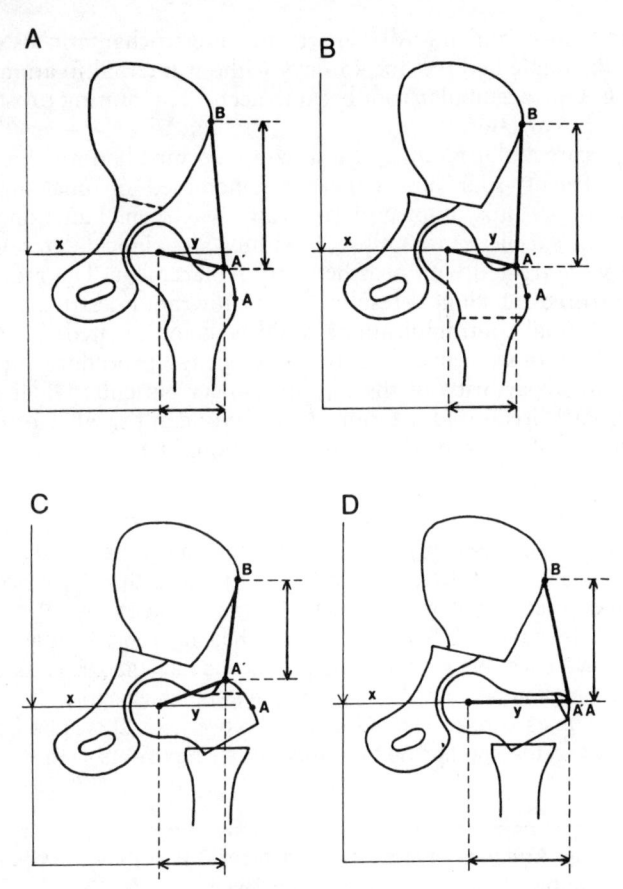

Fig 4–14.—Changes in mechanical relations within the hip joint after the Chiari pelvic osteotomy and lateralization and distal displacement of the greater trochanter. (Courtesy of Koržinek K, Muftić O: *Arch Orthop Trauma Surg* 103:112–115, February 1989.)

osteotomy. Such is the case whether or not varus and derotation osteotomies of the proximal femur are done at the same time.

▶ This is an excellent analysis of the changes in the biomechanics of the hip effected by Chiari pelvic osteotomy. Increasing the abductor level arm bilaterally and distal transposition of the greater trochanter improves function after a Chiari osteotomy.—R. Poss, M.D.

Intertrochanteric Osteotomy for Avascular Necrosis of the Femoral Head
Jacobs MA, Hungerford DS, Krackow KA (Johns Hopkins Univ)
J Bone Joint Surg [Br] 71-B:200–204, March 1989   4–76

The results of intertrochanteric osteotomy for avascular necrosis of the femoral head were reviewed in 22 patients followed up for an average of 63 months after operation. The procedures were designed to move the abnormal part of the femoral head out from under the weight-bearing acetabular dome. The average age of the 14 men and 8 women was 35 years. Seven patients had received steroid therapy, and 5 continued to receive steroids after osteotomy.

Sixteen patients (73%) had a good to excellent outcome when last seen. Six patients had had hip arthroplasty, including 4 who were receiving steroids. Range of movement was not significantly altered in the successful cases. Clinically, 2 patients had a moderate limp and 7 had a mild limp.

Survivorship analysis indicated that the chance of a satisfactory result was nearly 80% at 60 months, but fell to near 40% by 100 months. Six major orthopedic complications occurred, but there were no long-lasting significant medical complications.

Three fourths of these patients had satisfactory early results from intertrochanteric hip osteotomy for avascular necrosis. Good preoperative range of motion and a necrotic angle of less than 200 degrees are indications for this operation. Complications are frequent, but the procedure has a definite role in treating young, active patients. However, this role may change as other joint-preserving procedures are developed and the long-term results of arthroplasty become available.

▶ There is currently no best treatment option for the young active patient with progressive symptoms and stage II or III osteonecrosis of the hip. The authors report satisfactory results for the majority of patients undergoing intertrochanteric osteotomy for osteonecrosis in both stage II and stage III disease. The principle of osteotomy is to remove the affected segment from the weight-bearing sectors and achieve a necrotic angle measurement of less than 200 degrees on the combined anteroposterior and lateral radiographs. A joint preserving operation in the younger, more active age groups has substantial appeal, and these results suggest that this approach be considered as part of the treatment options for this problem.— R. Poss, M.D.

Infection in Total Joint Replacement

An Assessment of Published Trials on Antibiotic Prophylaxis in Orthopedic Surgery
Doyon F, Evrard J, Mazas F (Hôpital Cochin; Hôpital de Bicêtre, Paris)
Fr J Orthop Surg 3:49–53, March 1989   4–77

All trials of antibiotic prophylaxis in orthopedic surgery that were reported in leading international journals since 1970 were reviewed. The trials, involving various orthopedic procedures but not the treatment of compound fractures, compared prophylaxis with no treatment, a placebo, or another prophylactic antibiotic.

Among the 14 trials reviewed, those comparing prophylaxis against a placebo or no treatment suggested that prophylaxis is effective. The results obtained by Hill were most definitive. In most trials an inadequate number of patients were enrolled. Hill's study, which was well conducted, showed that antibiotics given for 5 days prevented both early and late infections after total hip arthroplasty.

The duration of prophylaxis has been quite variable in these trials. No results, however, have argued against a short duration of treatment. Such treatment involves fewer adverse effects, lower costs, and less bacterial resistance.

▶ The authors have reviewed all publications since 1970 that study the efficacy of prophylactic antibiotics in orthopedic surgery. Although the majority of these studies can be criticized in some regard, and none demonstrated superiority of 1 protocol over another, the results are unequivocal: prophylactic antibiotics are effective in reducing the incidence of perioperative infection, and they must be instituted slightly before the commencement of the operation.— R. Poss, M.D.

Shortwave Ultraviolet Radiation in Operating Rooms
Berg M, Bergman BR, Hoborn J (Univ of Gothenburg; Mölnlycke Health Care AB, Mölnlycke, Sweden)
J Bone Joint Surg [Br] 71-B:483–485, May 1989   4–78

A reduced incidence of wound infection was reported after using shortwave ultraviolet radiation (UVC) in the operating room. The effect of UVC on bacterial levels in an operating room was evaluated under experimental conditions. Twenty hip operations also were performed either under UVC or sham blue lights.

Compared with sham blue light, UVC produced a significant reduction in the number of bacteria. An ultraclean-air ventilation system can reduce the bacterial number to a recommended level of 0 to 10 colony-forming units (CFU)/m^3. The UVC system tested could reduce the bacterial count to about 15 CFU/m^3. In contrast, an operating room with a conventional ventilation system has a bacterial count of about 100 CFU/m^2.

In 1986, the cost of an ultraclean-air ventilating system was about $100,000. The UVC lights are much cheaper: about $2,000. A cost-benefit analysis has shown that a full ultraclean-air system is cost-effective only for facilities that perform more than 200 joint-replacement procedures per year.

Even though the UVC system studied was not quite as effective in reducing bacteria as an ultraclean-air system, the cost differential is large. Further studies are under way to evaluate the effectiveness of UVC in combination with different types of clothing.

▶ Numerous methods for decreasing the incidence of perioperative infection have been introduced since the laminar flow room developed by Sir John

Charnley: prophylactic antibiotics, ultraviolet radiation, body exhaust, etc. This paper demonstrates that ultraviolet light in the operating room is a cost-effective method of preventing intraoperative wound contamination and compared favorably with results produced by laminar flow ultraclean air ventilation.—C.B. Sledge, M.D.

Two-Stage Reconstruction of a Total Hip Arthroplasty Because of Infection
McDonald DJ, Fitzgerald RH, Ilstrup DM (Mayo Clinic, Mayo Found, Rochester, Minn)
J Bone Joint Surg [Am] 71-A:828–834, July 1989   4–79

Controversy surrounds treatment of an infection after a total hip arthroplasty. Most surgeons agree that the component must be removed and the area thoroughly débrided, but beyond that, the most effective means of restoring a painless functional hip is not agreed upon.

Resection arthroplasty was used to treat 82 hips that had become infected after previous total hip arthroplasty. Resection arthroplasty was followed by delayed repeat total hip arthroplasty using cement not containing antibiotics to fix femoral and acetabular components to bone.

At average 5.5-year follow-up after reimplantation, infection had recurred in 13% of hips. The presence of retained cement at the time of resection arthroplasty seemed to be associated with recurrent sepsis: 3 of 7 patients with retained cement had reinfection, whereas only 8 of 75 patients without retained cement had recurrent infection. Twenty-seven percent of patients who had reimplantation less than 1 year after resection had recurrent infections. Only 7% of hips reimplanted more than 1 year after resection arthroplasty became reinfected. Patients given antimicrobial therapy for highly virulent infection for fewer than 28 days had a high rate of recurrent infection, whereas those having treatment for more than 28 days did not.

Overall, results with 2-stage reconstruction compared favorably with other reports. Patients with highly virulent infections should receive at least 4 weeks of antimicrobial therapy, and reconstruction should be delayed for at least 1 year.

▶ Deciding when to perform reimplantation of a total hip arthroplasty after infection defies a simple algorithm because of the multiple variables that are involved. Such factors as the virulence of the infecting organism, the immune competence of the patient, the adequacy of surgical débridement, and the duration and appropriateness of the antibiotic regimen are among the major factors that must be considered. In this paper further documentation is offered to the proposition that all cement must be removed at the time of the resection arthroplasty. Newer information about bacterial resistance—in particular, the ability of microorganisms to survive antimicrobial therapy by the formation of a glycocalix—helps to explain the persistence of infection in the face of seemingly adequate antimicrobial therapy.

The authors suggest that with adequate débridement and cement removal at the time of resection arthroplasty, intravenous antimicrobial therapy for at least 28 days is sufficient. When the combination of risk factors is assessed, those patients at greatest risk of reinfection should have their second procedure delayed for longer periods.—R. Poss, M.D.

The Diagnostic Value of C-Reactive Protein in Infected Total Hip Arthroplasties
Sanzén L, Carlsson ÅS (Lund, Univ, Malmö, Sweden)
J Bone Joint Surg [Br] 71-B:638–641, August 1989   4–80

C-reactive protein (CRP) is an acute-phase protein that normally is present only in trace amounts in the plasma, but rises rapidly at the onset of acute inflammation. Whether CRP can help detect deep infections after total hip arthroplasty was investigated in 23 patients who had revision of total hip arthroplasty because of deep infection. Fifty control patients had had uneventful primary arthroplasty for osteoarthritis, and 35 had revision surgery for mechanical loosening.

Infected patients had higher prerevision levels of CRP and higher sedimentation rates than the patients with mechanical loosening. Five patients with infection had CRP values not exceeding 20 mg/L, but 4 of them had sedimentation rates of 30 mm/hour or more. Very few control patients had CRP values greater than 20 mg/L; for those who did there usually was a likely explanation.

Estimates of CRP can, along with the sedimentation rate, be of use in monitoring patients having hip arthroplasty for the development of infection. Moderate increases in either parameter are consistent with deep infection.

▶ C-reactive protein may be a valuable adjunct to the erythrocyte sedimentation rate in identifying those patients with deep infection after total joint replacement.—R. Poss, M.D.

Eikenella corrodens Cellulitis and Arthritis of the Knee
Flesher SA, Bottone EJ (Mount Sinai Hosp, New York)
J Clin Microbiol 27:2606–2608, November 1989   4–81

Eikenella corrodens is a gram-negative microorganism that produces a variety of systemic, local, and cutaneous infections. This report discusses a case of severe cellulitis and septic arthritis of the knee caused by *E. corrodens*.

Man, 22, with a history of a bleeding tendency and previous injury to his left medial meniscus, was admitted with 1 day of burning pain in his left knee and an overlying erythematous area. Four weeks before admission the patient had discomfort and swelling in his left knee similar to his previous knee problems. While the knee was still painful, the patient had undergone tooth cleaning without antibiotic prophylaxis. One week later the condition that led to his admission developed. The knee was hot, tender, red, and swollen on physical examination. Range of motion was limited by pain and swelling. The initial clinical impression was septic arthritis or cellulitis with a sympathetic effusion. The knee was aspirated, and the patient was given penicillin and oxacillin, which were discontinued when *E. corrodens* was identified with a culture. Ampicillin was started, and the patient had rapid improvement.

Eikenella corrodens should be regarded as a potential incitant in patients with similar signs and symptoms in an infection process originating from interactions with oral microflora, either through injury or dental manipulation. Early detection and prompt treatment with specific antimicrobial therapy will decrease morbidity.

▶ It has long been suspected that mouth organisms are capable of causing hematogenous seeding of prosthetic joints. This paper documents infection of a previously injured knee after tooth cleaning and adds further support to the use of prophylactic antibiotics when patients with prosthetic joints undergo dental procedures.—C.B. Sledge, M.D.

Urinary Tract Catheterization Protocols Following Total Joint Arthroplasty
Ritter MA, Faris PM, Keating EM (Ctr for Hip and Knee Surgery, Mooresville, Ind; Indiana Univ)
Orthopedics 12:1085–1087, August 1989   4–82

Three different catheterization protocols were compared in patients having total joint arthroplasty in 1986–1987. The numbers of hip and knee replacements in each group were roughly comparable. A large majority of operations were done for osteoarthritic disease.

Of 165 patients assigned to intermittent catheterization as needed, 64% needed at least 1 catheterization. The mean number of procedures per patient was about 2.5. This group had 1 postoperative urinary tract infection. Another 295 patients had in-and-out catheterization on 1 occasion, followed by anchoring of a closed drainage system if required. Of the 181 patients in this group who needed catheterization, 69% also needed anchoring of a closed system. Two patients had postoperative urinary tract infection. In group 3, 140 patients had intraoperative sterile anchoring of a closed drainage system, which was maintained for 48 hours or less. Ten of these patients later needed in-and-out catheterization. No urinary tract infections developed.

Any differences in infection rate between these groups were not important. Placement of a short-term anchored catheter in an operating room involves less patient trauma and allows postoperative monitoring of urine output. Most patients rapidly resume normal micturition after the system is discontinued.

▶ The possibility of hematogenous spread of organisms from the urinary tract to a recent joint implant is a concern. In this paper the authors examine 3 different protocols for catheterization of patinets undergoing total joint arthroplasty: intermittent catheterization; 1-time catheterization followed by indwelling catheter, if required; and intraoperative placement of an indwelling catheter. The authors demonstrated no difference in infection among 3 protocols and suggest that the placement of a catheter in a patient under anesthesia in an operating room before the procedure is less traumatic to the patient.—C.B. Sledge, M.D.

Total Knee Arthroplasty in Patients With Psoriasis
Stern SH, Insall JN, Windsor RE, Inglis AE, Dines DM (Hosp for Special Surgery, New York)
Clin Orthop 248:108–111, November 1989   4–83

Patients with progressive psoriasis have a greater risk of infection in conjunction with total joint arthroplasty because bacterial pathogens are harbored in their skin. Twenty-seven total knee arthroplasties were done in 18 patients, 10 with predominantly inflammatory disease and 8 with psoriasis with a chiefly osteoarthritic picture.

Two thirds of operations produced excellent results; 29% had poor results. Five of the latter patients went on to revision arthroplasty. Four failures were in knees with deep infection. These infections occurred up to 5 years after surgery. Three knees were successfully reimplanted after prostheses were removed and antibiotics were given intravenously. Active psoriatic lesions were controlled with a topical steroid. Three other patients had wound complications in the immediate postoperative period. In 1 of them psoriatic disease of the extremity was exacerbated.

Deep infection occurred in 17% of evaluable patients in this series. General infection rates ranged up to 2% after total knee arthroplasty. Skin care is especially important in this setting. Use of a topical steroid or other dermatologic treatment should be considered when total joint arthroplasty is planned.

▶ Every effort must be made to avoid incising through skin involved with psoriasis. Either alternative incisions must be used or the skin lesions must be cleared by medical management before surgery.—C.B. Sledge, M.D.

Salvage of Jeopardized Total-Knee Prosthesis: The Role of the Gastrocnemius Muscle Flap
Greenberg B, LaRossa D, Lotke PA, Murphy JB, Noone RB (Univ of Pennsylvania, Philadelphia)
Plast Reconstr Surg 83:85–89, January 1989   4–84

Total knee replacement requires adequate wound healing to be functionally successful. Infection, exposure, or both will jeopardize the knee prosthesis. It previously has been estimated that persistent drainage and delayed wound healing may occur in up to 17% of all primary total knee replacements. The reported overall risk of implant loss ranges between 1% and 12%. Experience with early surgical intervention is presented: gastrocnemius muscle and myocutaneous flaps were used to salvage prostheses in 10 patients with wound complications after total knee arthroplasty.

Technique.—After excisional wound débridement, the joint is entered and thoroughly irrigated with antibiotic solution. Joint fluid and excised tissues are cultured for pathogens. Size and location of the defect determine whether to use the medial or lateral head of the gastrocnemius muscle or the entire muscle unit. Dissection can be carried proximally to the level of the femoral condyles, and the muscle can be converted into a true island flap by division of its origin from the femur. After the operation, the knee is immobilized for 7–14 days with a well-padded, posteriorly placed knee immobilizer.

Eight of the 10 salvage operations were successful. All 8 patients underwent definitive débridement and muscle coverage between 3 and 7 days after skin necrosis was first noted. The 2 patients whose prostheses were ultimately unsalvageable had treatment more than 2 weeks after skin necrosis was noted. The importance of early restoration of a well-vascularized soft tissue cover to salvage a jeopardized knee prosthesis after total knee arthroplasty cannot be overemphasized.

▶ Failure of primary wound healing after total knee arthroplasty is uncommon, but usually results in disastrous consequences with infection, removal of the implant, reconstructive plastic surgery, and perhaps, successful reimplantation. The authors of this paper document the effectiveness of early surgical intervention with wide excision of necrotic tissue and rotation of a myocutaneous flap, with salvage of the prosthesis in 8 of the 10 patients so treated. All successful cases involved treatment within the first week after skin necrosis was first noted; delay beyond 2 weeks was universally unsuccessful.—C.B. Sledge, M.D.

Long-Term Results of Various Treatment Options for Infected Total Knee Arthroplasty
Morrey BF, Westholm F, Schoifet S, Rand JA, Bryan RS (Mayo Clinic, Rochester, Minn)
Clin Orthop 248:120–128, November 1989   4–85

Seventy-three infected total knee arthroplasties were treated in various ways in 1973–1984. Antibiotics alone are no longer generally accepted. Débridement is not an effective approach to chronic infection. Other options include resection arthroplasty, arthrodesis, and reimplantation. In this series 10 patients had aggressive débridement; 5 had resection arthroplasty; 43 had implant removal and attempted fusion; and 15 had implant removal and reimplantation. The average follow-up was 4.5 years.

Solid arthrodesis was achieved in 70% of cases, but 15% of patients with solid fusion had residual pain or recurrent infection. Débridement alone succeeded in 80% of cases. Reimplantation succeeded in 53% of cases, but only 33% had functionally successful results. Only 1 of 5 patients had a successful outcome after resection arthroplasty.

Leaving the prosthesis in place is preferred if infection occurs within a month of surgery and the organism is not gram-negative. Loosening precludes this approach. Acute infection is managed with aggressive débridement and primary closure over an antibiotic-soaked pack. Débridement is repeated every 2–3 days, and antibiotic beads are inserted. Rehabilitation may begin if 2 successive débridements fail to show a positive culture. Chronic infection is managed with antibiotic-impregnated beads and spacers with staged débridements.

▶ Should an infected knee arthroplasty be treated with débridement alone, fusion, or reimplantation? This large series of 73 infected total knee arthroplasties at the Mayo Clinic provides some answers to that question. Not all patients in whom fusion was attempted had a solid fusion, nor did solid fusion preclude residual pain or recurrent infection. Débridement alone, if done in the early postoperative period, succeeded in 80% of the cases. It is surprising that reimplantation was successful only 53% of the time and produced a functionally successful result only one third of the time. Our experience and that of others (1, 2) suggest greater likelihood of success with reimplantation, but delay between diagnosis and initial débridement clearly influences the success rate, as does the organism involved.—C.B. Sledge, M.D.

References

1. Wilde, Ruth: *Clin Orthop* 236:23, 1988.
2. Insall et al: *J Bone Joint Surg [Am]* 65-A:1087, 1983.

The Results of Spacer Block Technique in Revision of Infected Total Knee Arthroplasty
Booth RE Jr, Lotke PA (Rothman Inst, Philadelphia)
Clin Orthop 248:57–60, November 1989   4–86

Few options exist for a chronically, deeply infected total knee arthroplasty. Because reimplantation arthroplasty may be advantageous in selected cases, antibiotic-impregnated polymethyl methacrylate spacer blocks were used during the exchange interval in 25 patients with chronically infected knee arthroplasties. An 80-g mass of acrylic bone cement is mixed with tobramycin powder and shaped like a tibial trial—or like 2 flat bearing components—to fill the knee extension gap. The spacer block is retrieved at the time of reimplantation; little if any intracapsular soft tissue dissection is needed.

The interval between arthroplasties averaged 16 weeks, and the average follow-up was 25 months. Five patients had severe wound healing problems that ultimately healed. Twenty-one patients had excellent subjective results, and 2 others had good results. One patient had a fair outcome, and 1 failure was fused. An unexpectedly large number of patients had functional knees and were quite pleased with their outcomes. Flexion averaged 100 degrees. Seven knees lost up to 5 degrees of extension. Loss of motion was not proportional to the time of spacer block immobilization.

The timing of reimplantation is dependent in part on the appearance of the soft tissues and a patient's general health. Antibiotic use in this setting remains empirical. Little is gained from suction irrigation systems.

▶ The management of an infected knee arthroplasty is difficult. One of the most difficult aspects is how to manage the interval between removal of the infected implant and reimplantation. Most authors have recommended a delay between removal and reimplantation of at least 6 weeks to 3 months. During that time, a patient may have difficulty ambulating with an unstable knee. In addition, delivering an appropriate level of antibiotics into the scar tissue around the implant may be difficult. In an attempt to combine high local delivery of antibiotic and improve stability to the knee in the interval between removal and reimplantation, the authors recommend the use of an antibiotic-impregnated cement spacer. Using that technique in 25 patients, the authors report an excellent outcome with an average of 100 degrees of flexion after the reimplantation, 21 excellent subjective results, and 2 good results. Only 1 patient had a failure requiring fusion.

These excellent results undoubtedly result from a variety of factors such as the long interval between removal and reimplantation, the organisms involved, and surgical technique. The use of spacer block with antibiotics apparently improves the results and certainly improves the comfort and function of a patient between operations. In addition, the use of a spacer maintains an adequate gap between the resected bone ends so that subsequent reimplantation is technically easier.—C.B. Sledge, M.D.

Total Knee Reconstruction

Bone Ingrowth Into the Tibial Component of a Canine Total Condylar Knee Replacement Prosthesis
Turner TM, Urban RM, Sumner DR, Skipor AK, Galante JO (Rush-Presbyterian-St Luke's Med Ctr, Chicago)
J Orthop Res 7:893–901, October 1989

The use of porous metallic materials to achieve fixation by bony ingrowth in total joint replacement is an attractive alternative to acrylic cement. Bone ingrowth was studied in the tibial component of an unconstrained total condylar-type prosthesis designed for the canine knee, or stifle.

The tibial component consisted of a contoured surface of ultra-high-molecular-weight polyethylene bonded to a 1-mm perforated reinforcing plate of pure titanium. A 2-mm pad of 50% dense fiber metal composite was sintered to the underside of the device. Three fiber metal-coated cylindrical pegs 4 mm in diameter and 5 mm long projected from the pad surface. A posterior screw helped stabilize the device. The femoral prosthesis is cast from cobalt-chromium apply.

Six dogs had total knee replacements, which were examined 6 months afterward. All pegs of each tibial component had extensive bony ingrowth involving 12% to 81% of the pad area. In other areas the void spaces were filled with fibrous tissue or, peripherally, with fibrocartilage. Bone ingrowth in regions not adjacent to the pegs was variable. Granulomatous foci limited to the joint capsules were found in 3 animals.

The pegs of this implant strongly influence the pattern of bone ingrowth. The chief factors accounting for variable bone ingrowth in the tibial component probably are relative bone–implant motion and intimate contact.

▶ Does bone grow into porous coated tibial components of total knee arthroplasty? This experimental paper examining tibial components in a canine model showed consistent ingrowth into porous coated pegs but variable ingrowth into the plateau itself. When seen, this ingrowth usually was immediately adjacent to the fixation peg. The authors point out that the major factor contributing to variability in ingrowth probably is relative motion between the implant and the supporting bone and suggest that the techniques and the components used in cementless knee implants will be different from those used for cemented designs. The results also suggest that, when bone is particularly weak, as in rheumatoid arthritis, relative motion between the rigid implant and the weak supporting bone may be inescapable.— C.B. Sledge, M.D.

The Influence of the Surface Energy and Roughness of Implants on Bone Resorption
Murray DW, Rae T, Rushton N (Addenbrooke's Hosp, Cambridge, England)
J Bone Joint Surg [Br] 71-B:632–637, August 1989   4–88

Macrophages that adhere to bone implants might release mediators that stimulate bone resorption and thereby cause loosening. In vitro studies indicate that macrophage migration and spreading are affected by the surface energy and roughness of the material on which they are cultured. In this study, peritoneal macrophages from mice were cultured on various orthopedic materials, and conditioned media were evaluated with the neonatal mouse calvaria bone resorption assay.

The findings indicated that macrophages do release mediators that stimulate bone resorption. When the macrophages adhered to a foreign surface, the amount of bone resorption was increased up to tenfold. Bone resorption varied with the surface energy and roughness of the foreign surface but not with the chemical nature of the material. The materials used in the study included glass, stainless steel, polytetrafluoroethylene, epoxy resin, high-density polyethylene, and polymethyl methacrylate. Significantly more prostaglandin E_2 was released on a rough surface than on a smooth one.

Macrophages that adhere to bone implants release substances that stimulate local bone resorption. This may be a mechanism by which implant loosening is initiated. The roughness and surface energy of the implant appear to be more important than its chemical nature with respect to the amount of bone resorption that occurs, and therefore the risk of implant loosening.

▶ There is a great deal of discussion these days about the ideal surface for an uncemented implant. In spite of very few controlled experiments, 1 surface or the other and 1 material or the other are touted as more conducive to bone ongrowth or in-growth. This paper demonstrates that the composition of a material as well as its surface treatment influences the response of macrophages and, presumably, other cells. The results of this paper suggest that clinicians and investigators should look at the material, its coating, and its surface texture to understand the response of cellular elements to the implant.—C.B. Sledge, M.D.

Osseointegration of Metallic Implants: I. Light Microscopy in the Rabbit
Linder L (Univ of Lund, Malmö, Sweden)
Acta Orthop Scand 60:129–134, April 1989   4–89

To learn whether predictable osseointegration is dependent on the use of pure titanium, each of 38 adult rabbits was given a pure titanium implant and another implant of titanium-aluminum-vanadium alloy, chrome-cobalt alloy, or stainless steel. Follow-up times were 4 and 11 months.

New bone typically covered half to three fourths of implant circumference without an intervening soft tissue membrane. The extent of endosteal proliferation was similar with all implant materials. Only with 2 pure titanium implants and 1 of stainless steel were there only small areas of direct contact between the bone and implant surface.

Osseointegration appears to represent a basic, nonspecific healing potential of bone, not a particular reaction to a specific implant material. Failure to obtain osseointegration of a joint prosthesis reflects the inability to create a biologic environment suitable for bone formation. A tissue-oriented approach to bone implant surgery will give the surgeon more control over healing conditions and make creation of a predictable interface more likely.

Osseointegration of Metallic Implants: II. Transmission Electron Microscopy in the Rabbit
Linder L, Obrant K, Boivin G (Univ of Lund, Malmö, Sweden; Faculté Alexis Carrel, Lyon, France)
Acta Orthop Scand 60:135–139, 1989   4–90

Electron microscopic studies were carried out on 10 osseointegrated implants of pure titanium, Tivanium, Vitallium, and polished stainless steel. All implants were examined 11 months after their placement in the upper tibias of mature rabbits.

A cellular reaction was lacking but, even in cases of seemingly uniform osseointegration, unpredictable variation in the interface ultrastructure within 500–1,000 nm of the metal surface was noted with all the materials. No structural features were specific to particular implant materials. In some instances, more or less regularly arranged collagen fibrils approached to within 50 nm of the metal surface. In others, type I collagen fibrils were separated from implants by a zone of thin filamentous structures or by a zone of indistinct structures.

It is not likely that the quality of osseointegration can be determined on morphological grounds alone. True osseointegration is believed to be possible through improved tissue handling and controlling of the interface mechanics.

▶ To examine whether pure titanium is necessary for bone apposition (osteointegration), the authors of these papers (Abstracts 4–89 and 4–90) looked at the histology of implants composed of pure titanium, a titanium alloy, chrome cobalt, or stainless steel. No significant differences were seen in the degree of osteointegration with any of the materials, and it is suggested the process of osteointegration is nonspecific and not related to the chemical nature of the metal.—C.B. Sledge, M.D.

Effect of Knee Component Alignment on Tibial Load Distribution With Clinical Correlation
Hsu H-P, Garg A, Walker PS, Spector M, Ewald FD (Harvard Med School)
Clin Orthop 248:135–144, November 1989   4–91

The proper way to align the tibial component of a total knee prosthesis with respect to the long axis of the tibia in the frontal plane is uncertain. In an attempt to find the ideal position of tibial components, a test rig for force transmission to the prosthetic tibial interface was designed. Tibial components of both kinematic and total condylar prostheses were placed into artificial tibias without cement. The data were compared with postoperative roentgenograms showing radiolucent lines associated with total knee prostheses.

An even distribution of the vertical 1,500-newton load on the medial and lateral regions of the kinematic tibial component occurred at 9 degrees of valgus tilt of the femoral component and 2 degrees of varus tilt of the tibial component. For the total condylar device the figures were 7 degrees of valgus and zero varus tilt. Misalignment by 5 degrees led to a 7% change in load distribution under the kinematic prosthetic plateau, and a 40% change with the total condylar device. Misalignment by 10 degrees produced changes of 34% and 62%, respectively. In the radiographic series, radiolucent lines were least frequent with the kinematic prosthesis at 7 degrees of knee valus; the femoral component at 9 degrees of valgus; and the tibial component at 2 degrees of varus.

The clinical findings were correlated with the ideal bench-test findings for the kinematic prosthesis.

▶ Numerous papers have reported a relationship between mechanical alignment of the leg (and alignment of the implant components) and failure of total knee arthroplasty. The authors of this paper have carefully analyzed load distribution in vitro with 2 implants. Minor degrees of misalignment produce significant changes in load distribution under the tibial plateau. The total condylar implant appeared to be more sensitive to angular malalignment. The authors concluded from the in vitro portion of the study that the ideal position of a total knee arthroplasty was achieved with the femoral component in 9 degrees of valgus and the tibial component in 2 degrees of varus. They then compared the in vitro results with radiographic assessment of 21 total condylar and 532 kinematic total knee arthroplasties and showed good correlation with the in vitro study.

Failures of total knee arthroplasties are infrequent enough at 10 years to suggest that some predictor of impending failure is needed. This paper suggests that assessment of static alignment of components might be 1 such predictor of long-term success or failure.—C.B. Sledge, M.D.

Osteotomy of the Tibial Tubercle During Total Knee Replacement: A Report of Twenty-Six Cases
Wolff AM, Hungerford DS, Krackow KA, Jacobs MA (Good Samaritan Hosp, Baltimore)
J Bone Joint Surg [Am] 71-A:848–852, July 1989   4–92

Osteotomy of the tibial tubercle has been proposed for achieving exposure during total knee replacement surgery if adequate lateral retraction of the patella cannot be achieved safely. Among 24 patients who had 26 osteotomies of the tibial tubercle in conjunction with total knee replacement, the average age at surgery was 61 years. Twenty-two patients were followed up for an average of about 3.5 years.

The average range of motion was increased from 48 to 77 degrees at follow-up, and four fifths of all knees had increased motion. Four knees had an extension lag averaging 24 degrees at last follow-up. Complications occurred in 35% of osteotomies. Four knees had mechanical complications. Patients with rheumatoid arthritis and those having previous knee surgery were the most likely to have complications.

The use of at least 2 cortical lag screws promotes union without displacement. An osteotomized segment should be long enough to allow adequate space between adjacent screws, and between the screws and the edges of the osteotomy. Screws should be avoided at the distal junction of the tubercle osteotomy and the anterior part of the tibial cortex. Beveling of the distal edge of the osteotomy may lower the risk of tibial fracture at that site.

▶ Two major surgical techniques improve exposure during total knee arthroplasty if decreased motion or extensive scarring make routine measures inadequate. The more common technique is the patellar turndown described by Insall (1) and Scott (2). An alternative technique, elevation of the tibial tubercle, has been proposed (3) and is evaluated in this paper. Twenty-four patients who had that procedure were followed an average of 3.5 years. The complication rate of 35% is higher than seen with the quadriceps turndown.—C.B. Sledge, M.D.

References

1. Insall: *Surgery of the Knee.* New York, Churchill Livingstone, 1984, p 47.
2. Scott: *Orthopedics* 8:45, 1985.
3. Dolin: *J Bone Joint Surg [Am]* 65-A:704, 1983.

Autogenous Bone Grafting for Severe Angular Deformity in Total Knee Arthroplasty
Altchek D, Sculco TP, Rawlins B (Hosp for Special Surgery, New York)
J Arthroplasty 4:151–155, June 1989   4–93

Tibial deficiency associated with severe angular knee deformity causes difficulty in total knee reconstruction because reconstitution of this defect is needed for prosthetic support. A technique of tibial autografting in conjunction with total knee arthroplasty was evaluated in 14 patients with severe angular knee deformities. All tibial defects represented more than 25% of the tibial component support surface and were more than 10 mm deep. The tibial bone grafts involved bone resected from the distal femur during arthroplasty. Twelve knees received Insall-Burstein posterior stabilized total condylar knee implants. Two received constrained total condylar III implants.

Postoperative rehabilitation was uneventful, and weight bearing usually began on the third postoperative day. All grafts consolidated without evidence of resorption, collapse, or prosthetic subsidence. Clinical results were good or excellent in all cases. The average arc of motion after surgery was 90 degrees. There were no infections, and no implant had to be removed.

After an average 4.3 years, there is both clinical and radiographic evidence of graft union. Autogenous tibial bone grafting has the advantages of technical ease, no increased incidence of cement–bone radiolucency, addition to existing bone stock, and recreation of a biologic prosthetic support surface.

▶ In knees with severe angular deformity undergoing arthroplasty, several methods for managing the bony defect have been proposed: deeper bone resection, prosthetic replacement of the bony defect, allograft bone, and autograft bone. This study demonstrates excellent results achieved with autogenous tibial bone grafting in a small series of knees followed 4 years. For small defects that can be filled adequately by the small amounts of autogenous bone available, this technique is recommended.—C.B. Sledge, M.D.

Bone Grafting for Tibial Defects in Grossly Deformed Knees in Total Knee Arthroplasty
Nawalkar RR, Soudry M, Mendes DG (Haifa Med Ctr; Rappaport Family Inst for Research in the Med Sciences, Haifa, Israel)
J Orthop Surg Tech 4:95–98, 1989   4–94

Subchondral bone of good quality must be retained to achieve good results with surface replacement but, in a grossly deformed knee, this involves accepting a posteromedial or posterolateral bone defect. A simple bone grafting technique was used to correct proximal tibial bone deficiency in 14 patients having 15 total knee arthroplasties. All the implants were cemented, and autologous bone from resected parts of knees was used in all cases.

Technique.—After appropriate medial or lateral release the bony defect in the tibial condyle is assessed (Fig 4–15). No more than 5–8 mm of the height of the proximal tibia are resected, preserving the floor of the defect. The proximal tibial cut usually extends beyond the tibial midline. The area of the defect is shaped in a steplike pattern (Fig 4–16). Bone from the tibial condyle and femoral condyles has been used for grafting, but iliac bone may be used if necessary. The grafts are fixed with 1 or 2 cancellous miniscrews, countersinking the screw heads, and are roughened before cementing.

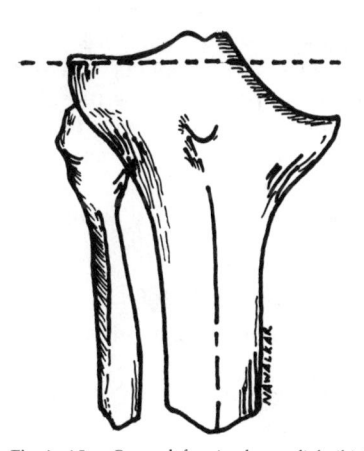

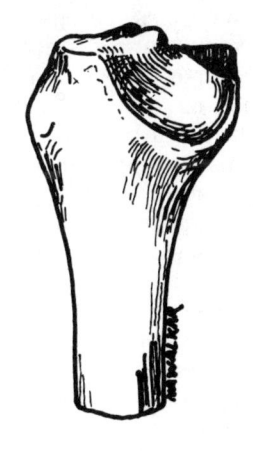

Fig 4–15.—Gross defect in the medial tibial condyle, as seen from the front and side. It usually slopes medially and backward and starts close to the anterior margin of the condyle. *Dotted line* indicates the proposed level of bone section. (Courtesy of Nawalkar RR, Soudry M, Mendes DG: *J Orthop Surg Tech* 4:95–98, 1989.)

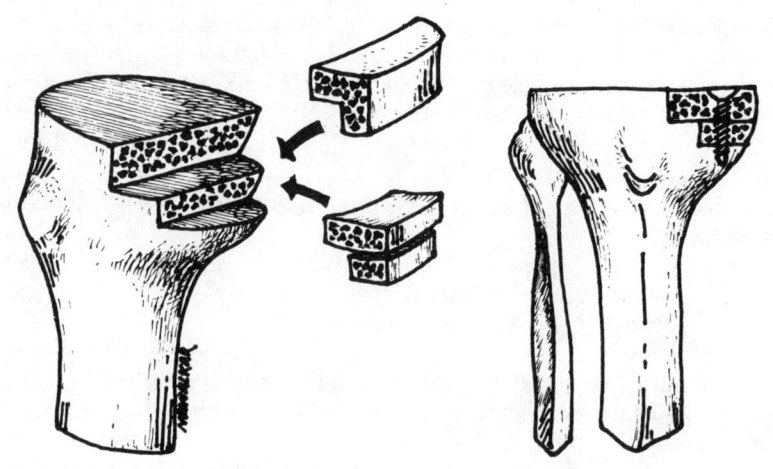

Fig 4–16.—Perspective of the proximal after preparation. Note the different shape of grafts that can be used *(left)*. Note that after fixation of the grafts with a screw or screws, they do not encroach on the area required for tibial stem fixation. (Courtesy of Nawalkar RR, Soudry M, Mendes DG: *J Orthop Surg Tech* 4:95–98, 1989.)

Seven operations yielded excellent results and 2 had good results on follow-up averaging 2.5 years. None of the 9 knees followed had radiologic signs of loosening. In no case was there tilting or subsidence of the tibial component.

When steplike cuts are used, the compressive stresses on the graft promote its incorporation. The screws used to fix the graft should not interfere with introducing the tibial stem. This is a satisfactory approach to knees with gross bone deficiency, but the method may be used in any type of surface replacement procedure.

▶ The optimal management of tibial bone defects in patients undergoing total knee arthroplasty is controversial; some authors recommend bone grafting, others recommend filling the defect with cement with or without screws and others recommend custom implants or metallic devices to fill the defect. The authors of this paper demonstrate excellent results obtained by using bone resected during preparation of the other surfaces to receive the implant. They emphasize the importance of making step cuts so that the grafts are placed under compression load. The results in this 2.5 year follow-up appear to be quite excellent.—C.B. Sledge, M.D.

Stiffness of Bone Underlying the Tibial Plateaus of Osteoarthritic and Normal Knees
Finlay JB, Bourne RB, Kraemer WJ, Moroz TK, Rorabeck CH (Univ of Western Ontario, London, Ont)
Clin Orthop 247:193–201, October 1989

Total knee arthroplasty (TKA) is an effective treatment for osteoarthritis of the knee when more conservative measures have failed. The mechanical properties of normal cancellous bone in the proximal tibia supporting TKA have been reported, but little is known about these mechanical properties in the osteoarthritic (OA) state.

Fifteen normal and 28 OA tibial plateaus were obtained at autopsy or TKA. The tibial plateaus were mechanically tested with an indentor technique to assess variations in stiffness patterns.

The ratio of medial to lateral stiffness calculated for normal plateaus was significantly different from ratios computed for specimens with either medial compartment or lateral compartment OA. The ratio was unchanged in tricompartment OA, however.

The design of TKA traditionally has been predicated on the mechanical properties of normal cancellous bone in the proximal tibia. These findings suggest that greater consideration should be given to the properties of OA bone when designing total knee replacements.

▶ The ideal prosthesis should have mechanical properties similar to those of the replaced skeletal components. This design goal is made difficult if the mechanical parameters are not known. This paper reports the stiffness of bone in the tibial plateau in osteoarthritis and compares those findings with stiffness of bone in normal knees. Wide variation was found, with all arthritic specimens showing areas of stiffness greater than those in normal bone.—C.B. Sledge, M.D.

The Cruciate Ligaments in Knee Replacement
Hagena F-W, Hofmann GO, Mittlmeier T, Wasmer G, Bergmann M (Univ of Munich)
Int Orthop 13:13–16, 1989   4–96

Little is known of how the severity of knee arthritis is correlated with the state of the ligaments. The biomechanical properties of cruciate ligaments were examined in 12 patients with severe rheumatoid arthritis or osteoarthritis in whom such ligaments were resected with their bony insertions at total knee arthroplasty. Ten specimens from healthy adults were used as controls.

Both groups had considerable variability in the lengths of the cruciate ligaments. The arthritic ligaments had degenerative changes resembling chondroid metaplasia. Ligaments in rheumatoid knees had distinctly less tensile strength than those in osteoarthritic knees. Studies of the viscoelastic behavior of the ligaments showed that damaged ligaments recovered only to about 50%, implying that their ability to absorb peak loads and dampen shocklike impulses is impaired.

It is not likely that any prosthesis can protect the cruciate ligaments, and it seems best to resect these ligaments in knee replacement surgery, at least in patients with severely damaged rheumatoid joints.

▶ The authors of this paper examine the mechanical properties of the cruciate ligaments in patients with osteoarthritis and rheumatoid arthritis with respect to the preservation or excision of these ligaments during total knee arthroplasty. The study shows that the mechanical behavior of the ligaments in these arthritic knees is highly abnormal, which suggests to the authors that resection of the ligaments during knee arthroplasty is desirable, at least in patients with severely damaged rheumatoid joints. This in vitro analysis differs, however, from the long-term clinical results reported in the literature.—C.B. Sledge, M.D.

Gait Laboratory Analysis of a Posterior Cruciate-Sparing Total Knee Arthroplasty in Stair Ascent and Descent
Kelman GJ, Biden EN, Wyatt MP, Ritter MA, Colwell CW Jr (Scripps Clinic and Research Found, La Jolla, Calif; Univ of New Brunswick, Fredericton; Children's Hosp and Health Ctr, San Diego; Center for Hip and Knee Surgery, Mooresville, Ind)
Clin Orthop 248:21–26, November 1989   4–97

Retention of the posterior cruciate ligament (PCL) during knee arthroplasty provides anteroposterior stability to the joint and aids femoral roll-back, which is critical to proper function of the extensor mechanism. Gait analysis of a PCL-sparing implant on 1 side and an opposite normal limb was carried out in 8 elderly patients who had excellent clinical results of knee arthroplasty.

Symmetric gait patterns were observed on stair descent. The sagittal angles of the hip, knee, and ankle were comparable, and dynamic ranges of motion were nearly identical in both the leading and trailing modes. Studies of stair ascent yielded similar findings, though symmetry was somewhat less than in descent. Leg angle and effective leg-length estimates compared very well under all conditions. Electromyographic studies showed a greater duration of muscle activity on the operated side; the medial hamstrings were almost continuously active. Force loads at the foot were comparable on both sides.

A highly symmetric gait pattern is observed after unilateral total knee arthroplasty. Sagittal plane measurements during stair ascent and descent are close to normal values.

▶ The theoretic argument about whether to retain the posterior cruciate ligament in knee arthroplasty continues with little evidence backing either side of the argument. In this gait analysis of 8 patients who underwent posterior cruciate-sparing unilateral knee arthroplasty, nearly normal gait in level walking, as well as in stair ascent and descent, was demonstrated. These results confirm those reported by Simon et al. (1) and Dorr (2). Whether these improved functional results will be accompanied by greater longevity of the implant remains to be seen, as failure rates for the 2 approaches are comparable at 10 years.—C.B. Sledge, M.D.

References

1. Simon et al: *J Bone Joint Surg [Am]* 65-A:605, 1983.
2. Dorr: *Clin Orthop* 236:26, 1988.

The Total Condylar Prosthesis: 10- to 12-Year Results of a Cemented Knee Replacement
Vince KG, Insall JN, Kelly MA (Cornell Univ, New York)
J Bone Joint Surg [Br] 71-B:793–797, November 1989   4–98

The total condylar knee prosthesis was introduced in 1974. This report describes results of the earliest arthroplasties and analyzes the survivorship in a series of patients.

During the first year, 104 consecutively seen patients had 130 primary knee arthroplasties using the total condylar knee prosthesis. Before surgery, 63 knees had varus angulation; 15 knees had valgus angulation; and 52 knees had femorotibial alignment between 0 and 9 degrees of valgus.

At 10- to 12-year review, 58 patients with 74 knee replacements survived and were available for radiographic and clinical evaluation. Thirty-eight knees had excellent results, 27 had good results, 3 had fair results, and 6 had poor results. Five of 6 patients with poor results had had revision surgery. In these results, the lack of an intact posterior cruciate ligament did not cause loosening of the components.

On the basis of these results, no need to develop cementless fixation of knee arthroplasties for patients similar to those of the study group is apparent. The success of this early type of prosthesis supports the continued use of methacrylate cement for knee arthroplasties.

▶ A total condylar knee prosthesis, now only rarely used, continues to demonstrate remarkable longevity as illustrated by this 10–12-year review. The authors point out that the quality of these long-term results argues strongly against cementless fixation for knee arthroplasty.—C.B. Sledge, M.D.

Mechanisms of Failure of the Femoral and Tibial Components in Total Knee Arthroplasty
Windsor RE, Scuderi GR, Moran MC, Insall JN (Hosp for Special Surgery, New York)
Clin Orthop 248:15–20, November 1989   4–99

Of 1,430 cemented primary total knee arthroplasties done in 1974–1986, 224 total condylar prostheses with a polyethylene tibial component, 289 posterior stabilized prostheses with a polyethylene tibial component, and 917 posterior stabilized prostheses with a metalbacked tibial component were implanted. The average age of patients at arthroplasty was 67 years.

Twelve failures occurred in the total condylar group, including 7 component loosenings, 3 infections, and 2 unstable arthroplasties. Six operations done with a posterior stabilized prosthesis and polyethylene tibia failed, 4 because of component loosening. Seven posterior stabilized prostheses with metal-backed tibial components failed, 6 because of infection and 1 because of femoral loosening. None of the metal-backed tibial components have been revised for loosening.

The overall failure rate in this series was 1.7%, and the overall rate of infection was 0.6%. Mechanical failures were caused chiefly by technical error and mechanical misalignment of the tibial component. A well-aligned total knee arthroplasty with balanced ligaments can be expected to serve for a long time with a low risk of mechanical failure at the femorotibial articulation.

▶ Modern knee arthroplasties fail so infrequently that a careful analysis of a large series is necessary to understand failure mechanisms. This report from the Hospital for Special Surgery analyzes 25 failures and attributes most failures to technical error with mechanical misalignment. Although the authors have used a metal-backed tibial component only since 1981, they report no failures, which is consistent with other reports of improved results in prostheses with metal support for the polyethylene tibial component.—C.B. Sledge, M.D.

Total Knee Arthroplasty for Patients Younger Than 55 Years
Ranawat CS, Padgett DE, Ohashi Y (New York Hosp; Cornell Univ; Hosp for Special Surgery, New York)
Clin Orthop 248:27–33, November 1989   4–100

Ninety-three knee arthroplasties were done in 62 patients aged less than 55 years in 1974–1982, all by the same surgeon. The mean age of patients at surgery was 49 years. A total condylar knee prosthesis was used. All but 8 patients had patellar resurfacing. Tibial plateau defects were repaired in 13 extremities.

Follow-up of 60 patients for an average of 6 years showed excellent results in 70% of cases and good results in 28%. One patient each had a fair and a poor outcome. Two thirds of operations in patients with rheumatoid disease yielded excellent results. The rate of radiolucency was 30%. Two implants were considered to be loose. There were no deep infections. Complications included 1 case each of transient peroneal nerve palsy, adynamic ileus, thrombophlebitis, and postoperative bleeding caused by coagulopathy.

These results are comparable to those obtained in older patients, and they are superior to the results of total hip arthroplasty in younger patients. Nevertheless, total knee arthroplasty is not often indicated in the young. In both young and elderly patients, good results are dependent on achieving a close cement–bone microinterlock on a wide area of cancellous bone.

▶ Total joint arthroplasty has long been reserved for older patients with reduced levels of activity for fear that the longevity of the prosthesis would be jeopardized by the activities of the younger patient. This series demonstrates that excellent long-term results of knee arthroplasty can be obtained in patients aged less than 55 years: 2 loose implants in 60 patients followed an average of 6 years.—C.B. Sledge, M.D.

Arthroplasty for the Stiff or Ankylosed Knee
Aglietti P, Windsor RE, Buzzi R, Insall JN (Univ of Florence, Italy; Hosp for Special Surgery, New York)
J Arthroplasty 4:1–5, March 1989   4–101

Results of knee arthroplasty with the posterior stabilized condylar prostheses were reviewed for 20 knees that had less than 50 degrees of motion and 6 others that were ankylosed. The average age of patients at surgery was 66 years, and the average follow-up was 4.5 years. Three fourths of the knees had osteoarthritis, and the rest had rheumatoid disease. Care was taken to avoid excessive tension on the suture line; the lateral retinacular release was left open. Where V-Y quadricepsplasty was required, the rectus tendon was joined at the apex of the V.

Twenty-one knees had excellent or good results, 3 had fair results, and 2 had poor outcomes. Two fair results were in a rheumatoid patient with bilateral involvement. Pain was absent from most patients with excellent or good outcomes and, for one third of these knees, walking was unlimited. About 40% of knees had more than 90 degrees of flexion at followup. Stiff knees did better than those that were ankylosed.

Good results can be obtained consistently when knee arthroplasty is done for a stiff or even an ankylosed knee. Motion can be improved if both cruciate ligaments are removed. The posterior stabilized condylar prosthesis will help ensure stability in flexion.

▶ Total hip arthroplasty for ankylosed hips is a fairly common procedure with good results. In contrast, there have been very few reports of arthroplasty in patients with ankylosed knees. Although 20 of the 26 patients in this study had limited motion before surgery, rather than ankylosis, the results are nonetheless worthy of study. Twenty-one of the 26 patients had excellent or good results, and only 2 had poor outcomes. The overall average arc of motion was 78 degrees, and those patients who had ankylosed knees before surgery averaged 68 degrees arc of motion after surgery. As 65 degrees of knee flexion are adequate for normal level gait, these results would appear to be quite encouraging and suggest that, with experience and careful technique, knee arthroplasty in the stiff or ankylosed knee can be rewarding with appropriate indications.—C.B. Sledge, M.D.

Bilateral Total Hip and Knee Replacement in Rheumatoid Arthritis Patients
Hoekstra HJ, Veth RPH, Nielsen HKL, Veldhuizen AG, Visser JD, Nienhuis RLF, Hoekstra AJ (Univ of Groningen; Beatrixoord, Haren, The Netherlands)
Arch Orthop Trauma Surg 108:291–295, 1989   4–102

Fourteen patients with rheumatoid arthritis underwent bilateral total hip and knee replacements in 1978–1983. The average age at the first arthroplasty was 45.5 years, and the average time from the onset of disease was nearly 13 years. There was a minimum of 2 weeks between operations. The Harris prosthesis was most often used at the hip, and the total condylar prosthesis, at the knee. Thirteen patients were followed up for an average of 6 years. All had marked relief of pain and good function. Walking ability was not always improved, but all patients were enthusiastic about the overall results of joint replacement surgery. Only 4 of 11 patients remained completely dependent after the last arthroplasty. Four patients became capable of sexual intercourse after surgery. Seven patients had no complications.

Quadruple arthroplasty is not done if severe concomitant disease is present or if the patient is poorly motivated. Severe upper extremity involvement and atlantoaxial subluxation are not absolute contraindications.

▶ The combination of involvement of both hips and both knees seen in juvenile rheumatoid arthritis has a devastating effect on function of these unfortunate young patients. This paper, like several earlier papers, demonstrates the relative efficacy of replacing all 4 involved joints in properly motivated patients. All patients in this series had improvement, although only 5 of the 14 patients achieved "excellent" results. There were no major complications.—C.B. Sledge, M.D.

Hip Fractures

Risk Factors for Falls in a Community-Based Prospective Study of People 70 Years and Older
Campbell AJ, Borrie MJ, Spears GF (Univ of Otago, Dunedin, New Zealand)
J Gerontol (Med Sci) 44:M112–M117, July 1989   4–103

Factors to distinguish elderly persons at risk of falling have not been identified clearly. A better insight into what causes elderly persons to fall not only would be helpful in patient management, but also would be useful for the development of public health programs aimed at prevention. To identify factors associated with falls by elderly persons, a community population of persons aged 70 years and more was monitored prospectively for 1 year.

The study population consisted of 761 persons who were living in the community or in residential homes. Patients in continuing hospital care were excluded from the study. All participants completed 3 assessments, including an initial assessment at home by a research nurse, an assessment at home by an occupational therapist, and an assessment at a health center by 2 physicians specializing in geriatric medicine. When a fall was preceded by loss of consciousness, cardiovascular and neurologic examinations were performed as indicated. To analyze the risk factors for falls, the circumstances of each fall were examined. Falls were divided into internal and external falls.

During the year of the study, 58 participants died and 19 left the area. The total months of observation were 5,483 for women and 3,431 for men. A total of 507 falls were reported during the monitoring period.

Persons with high rates of alcohol intake were not at increased risk of falling. No strong association was found between impaired vision and increased risk of falling. Neither was impaired memory an independent risk factor for falls. However, a history of stroke was strongly associated with an increased risk of falling.

Variables associated with increased risk of falling differed between men and women. In men, decreased levels of physical activity, stroke, arthritis of the knees, impairment of gait, and increased body sway were associated with an increased risk of falls. In women, the total number of drugs, psychotropic drugs, and drugs that can cause postural hypotension, standing systolic blood pressure of less than 110 mm Hg, and evidence of muscle weakness were associated with an increased risk of falling.

Most falls in elderly persons are associated with multiple risk factors. However, many of the risk factors identified are potentially remediable.

A Hypothesis: The Causes of Hip Fractures
Cummings SR, Nevitt MC (Univ of California, San Francisco)
J Gerontol (Med Sci) 44:M107–M111, July 1989   4–104

The incidence of hip fractures increases exponentially with age. This dramatic increase commonly is thought to be a consequence of age-related osteoporosis, which has an important role in the pathogenesis of hip fractures. However, mathematical models have not been able to explain the exponential increase in hip fractures with age on the basis of bone density alone. About 80% to 90% of all hip fractures in elderly persons are caused by falls. In addition to osteoporosis and falling, hip fractures may be the result of several age-related changes in neuromuscular function that increase the likelihood that a fall will lead to a hip fracture.

A simple fall from a standing height has several times the potential energy needed to fracture even a normal hip. To transmit this energy to the proximal femur, the primary impact of the fall must occur near the hip. Protective responses might absorb part of the energy of a fall. If the residual energy of the fall transmitted to the proximal femur exceeds a critical threshold, the proximal femur will fracture. This threshold is dependent on the strength of the bone in the proximal femur for the particular direction and rate of the force that is applied.

For a fall to cause a hip to fracture, 4 conditions must be satisfied: The falling person must be oriented to have an impact near the hip, protective responses must fail, local soft tissues must absorb less energy than required for preventing the fracture, and the bone strength must be insufficient to withstand the force of the fall. When these 4 conditions are met, the residual energy of the fall applied to the proximal femur will cause the femur to fracture.

All these factors become more pronounced with aging, which explains the exponential increase in the risk of hip fracture with advancing age. The combined measurement of neuromuscular function and bone strength may be the most accurate approach to assessing the risk of hip fractures in elderly persons.

▶ A body of thought is being developed in which hip fractures are seen as a sign of more global functional deficiencies in elderly patients. The increasing incidence of fracture of the hip cannot be explained by depletion of mineral bone content alone. These 2 studies (Abstracts 4-103 and 4-104) point to the roles of diminished neuromuscular function, decreased sensory input, associated joint and gait impairment, and the adverse affects of numerous medications taken by this age group in contributing to the high and rising incidence of fracture in the elderly.—R. Poss, M.D.

The Tension-Stress Effect on the Genesis and Growth of Tissues: Part I. The Influence of Stability of Fixation and Soft-Tissue Preservation
Ilizarov GA (USSR Academy of Sciences; Kurgan All-Union Ctr for Restorative Traumatology and Orthopaedics, Kurgan, USSR)
Clin Orthop 238:249-281, January 1989   4-105

Gradual traction on living tissues creates stresses that can stimulate and maintain the regeneration and active growth of certain tissue structures. This principle is called the Law of Tension-Stress. The application of this principle allows control of osseous healing and the shaping processes of bone and soft tissue. To determine the optimal conditions for osteogenesis during limb lengthening, and to assess the changes in soft tissues undergoing elongation, 3 series of experiments were performed on canine tibia.

The experiments were done with 480 adult dogs divided into 5 groups. In the first 3 groups, open transverse osteotomy of the tibial diaphysis, periosteum, and bone marrow was performed, and longitudinal distraction was achieved with the transfixion-wire Ilizarov circular external skeletal fixator used in configurations of differing stability. The last 2 groups of dogs were stabilized with the same Ilizarov fixator, but with two thirds and total preservation of bone marrow, periosteum, and intramedullary nutrient blood vessels at the osteotomy level.

Osteogenic activity was least in the group with the most mobility between bone ends. Osteogenesis overtook distraction and consolidated bone prematurely in the group of maximal preservation of bone marrow, blood vessels, and periosteum. In the group with two thirds preservation, osteogenesis proceeded more actively than in any of the 3 groups with complete transverse osteotomy.

The second set of experiments was done to assess the role of the direction of the elongation vector in osteogenesis by widening rather than lengthening bones, using a Ilizarov system modified for lateral distraction. Osteogenesis occurred parallel to the tension vector even when perpendicular to the bone's mechanical axis. As with longitudinal distraction, damage to the bone marrow inhibited osteogenesis.

The third set of experiments involved creating half- and full-circumference cortical defects in the tibia. In dogs with a half-circular cortical defect, new cancellous bone formed rapidly and spread far beyond the limits of the original bone marrow canal. In dogs with complete cortical diaphyseal defects, intact marrow, and uninterrupted blood vessels, the defect also filled rapidly.

The level of osteogenic activity within the distraction zone is dependent on the degree of stability and the amount of damage to the bone marrow, periosteum, and nutrient vessels at the time of osteotomy.

The Tension-Stress Effect on the Genesis and Growth of Tissues: II. The Influence of the Rate and Frequency of Distraction
Ilizarov GA (Kurgan All-Union Ctr for Restorative Traumatology and Orthopaedics, Kurgan, USSR)
Clin Orthop 239:263-285, February 1989   4-106

The quality of osteogenesis during limb elongation is dependent on the stability of external fixation and on the degree of preservation of periosteal and marrow tissues and the nutrient vessels at the level of the osteotomy. Because different rates of distraction may influence both the bone and soft tissues, these effects were examined in a canine tibia model at daily distraction rates of 0.5, 1.0, and 2.0 mm and distraction frequencies of 1, 4, or 60 steps per day. Distractions were done after both open osteotomy and closed osteoclasis.

Distraction at a rate of 0.5 mm per day frequently led to premature consolidation of the bone; a rate of 2 mm daily often resulted in undesired changes in the elongating tissues, such as a tendency for the distraction zone to fill with fibrous tissue rather than bone. Distraction of 1 mm per day produced the best results. A better outcome was achieved with a higher distraction frequency.

Osteogenesis ideally takes place in an elongating bone through formation of a physislike structure. New bone forms in parallel columns that extend in both directions from a central growth zone. The growth plate has features of both physeal and intramembranous ossification. Many types of orthopedic disorders and injuries are amenable to treatment using the tension-stress effect combined with the circular external fixator.

▶ The theory and experimental results that form the basis of this method are presented. Those interested in applying these principles in a clinical setting should be familiar with the thinking and experiments that form the scientific basis of this new treatment modality.—R. Poss, M.D.

Osteoporosis

Reduced Bone Mass in Daughters of Women With Osteoporosis
Seeman E, Hopper JL, Bach LA, Cooper ME, Parkinson E, McKay J, Jerums G (Univ of Melbourne)
N Engl J Med 320:554-558, March 2, 1989   4-107

A family history of osteoporosis often has been cited as an important risk factor, but little evidence in the literature supports this view. Whether premenopausal daughtes of women with postmenopausal osteoporosis have lower bone mass than other women of similar age was assessed in 25 mothers and 32 of their premenopausal daughters, and in 20 normal postmenopausal mothers and 22 of their premenopausal daughters. All participants were white women. Bone mineral content of the lumbar spine and femoral neck and midshaft was measured with dual-photon absorptiometry. A reference sample of 133 premenopausal and 386 postmenopausal healthy volunteers served as a control for the establishment of age- and sex-specific normative bone mineral content data.

The mothers with osteoporosis were shorter and tended to be older and weigh less than the normal mothers. The daughters of the mothers with osteoporosis did not differ in age, height, or weight from the daughters of the normal mothers. The bone mineral content in the normal mothers did not differ significantly from that in the reference sample of the postmenopausal controls. Similarly, the bone mineral content in the normal daughters did not differ significantly from that in the reference sample of the premenopausal controls. Compared with the normal postmenopausal women, the bone mineral content in the mothers with osteoporosis was lower by 33% in the lumbar spine, by 23% in the femoral neck, and by 15% in the femoral midshaft. Compared with the normal premenopausal women, the bone mineral content in daughters of mothers with osteoporosis was lower by 7% in the lumbar spine, by 5% in the femoral neck, and by 3% in the femoral midshaft.

Premenopausal daughters of women with postmenopausal osteoporosis have lower bone mass in the spine and femoral neck than do daughters of normal women and a reference population of premenopausal women, both before and after adjustment for age, height, and weight.

Ethnic and Genetic Differences in Bone Mass: A Review With a Hereditary vs. Environmental Perspective
Pollitzer WS, Anderson JJB (Univ of North Carolina, Chapel Hill)
Am J Clin Nutr 50:1244–1259, December 1989   4–108

A review of the literature indicates the significance of genetic and ethnic factors in determining bone mass, as well as dietary factors and physical activity. Real differences in bone density exist between whites and blacks, even after adjustment is made for body mass. Blacks have greater muscle mass, total body potassium, and skeletal calcium content. In genetic studies of parent–offspring pairs and twins, bone density is strongly associated with bone mineral content at specific skeletal sites.

Bone mass in females during adolescence is related to maternal bone mass and then is influenced by reproductive events until menopause, when other environmental factors become more important. Knowledge of environmental factors, such as nutritional status, physical activity and lifestyle is necessary before family resemblance and true hereditary determinants can be separated.

Hereditary factors play a strong role in bone density and mineral content. Environmental factors, such as exercise and dietary calcium, have less significance for bone mass than heredity but exert modulating influences. Further research is necessary to understand the relative contributions of genetic, hormonal, exercise, and dietary influences.

▶ These 2 articles (Abstracts 4–107 and 4–108) point to the importance of both genetic and environmental factors in the development of symptomatic osteoporosis. Two important conclusions may be derived from the paper that demonstrates decreased bone mass in the daughters of women with osteoporosis: first, that a subgroup of premenopausal women can be identified to be at increased risk of development of subsequent fracture; and second, that a likely contributory cause to their subsequent osteoporosis is their failure to obtain a sufficiently high bone mass at skeletal maturity.

The second paper corroborates the findings of genetic and ethnic differences in bone mass and stresses, properly, that after menopause, factors under the control of the patient, such as dietary calcium intake and physical activity, are significant in the control of bone mass.—R. Poss, M.D.

Prevention of Osteoporosis by Pulsed Electromagnetic Fields
Rubin CT, McLeod KJ, Lanyon LE (State Univ of New York, Stony Brook)
J Bone Joint Surg [Am] 71-A:411–417, March 1989   4–109

Can pulsed electromagnetic fields prevent disuse osteoporosis? The functionally isolated ulna of the turkey, a bone about twice the width and length of a human metacarpal, served to test the effects of 1 hour a day of pulsed electromagnetic fields. The preparation consisted of a 100-μm diaphyseal section of mature bone deprived of mechanical function, but with intact musculature, nerves, and nutrient supply. The contralateral ulna served as a control.

Cross-sectional bone area declined by 11% when the functionally isolated ulna was exposed to an inactive coil. Both endosteal resorption and intracortical porosis were noted. Bone mass was increased substantially when the ulna was exposed to a pulsed electromagnetic field (Fig 4–17). The osteogenic effect was maximal at 0.01–0.04 tesla^2/sec. Endosteal resorption was inhibited, and both periosteal and endosteal new bone formation were stimulated. The new bone was well mineralized and consisted chiefly of primary osteons.

Exposure of functionally isolated bone tissue to a pulsed electromagnetic field can maintain bone mass. In this study, exposure for 1 hour a day at physiologic intensity and frequency was effective. This approach might prove useful for immobilized patients, postmenopausal women,

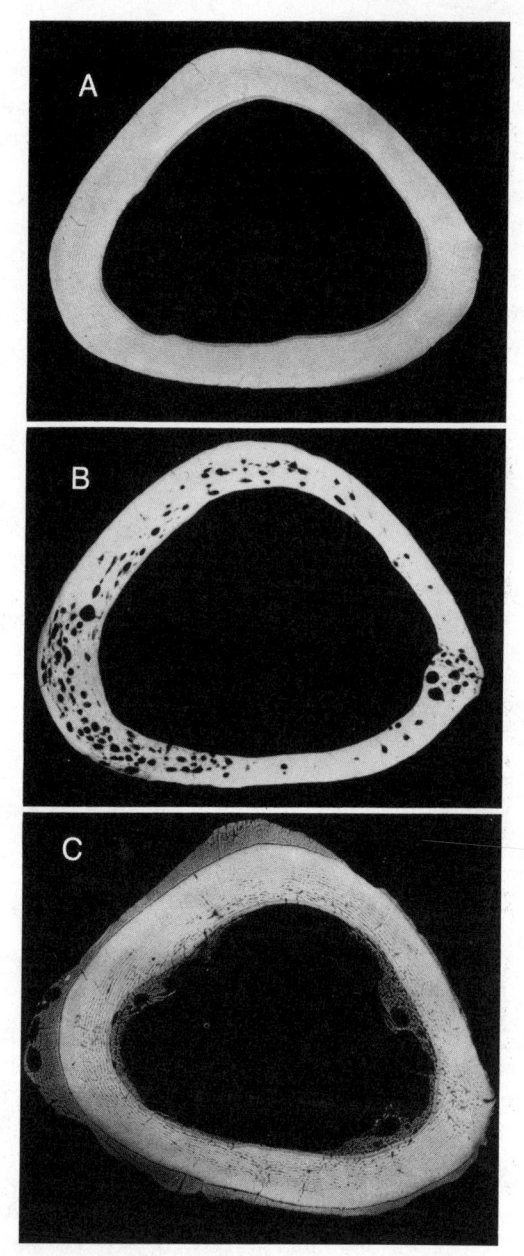

Fig 4–17.—Transverse microradiographs of the middle of the diaphyseal shaft of the ulna of the turkey after 8 weeks of treatment. **A,** intact control, showing a quiescent, uniformly mineralized cortex (scale mark, 2.0 mm). **B,** ulna that was functionally isolated and was exposed to a dummy coil. Compared with its intact contralateral control (A), the functionally isolated ulna has lost 13.1% of its bone. Activity in the cortex shows remodeling that is typical of disuse osteoporosis: cortical thinning by endosteal resorption and porosis caused by incompletely infilled haversian remodeling. **C,** ulna that was functionally isolated and was treated with 1 hour a day of a pulsed electromagnetic field, engendering an average power to proportional to 0.04 tesla^2/second. There is an increase in bone mass of 23%. This remodeling activity represents a net increase, compared with the functionally isolated ulna that was exposed to inactive coils, of approximately 33%. Periosteal and endosteal new-bone formation was substantial, but there is very little remodeling activity in the cortex. Despite the disuse, osteoporosis has been prevented and bone mass has increased. (Courtesy of Rubin CT, McLeod KF, Lanyon LE: *J Bone Surg [Am]* 71-A:411–417, March 1989.)

and even astronauts who are exposed for some time to a microgravitational milieu.

▶ In this elegant experiment, bone mass in a functionally isolated turkey ulna is maintained by the application of a pulsed electromagnetic field. Further confirmation of these findings would have obvious implications in the treatment of those patients at risk of disuse osteopenia.—R. Poss, M.D.

5 Hand

Introduction

This chapter focuses on significant contributions to reconstructive surgery of the hand and upper extremity over the past year, with emphasis on the treatment of scaphoid fractures and the complications associated with their treatment. Relevant clinical studies and basic research dealing with carpal kinematics present with scaphoid abnormalities are presented. Contributions to the treatment of the rheumatoid wrist with the Swanson implant provide insight into the long-term results and complications associated with the use of the prosthesis. The long-term results of synovectomy of the rheumatoid wrist and the role of soft tissue interposition arthroplasty of the metacarpophalangeal joint are clinically relevant contributions.

New methods of diagnosis of Kienböck's disease and the treatment of difficult fractures of the distal radius by open reduction and internal fixation are timely articles, as are studies dealing with the efficacy of repair of the triangular ligament in Colles' fracture and the role of early active mobilization of flexor tendon injuries in zone 2. Two interesting articles about congenital hand deformities contribute significantly to this difficult field, as do discussions about the prediction of recurrence of Dupuytren's disease. Finally, the treatment of unstable distal radial ulnar joint injuries, diagnosis of wrist pain in the adolescent gymnast, and corrective osteotomies of metacarpal and phalangeal malunions with AO plate and screws provide meaningful information. The material presented in this chapter is representative of recent advances in the field of hand surgery and should be informative to the reader.

Andrew J. Weiland, M.D.

Comparison of Short and Long Thumb-Spica Casts for Non-Displaced Fractures of the Carpal Scaphoid
Gellman H, Caputo RJ, Carter V, Aboulafia A, McKay M (Univ of Southern California)
J Bone Joint Surg [Am] 71-A:354–357, March 1989   5–1

In a prospective randomized study, each of 51 patients were treated with a short or long thumb-spica cast for a nondisplaced fracture of the carpal scaphoid. Follow-up averaged 1 year.

Two of 28 patients treated with a long thumb-spica cast had delayed union, but there were no nonunions. Average time to bony union was 9.5 weeks, and average time to clinical union was 9.3 weeks. Two of 23 fractures treated with a short thumb-spica cast failed to unite. Average time to union in the remaining cases was 12.7 weeks. Six patients had delayed union. Avascular necrosis was identified in 3 patients with a long thumb-spica cast and 4 with a short cast. Average duration of immobilization in these 7 cases was 15.3 weeks. No long-term disability resulted from immobilizing the elbow in a long thumb-spica cast.

An initial immobilization period of 6 weeks in a long thumb-spica case followed by use of a short cast is recommended for nondisplaced fractures of the proximal or middle third of the scaphoid. When pronation-supination of the forearm is eliminated, shear stresses across the fracture site are reduced, and union occurs more rapidly.

▶ The authors have conventionally demonstrated the superiority of long-arm thumb-spica cast immobilization in the treatment of nondisplaced fractures of the scaphoid involving the proximal or middle third for the initial 6 weeks. Time to union was decreased, as well as the incidence of nonunion, with no loss of elbow motion. This study provides useful clinical information about the treatment of this difficult problem.—A.J. Weiland, M.D.

Scaphoid Malunion
Amadio PC, Berquist TH, Smith DK, Ilstrup DM, Cooney WP III, Linscheid RL
(Mayo Clinic; Mayo Found, Rochester, Minn)
J Hand Surg [Am] 14A:679–687, July 1989   5–2

Scaphoid fractures usually heal with cast immobilization; however, displaced fracture and those with carpal instability may proceed to malunion. A technique for evaluation of the anatomy and function of scaphoid fractures with the use of trispiral tomography and the relationship of malunion to final functional result were described.

Forty-five patients with 46 scaphoid fractures were examined clinically more than 6 months after union. Examination assessed pain status, wrist range of motion, and measurement of grip strength in injured and uninjured hands. Affected wrists were also studied with trispiral tomography to determine the extent of scaphoid malunion.

Twenty patients had normal scaphoid anatomy; 26 had malunion. Univariate analysis showed that decreasing capitolunate angle, decreasing carpal height ratio, increasing radiolunate angle, increasing lateral intrascaphoid angle, and increasing scapholunate angle were significantly associated with the presence of posttraumatic arthritis. On multivariate analysis, increasing radiolunate angle, decreasing capitolunate angle, and decreasing carpal height ratio all remained significant factors. Decreasing carpal height ratio was significantly associated with a decreasing total score and increasing pain. Increasing lateral intrascaphoid angle was significantly associated with decreasing relative grip (Fig 5–1). Of those patients with normal scaphoid anatomy, 83% had satisfactory clinical outcomes; only 22% had posttraumatic arthritis. Of those with more than

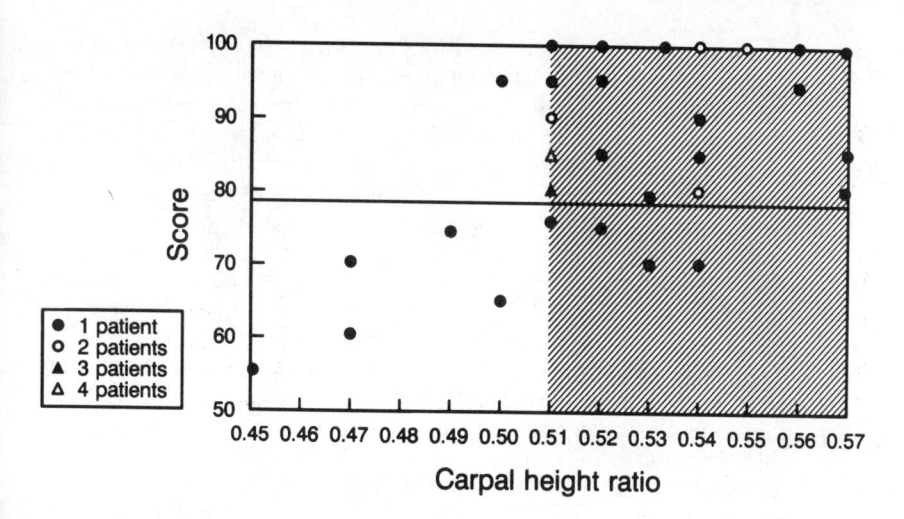

Fig 5–1.—Lateral intrascaphoid angle vs. total clinical score. Normal range for control group is shaded. Cutoff of 45 degrees *(dotted line)* successfully identifies 8 of the 13 fair and poor results, while including only 3 good or excellent results. (Courtesy of Amadio PC, Berquist TH, Smith DK, et al: J Hand Surg [AM] 14A:679–687, July 1989.)

45 degrees of lateral intrascaphoid angulation at union, 27% had a satisfactory outcome and 54% had post-traumatic arthritis.

Scaphoid malunion is an increase in the angle between the proximal and distal poles of the scaphoid, as measured by lateral tomography. Malunion is associated with an increased risk of functional impairment, especially with angulation of more than 45 degrees. Union alone does not ensure success in the treatment of scaphoid fractures. For optimal success, it is important that union occurs promptly and with normal scaphoid alignment.

▶ This clinical study provides significant evidence that patients with more than 45 degrees of lateral intrascaphoid angulation at union have a greater risk of posttraumatic arthritis than those with normal scaphoid anatomy. It provides impetus for the treating surgeon to correct malalignment in the acute scaphoid fracture and raises the interesting question of whether scaphoid osteotomies should be performed in a patient with a healed scaphoid fracture and greater than 45 degrees of angulation.—A.J. Weiland, M.D.

The Fate of Failed Bone Graft Surgery for Scaphoid Nonunions
Carrozzella JC, Stern PJ, Murdock PA (Cincinnati Hand Surgery Consultants)
J Hand Surg [Am] 14A:800–806, September 1989   5–3

Most scaphoid fractures unite if properly treated, but occasionally nonunion does occur. Causes for nonunion include inadequate immobilization, patient noncompliance, fracture instability, and treatment delay. The Russe technique for the treatment of nonunion of a scaphoid fracture, which involves inserting an inlay bone graft by a palmar approach, is usually successful in more than 80% of patients. Data on 20 patients with scaphoid fractures that failed to achieve union after bone grafting procedures were reviewed. The average follow-up was 30 months after the original fracture, and at least 1 year after the last surgery.

The dominant hand was involved in 14 patients; 19 patients had persistent wrist pain. Ten patients had a second bone grafting, of whom 8 had a repeat palmar inlay bone graft, 1 had an interpositional trapezoidal bone graft, and 1 had a vascularized pedicle graft from the distal radius. Six scaphoids united, and 4 continued with nonunions. One nonunion was treated with a third bone grafting, and the fracture healed. Six patients subsequently underwent salvage procedures, of whom 3 had silicone replacement arthroplasty, 1 underwent wrist fusion, 1 had a proximal pole excision, and 1 had an intercarpal fusion. Four of these 6 patients became asymptomatic. The other 2 patients became asymptomatic after undergoing wrist fusions.

Eight of the 20 originally grafted nonunions and 4 of the regrafted nonunions had avascular necrosis. After the first graft failure, 5 patients had external electrical stimulation for an average of 11 weeks, but none of the fractures went on to union. Thirteen of the 20 original nonunions showed either fracture displacement or instability on plain radiographs. Five fracture that appeared united on plain radiographs later showed persistent nonunion on tomographic examination.

Persistent scaphoid nonunions are extremely difficult to treat. Union after a second bone graft is less likely than union after a single bone graft. Despite scaphoid union after a second bone grafting, a high percentage of patients remain symptomatic. Fracture location, avascular necrosis, and instability do not adversely affect the success rate in obtaining union after a second bone graft. Electrical stimulation is useless for obtaining union. Salvage procedures were more successful than second bone grafts in obtaining an asymptomatic wrist. Plain radiography should be supplemented with tomography to determine whether union has taken place after bone grafting.

▶ The authors have evaluated critically the fate of failed bone graft surgery for scaphoid nonunions in 20 patients and emphasize the difficulty in obtaining union with a second or third bone grafting procedure. Of interest was the observation that, of the 7 patients who ultimately obtained union after a second or third bone grafting procedure, only 3 patients were asymptomatic. Salvage procedures were more successful in obtaining an asymptomatic wrist. These findings suggest that salvage procedures should be considered seriously for patients who have had failed bone grafting procedures for scaphoid nonunions. I agree with the authors' conclusions.—A.J. Weiland, M.D.

Fascial Implant Arthroplasty for Treatment of Radioscaphoid Degenerative Disease

Eaton RG, Akelman E, Eaton BH (St Luke's-Roosevelt Hosp, New York; Rhode Island Hosp, Providence)
J Hand Surg [Am] 14A:766-774, September 1989   5-4

Radioscaphoid arthritis is a degenerative complication of a malunited, nonunited, or hypermobile scaphoid after traumatic injury to the scaphoid. Although several procedures for treating radioscaphoid arthritis have been described, there is no agreement on the ideal reconstructive procedure.

During a 9-year study period, 26 patients with radioscaphoid arthritis underwent scaphoid hemireplacement with an implant of autogenous or allograft fascia. Twenty patients, aged 20-71 years, were available for follow-up examination. Twelve patients had a primary diagnosis of chronic scaphoid nonunion; 6, scapholunate advanced collapse pattern; and 2, irreducible transscaphoid perilunate dislocations. Treatment involved the replacement of the degenerated or impinging portion of the scaphoid by a slightly oversized fascial implant. Four implants were constructed of autograft, and 16, of allograft fascia lata.

After an average follow-up of 44.2 months, wrist range of motion was considerably improved. Overall, extension averaged 71 degrees, a gain of 30 degrees (73%), and flexion averaged 69 degrees, a gain of 19 degrees (38%). The greatest improvement occurred in the 6 patients with scapholunate advanced collapse who had the most limitation before operation. However, their final arc of motion was slightly less than that in patients treated for nonunion. Postoperative grip strength averaged 78 lb, a 17% improvement. However, specific grip strengthening exercises were avoided during the first 6 months after operation to prevent excessive compression of the fascial spacer. All patients were able to return to their preoperative occupations. The final results were rated excellent in 13 patients, good in 6 patients, and poor in 1 patient. It appears that subtotal fascial replacement of the scaphoid appears to hold up well with full wrist activity.

▶ Doctor Eaton and co-workers describe an interesting approach for the treatment of radioscaphoid arthritis secondary to chronic scaphoid nonunion and scapholunate advanced collapsed pattern. Of particular interest is the reduction in carpal height noted at follow-up, which averaged 3.8 years. I would be concerned about the possible further loss of carpal height with longer follow-up because of the disruption of scapholunate ligament. An alternative form of treatment would be limited arthrodesis such as scaphocapitate or triscaphe arthrodesis.—A.J. Weiland, M.D.

Effects of a Scaphoid Waist Osteotomy on Carpal Kinematics
Smith DK, An KN, Cooney WP III, Linscheid RL, Chao EY (Mayo Clinic, Mayo Found, Rochester, Minn)
J Orthop Res 7:590-598, July 1989   5-5

Among the most frequently fractured carpal bones is the carpal scaphoid. Unstable scaphoid fractures, which are not easily evaluated on routine radiographs, are predisposed to malunions or nonunions. The effects of a scaphoid osteotomy on the kinematics of the carpal bones were investigated.

Tests were undertaken on 5 freshly frozen wrist specimens with normal radiographic carpal anatomy. Carpal markers were inserted through limited arthrotomies into the distal radius and selected carpal bones. Care was taken to avoid injury to the intercarpal ligaments. By the application of a predetermined load to each of the 5 carpal tendons, the wrist specimens were placed into the extreme wrist positions of extension, flexion, and radial and ulnar deviation. With a biplanar radiographic device, simultaneous radiographs were obtained in the neutral and extreme positions, both before and after the scaphoid waist osteotomy. For each wrist position, the positions of each of the carpal markers and their corresponding bones were digitized and a computer-assisted motion analysis was performed for each specimen.

Significant alterations in carpal kinematics were noted after a simple transverse waist osteotomy. During wrist motion, increased motion of the distal scaphoid fragment and decreased motion of the proximal scaphoid fragment produced significant multiplanar interfragmentary motion. The scaphoid osteotomy had a tendency to collapse into a dorsally angulated deformity during each extreme wrist position. Also affected were the kinematics of the capitate and lunate bones and the trapezium. Treatment of scaphoid fracture must restore carpal stability to attain normal union and maintain normal carpal kinematics.

▶ This biomechanical study provides experimental documentation about alteration in the carpal kinematics produced by waist osteotomy of the scaphoid. The inherent instability of scaphoid fractures contributes to the frequency of malunion and nonunion observed clinically. I agree with the authors that this investigation provides a rational basis for the operative treatment of unstable scaphoid fractures.—A.J. Weiland, M.D.

Arthroplasty of the Rheumatoid Wrist With Swanson Implant: Long-Term Results and Complications
Haloua JP, Collin JP, Schernberg F, Sandre J (Centre Beaulieu, Chamalières; Centre Hospitalier de Reims, Reims, France)
Ann Chir Main 8:124–134, 1989   5–6

Flexible implant athroplasty of the metacarpophalangeal joint with a Swanson silicone implant has been used as an alternative to wrist arthrodesis in the treatment of severe rheumatoid polyarthritis. The 5-year results of 75 Swanson implant procedures were evaluated in 59 women and 6 men, aged 24–77 years, with radiologic Steinbrocker stage III and stage IV rheumatoid polyarthritis in 75 wrists. Ten patients had bilateral procedures. Thirty-seven of the 55 unilateral procedures were of the

	Late Complications		
Radial implants	62	Ulnar implants	12
Fractures	14	Fractures	1
Synovitis	13	Luxations	5

(Courtesy of Haloua JP, Collin JP, Schernberg F, et al: *Ann Chir Main* 8:124–134, 1989.)

dominant hand. Fifteen wrists received ulnar implants. Pain was the major indication for operation, with 49 patients having a preoperative pain score of 3, and 26 having a pain score of 2. After a mean follow-up of 5 years, 7 patients had died and 6 could not be located, leaving 52 patients with 62 Swanson implants for follow-up evaluation.

Clinical review showed significantly improved pain scores in all patients, as only 5 complained of intermittent wrist pain with recurrent synovitis. Functional evaluation showed that 80% of the patients had improved mobility in flexion-extension, and 87% had improved mobility in pronation-supination. Overall wrist function was rated good in 23 patients, average in 17, and poor in 21. Follow-up of 12 wrists with ulnar implants showed fracture in 1 and dislocation in 5 implants, yielding a 50% complication rate for ulnar implants (table). Four implants had to be removed, and the procedure was subsequently abandoned. There were 14 radial fractures between 1 and 4 years after implantation, yielding a 23% radial fracture rate. All fractures occurred at the junction of the lower stem of the implant. Seven fractures were not reoperated because of patient refusal, 4 were revised to arthrodesis, and 3 were replaced with new implants, which all refractured and had to be revised to arthrodesis. Foreign body synovitis or siliconitis was observed in 18 wrists (29%).

The 44% overall complication rate among patients with Swanson wrist implants after 5 years of follow-up suggests that silicone wrist replacement procedures as presently performed should be abandoned.

▶ The authors from France have confirmed the findings of hand surgeons in the United States that silicone wrist replacement procedures as presently performed should be abandoned. The 44% overall complication rate parallels my experience with this procedure, and I concur with the conclusion.—A.J. Weiland, M.D.

The Long-Term Results of Synovectomy of the Rheumatoid Wrist: A Report of 60 Cases
Allieu Y, Lussiez B, Asencio G (Hôpital Lapeyronie, Montpellier, France)
Fr J Orthop Surg 3:188–194, June 1989   5–7

Synovectomy of the wrist tendons has been the major procedure to relieve pain and restore function in the wrists of patients with rheumatoid polyarthritis. The long-term results of combined dorsal tenosynovectomy,

synovectomy of the wrist, and resection of the ulnar head were evaluated in 42 women (mean age, 50 years) and 7 men (mean age, 53 years) who underwent operations on 60 wrists. Eleven patients had bilateral procedures. Indications for operation included persisting pain in spite of medical treatment, and palpable synovitis on the back of the wrist persisting after 6 months of medical treatment and presenting a risk for tendon rupture. The average follow-up for the entire series was 5 years 4 months, and ranged from 13 months to 13.5 years. However, one third of the patients had a mean follow-up of 8 years and 8 months.

At the 5.5-year follow-up, 78% of the wrists were painless, and 22% of the patients had pain only on heavy use of the wrist. Synovitis had been present in 95% of the cases before operation, but was absent in 80% of the cases at follow-up. However, the mean active range of motion (ROM) had decreased by 28% of the inital postoperative ROM in the sagittal plane and by 21% in the frontal plane. Follow-up radiography revealed progressive radiologic deterioration of the carpal arthritis over time, confirming that synovectomy does not halt disease progression.

At the 8.5-year follow-up of 19 available patients, the mean active ROM had further declined to 33% of the initial active ROM in the sagittal plane and to 41.5% in the frontal plane. However, 67% of the patients were still pain free or had only intermittent wrist pain.

Although the long-term clinical results after synovectomy with resection of the ulnar head have been satisfactory, synovectomy alone has not prevented radiologic deterioration of the wrist over time. Therefore, synovectomy is now performed earlier as a prophylactic procedure, or supplemented by intracarpal arthrodeses or tendon transfers in cases of partial destruction of the carpus.

▶ The authors present the long-term results of synovectomy of the rheumatoid wrist in 49 patients followed for an average of 5 years 5 months. The significant information to be gained from this study is that the procedure will result in significant pain relief in 78% of the patients and no recurrence of tenosynovitis in 80% of patients. The majority of patients had improved function despite progressive loss of motion and radiographic evidence of progressive carpal arthritis over time. I agree with the authors' conclusion that synovectomy is a useful procedure in the treatment of the rheumatoid wrist. One, however, questions the recommendation about the efficacy of limited wrist arthrodesis for the patient with rheumatoid disease because the entire carpus and radiocarpal joint usually is involved.—A.J. Weiland, M.D.

Soft Tissue Metacarpophalangeal Reconstruction for Treatment of Rheumatoid Hand Deformity
Wood VE, Ichtertz DR, Yahiku H (Loma Linda Univ, Loma Linda, Calif)
J Hand Surg [Am] 14A:163–174, March 1989   5–8

Author	Year	Joints (No.)	Mean follow-up (yr)	Active Rom (°)	Drift (°)	Recurrence	Ext° lag (°)	Failure	
Beckenbaugh	1976	403	2.5	38		11.3%		26.27%	Swanson
		127				44%		38.2%	Niebauer
Bieber	1986	210	5.25	56	12		22	0	Swanson
Blair	1984	115	4.5	43	<30	43%	13	21%	Swanson
Hagert	1975	104	1.5-5.5					24%	Swanson
Madden	1977	92	2 Yr.	57			9		
Mannerfelt	1975	144	2.5	40	96%<30		10	2.8%	Swanson
Steffee	1981	503	2.4	42	7.7%>20		17	18%	Cemented
Vahvanen	1986	107	3.75	34	31%>10		7	14%	Swanson
Loma Linda U.	1987	64	6.75	56	6	12%	27	12%	Soft tissue realigned

Cross Comparison*

*Only series reporting active range of motion (Rom) were included for consistency.
(Courtesy of Wood VE, Ichtertz DR, Yahiku H: *J Hand Surg [Am]* 14A:163–174, March 1989.)

Silicone metacarpophalangeal joint (MP) arthroplasty offers pain relief and correction of hand deformity to patients with rheumatoid arthritis and systemic lupus erythematosis. A number of studies, however, report a high incidence of fracture in the silicone implants at long-term follow-up. The long-term results of soft tissue MP reconstruction without articular resection of 16 hands of 12 patients with painful ulnar deviation-subluxation deformity were reviewed.

Patients had a mean age at surgery of 66 years and a mean disease duration of 15.9 years. Most patients were in the American Rheumatoid Association Class II stage 3, and all had painful, subluxated, or severely deviated MP joints. The operative procedure, described and illustrated, included a thorough synovectomy.

No immediate complications occurred, although swan neck deformities worsened in 2 patients. Overall results were judged excellent in 6 hands, good in 7, fair in 1, and poor in 2 (table). Except for the 2 failures, the patients were satisfied with the results. At follow-up (mean, 81 months) complete pain relief had occurred in 88% of patients. The operated hands had a mean active MP range of motion of 56 degrees and a mean proximal interphalangeal range of motion of 64 degrees. Only 1 of the operated MP joints had a recurrence of synovitis.

These results suggest that the procedure should be performed before joint dislocation and fixed contractures occur. Many patients may be spared replacement arthroplasty, and the results of soft-tissue reconstruction compare favorably with those of silicone replacement. Patients with systemic lupus erythematosus, who have less articular destruction than those with rheumatoid disease, may especially benefit from this procedure.

▶ The authors have reintroduced the concept of soft tissue arthroplasty in the reconstruction of painful, sublux, or severely deviated metacarpal phalangeal joints with some articular cartilage remaining. The procedure as described is combined with crossed intrinsic transfer. The results achieved are impressive, with complete pain relief in 88% of the patients and 56% and 64% mean active range of motion of the metacarpophalangeal joints and proximal interphalangeal joints, respectively. The results achieved are comparable to those obtained with silicone metacarpophalangeal joint arthroplasty, and the procedure should be considered for those rheumatoid patients with some articular cartilage remaining at the metacarpophalangeal joint.—A.J. Weiland, M.D.

Application of Magnetic Resonance Imaging to Ischemic Necrosis of the Lunate
Sowa DT, Holder LE, Patt PG, Weiland AJ (Delaware Hand Ctr, Newark; Union Mem Hosp, Baltimore; Johns Hopkins Univ)
J Hand Surg [Am] 14A:1008–1016, November 1989   5–9

Ischemic necrosis of the lunate may be difficult to diagnose, particularly in its early stages. The role of magnetic resonance imaging (MRI) in the diagnosis and management of ischemic necrosis of the lunate was investigated in a prospective study of 20 patients (22 wrists) suspected of having ischemic necrosis of the lunate who also were evaluated by physical examination, conventional radiography, and radionuclide bone scintigraphy.

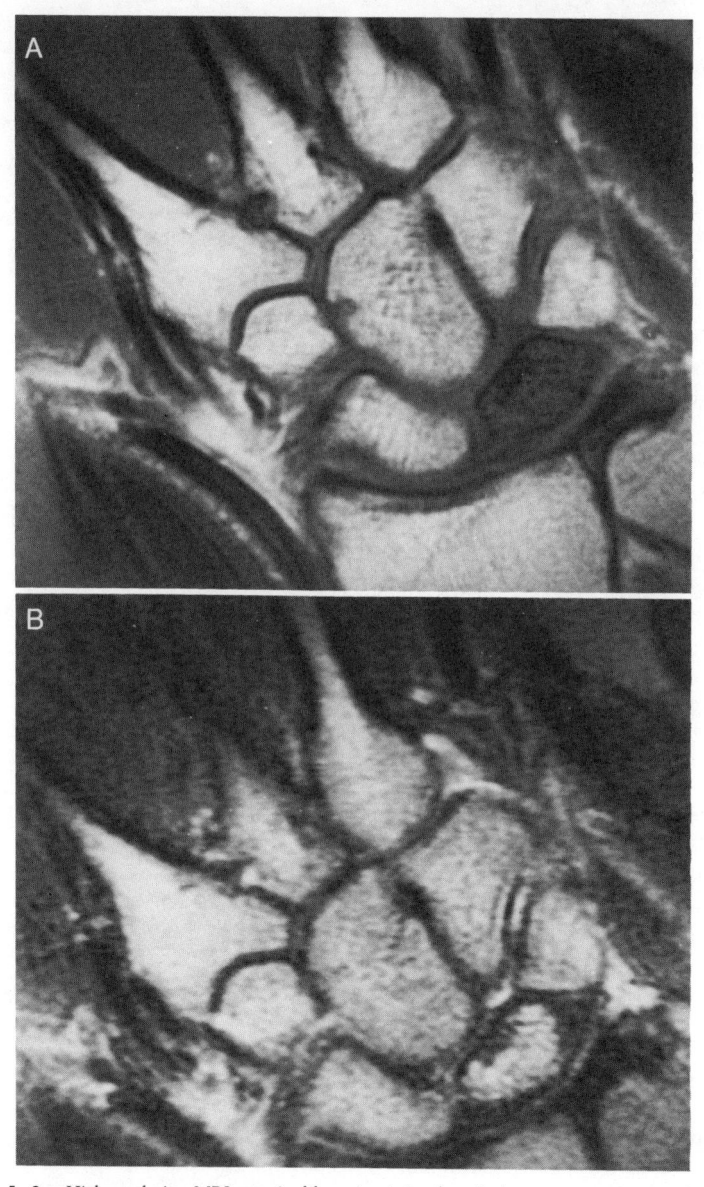

Fig 5-2.—High resolution MRI, acquired by using 1.5 tesla unit demonstrating **A**, generalized loss of lunate signal in T_1-weighted image, and **B**, generalized increase in lunate signal on T_2-weighted image. (Courtesy of Sowa DT, Holder LE, Patt PG, et al: *J Hand Surg [Am]* 14-A:1008–1016, November 1989.)

In 12 cases (14 wrists) the final diagnosis was ischemic necrosis of the lunate. Magnetic resonance imaging was more specific than radiography or radionuclide bone imaging in making the diagnosis. Two patterns of lunate signal defect were observed on MRI with focal or generalized loss

	Magnetic Resonance Imaging Subclassification of Radiographic Stage 2 Ischemic Necrosis of Lunate	
Stage	T_1 Image	T_2 Image
II A	Focal signal loss	Focal signal increase
II B	Focal signal loss	Focal signal loss
II C	Generalized signal loss	Generalized signal increase
II D	Generalized signal loss	Generalized signal loss

(Courtesy of Sowa DT, Holder LE, Patt PG, et al: *J Hand Surg [Am]* 14A:1008–1016, November 1989.)

of the lunate signal on T_1-weighted and T_2-weighted images (Fig 5–2). Generalized loss of the lunate signal on T_1-weighted images was diagnostic for ischemic necrosis of the lunate. In 1 patient with focal signal loss on the radial half of the lunate, microscopic findings were suggestive of ischemic necrosis of the lunate.

The MRI evaluation of the lunate may be useful for subclassification of Lichtman's radiographic stage 2 (table). Focal loss of T_1 signal in the radial half of the lunate suggests an ealier stage of ischemic necrosis than generalized loss of the lunate signal. Increased T_2-weighted signal in lunates with either focal or generalized lunate involvement suggests early revascularization and better prognosis.

Magnetic resonance imaging is the definitive test in evaluating ischemic necrosis of the lunate and can be used to follow lunate revascularization after treatment.

▶ In this interesting study, the authors have evaluated the application of MRI in Kienböck's disease. Magnetic resonance imaging showed more specificity than radiography or radionuclide bone imaging in making the diagnosis of ischemic necrosis of the lunate. A subclassification of stage II disease is proposed. The cost-effectiveness of MRI in the diagnosis and treatment of this disease must be evaluated carefully but there is no question that MRI is the definitive test in evaluating Kienböck's disease and can be useful as a means of serial follow-up in both treated and untreated patients.—A.J. Weiland, M.D.

Open Reduction and Internal Fixation of Displaced, Comminuted Intra-Articular Fractures of the Distal End of the Radius

Bradway JK, Amadio PC, Cooney WP (Mayo Clinic, Mayo Found, Rochester, Minn)
J Bone Joint Surg [Am] 71-A:839–847, July 1989   5–10

A closed method of treatment often brings unsatisfactory results in patients who have a displaced, comminuted intra-articular fracture of the distal end of the radius. Open reduction and internal fixation have been employed in an effort to improve treatment results. The records of 16 patients were reviewed to document the benefits of the latter approach.

The patient group was made up of 9 men and 7 women; their average age was 40 years. Many had concomitant ipsilateral injuries. On the basis of the AO classification system, all fractures were type C2 or C3, thus involving intra-articular extension and comminution. Articular incongruity was at least grade 1 in all cases; 12 patients had a grade of 2 or worse. Open reduction followed failure of closed reduction to achieve or maintain articular congruity and was performed at an average of 6.5 days after the injury.

The fractures were reduced under direct vision. Internal fixation was accomplished in most patients with Kirschner wires or an internal fixation plate. A plate and screws were used to fix larger fragments. On follow-up at a mean of 5.7 years, the wrist was evaluated for strength and range of motion, and radiographically were examined for evidence of arthritic changes, nonunion of the ulnar styloid process, and radial and dorsal-volar tilt of the distal radial surface.

With the criteria of Gartland and Werley, 81% of patients had excellent or good results and no wrist received a poor rating. By the modified system of Green and O'Brien, only 56% had excellent or good results, although none were judged poor. One patient expressed dissatisfaction with appearance of her wrist; all patients, however, had adequate function for their normal work and leisure activities. Age, osteoporosis, high-energy injuries, and an intra-articular incongruity of 2 mm or more persisting after closed or percutaneous treatment are associated with less satisfactory results or posttraumatic arthritis, or both.

▶ This study confirms the findings of others that open reduction and internal fixation of displaced comminuted, intra-articular fractures of the distal end of the radius are indicated when an intra-articular incongruity of 2 mm or more persists or recurs after closed or percutaneous treatment. Concomitant use of internal and external fixation may aid in obtaining and maintaining reduction. Bone grafting also may be indicated for patients with severely comminuted fractures. These fractures warrant a more aggressive surgical approach in view of the increased incidence of posttraumatic arthritis with poor reduction and intra-articular incongruity.— A.J. Weiland, M.D.

Repair of the Triangular Ligament in Colles' Fracture: No Effect in a Prospective Randomized Study
af Ekenstam F, Jakobsson OP, Wadin K (Uppsala Univ, Uppsala, Sweden)
Acta Orthop Scand 60:393–396, August 1989   5–11

Forty-one patients had treatment for closed, extra-articular, dislocated fractures of the distal radius. Patients were grouped according to whether their birthdays fell on odd or even days. Reduction and splinting of the fractured radius was the same for both groups. One group had closed manipulation followed by suturing of the triangular ligament and stabilization of the ulnar styloid. The other group had closed reduction and fixation with plaster casts only. Standard radiographs of forearms were obtained immediately before and after fracture treatment and at 1 week and 2 years. Two-year follow-up involved interviews with patients, evaluation of range of motion in both wrist joints and forearms, and measurement grip of strength. Fifty-four wrists—33 fractures and 21 controls—underwent arthrography.

Four of 19 patients in the surgical group and 7 of 21 in the conservative treatment group had painful restricted forearm rotation. There was no difference between the treatment groups for any part of the clinical examination. At 2-year follow-up radiography, alignment of the distal fragment of the radius had deteriorated equally in both groups. The ulnar styloid healed with the same frequency in both groups. Contrast material leaked into the distal radioulnar joint from the radiocarpal joint with equal frequency in treated patients and in controls, and contrast-medium concentration in the foveolar area at the base of the ulnar styloid was similar in the 2 treatment groups.

Triangle ligament repair did not improve the treatment of Colles' fracture. The lack of improvement might be explained by prolonged or inadequate healing. Although ligament healing was assessed with arthrography, problems in interpreting the films made it difficult to assess this parameter.

▶ This prospective randomized study evaluates the effect of repair of the triangular fibrocartilage in patients with Colles' fracture and associated ulnar styloid avulsions. Surgical repair did not improve the results obtained with respect to range of motion of the wrist and forearm, in addition to grip strength. Somewhat puzzling is the finding that on follow-up wrist arthrography, contrast material leaked into the distal radioulnar joint from the radiocarpal joint with equal frequency in the treated patients and controls. Perhaps the repair performed was not effective in maintaining the integrity of the triangular fibrocartilage.—A.J. Weiland, M.D.

Early Active Mobilisation Following Flexor Tendon Repair in Zone 2
Small JO, Brennen MD, Colville J (Northern Ireland Plastic and Maxillofacial Service, Belfast)
J Hand Surg [Br] 14B:383–391, November 1989   5–12

Active motion might be beneficial in repaired flexor tendons. In this prospective study, 114 patients who had 138 flexor tendon injuries in zone 2 had repair of both flexor tendons by suturing and closure of the sheath, covering of the wound with only paraffin and dry gauzes, and application of a plaster-of-Paris splint with the wrist in midflexion (Fig 5–3). Within 48 hours after operation, passive and active mobilization of the injured fingers was begun. Patients had assessment and instruction twice a week thereafter.

At review 6 months after repair, the active range of motion was graded good or excellent in 77% according to the American Society for Surgery

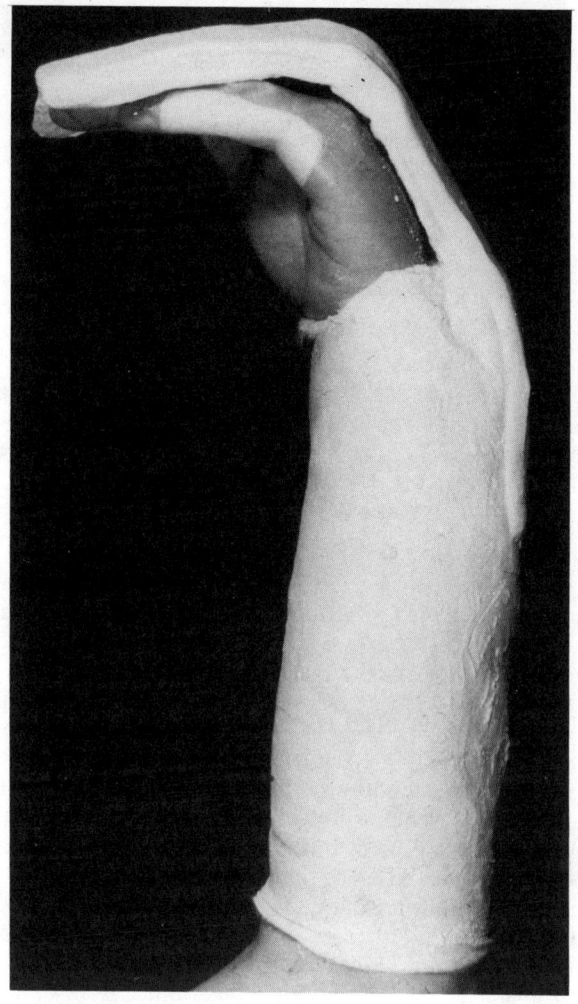

Fig 5–3.—The plaster-of-Paris splint. (Courtesy of Small JO, Brennen MD, Colville J: *J Hand Surg [Br]* 14B:383–391, November 1989.)

of the Hand criteria and in 75% according to Kleinert's criteria (table). Full extension was possible in 60.7%. Dehiscence of the repair occurred in 9.4% of digits, usually during the second week. Further repair and postoperative mobilization produced good or excellent results in 64% of these cases.

These early results are encouraging and are as good as or better than those of others who used the Kleinert dynamic splint and better than results with passive mobilization alone. Basic research on the histochemical effects of early active motion and controlled clinical testing of this method are recommended.

Results (Percentage of Digits) Assessed by
A.S.S.H. and Kleinert Criteria

	A.S.S.H.		Kleinert	
Excellent	46	} 77	60	} 75
Good	31		15	
Fair	14		8	
Poor	9		17	

(Courtesy of Small JO, Brennen MD, Colville J: *J Hand Surg [Br]* 14B:383–391, November 1989.)

▶ This study presents the authors' experience with early active mobilization after flexor tendon repair in zone 2 in 114 patients. The results achieved are similar to those achieved by Lister using Kleinert dynamic splinting and are better than those series employing passive motion. Although the results of this series are encouraging further clinical trials need to be carried out that include the appropriate controls to critically evaluate Kleinert traction, passive motion, and early active motion.—A.J. Weiland, M.D.

Perfusion of the Abductor Digiti Quinti After Transfer on a Neurovascular Pedicle
Dunlap J, Manske PR, McCarthy JA (Washington Univ, St Louis)
J Hand Surg [Am] 14A:922–995, November 1989   5-13

The abductor digiti quinti (ADQ) opponensplasty is a well-established procedure for restoring thumb opposition. The technique involves dissection of the muscle from the pisiform before its transfer and subcutaneous tunneling into the thumb area, but recent studies advocate maintenance of the attachment of the ADQ to the pisiform.

The hydrogen washout technique was used to determine blood flow to the ADQ both before and after opponensplasty transfer on its neurovascular pedicle in 6 monkeys. Measurements were compared with those obtained after transfer through a subcutaneous tunnel as an opponensplasty to the thumb and after proximal dissection of the muscle origin off the pisiform.

The muscle could be transferred as an opponensplasty without vascular compromise. However, dissection of the muscle off its origin from the pisiform significantly reduced blood flow to the muscle by 14% (Fig 5–4). Dissection of the neurovascular pedicle of the ADQ off the pisiform results in ischemia and may contribute to the postoperative fibrosis that has been seen as a complication of the procedure.

▶ In this clinically significant study the authors evaluated various techniques of transferring the abductor digiti quinti for an opponesplasty using the hydrogen washout technique to monitor blood flow. The finding that the musculocutaneous unit can be transferred without vascular compromise but that detachment

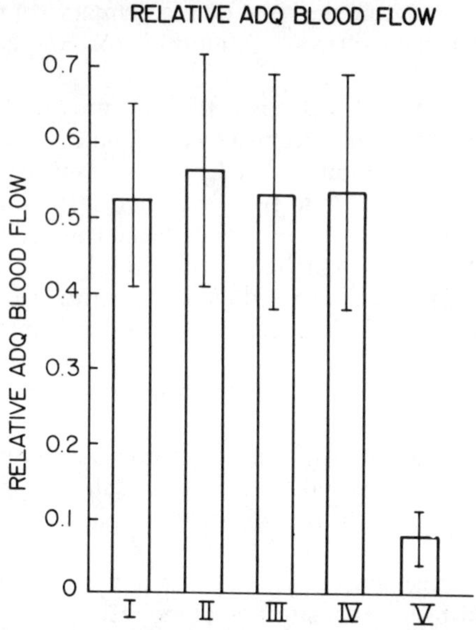

Fig 5-4.—Relative blood flows to the ADQ. Condition I: undissected ADQ (baseline); condition II: dissected ADQ left in anatomical bed; condition III: dissected ADQ transferred through subcutaneous tunnel; condition IV: distal ADQ tendon tied to abductor policis brevis; condition V: ADQ origin dissected off pisiform. (Courtesy of Dunlap J, Manske PR, McCarthy JA: *J Hand Surg [Am]* 14A:992-995, November 1989.)

from the pisiform results in ischemia is significant and provides meaningful information to the hand surgeon.—A.J. Weiland, M.D.

Treatment of Duplicated Thumb Using a Ligamentous/Periosteal Flap
Manske PR (Washington Univ, St Louis)
J Hand Surg [Am] 14A:728-733, July 1989   5-14

Duplication of the thumb is a relatively rare congenital anomaly. Several surgical reconstructions are available, but cosmetic and functional results are often not satisfactory. The reconstruction technique presented provides ablation of the less developed duplicated thumb and the use of a ligamentous/periosteal flap from the proximal bone to centralize and stabilize the retained thumb. The procedure also includes reduction osteotomy to narrow the widened proximal bone to improve cosmetic results.

Since 1975 this procedure has been used to reconstruct 22 duplicated thumbs in 21 skeletally immature children aged 6 months to 16 years. The average age at operation was about 4.5 years. Two patients had a common nailbed, requiring reconstruction of the radial nailfold. The radial digit was excised in 19 patients and the ulnar digit was excised in 2 patients. Five patients had angle-correcting osteotomies to obtain appropriate longitudinal alignment, 1 of whom required 2 osteotomies. Angle-correcting osteotomies used to be performed as secondary procedure, but they are now performed at the time of the primary thumb ablation procedure. Follow-up ranged from 3 months to 10 years (average, 22 months).

All 21 patients had excellent cosmetic and functional results with the retained thumb maintained in centralized alignment. Six patients with a follow-up of less than 6 months lived too far from the hospital for further follow-up, but all had good results at their last clinic visit. The 6 associated angle-correcting osteotomies all healed uneventfully. Three patients in whom the radial digit had been excised with restoration of the radial collateral ligament had residual postoperative laxity of the contralateral ulnar collateral ligament. Two of these patients have undergone arthrodesis; the third patient was awaiting a metacarpophalangeal joint fusion. There has been no interference with physeal growth, and nailbed defects have not been observed.

Treatment of a duplicated thumb using ablation with a ligamentous–periosteal flap yields functionally and cosmetically acceptable results and is technically not as difficult as some of the other available procedures.

▶ The authors have described a useful technique in the treatment of the duplicated thumb that involves reconstruction of the radial collateral ligament with a ligamentous periosteal flap. The procedure results in a more acceptable cosmetic result and greater ligamentous stability as evidenced by the results in the 21 patients treated.—A.J. Weiland, M.D.

Prediction of Recurrence in the Treatment of Dupuytren's Disease: Evaluation of a Histologic Classification
Rombouts J-J, Noël H, Legrain Y, Munting E (Saint-Luc Univ Hosp; Univ of Louvain, Brussels)
J Hand Surg [Am] 14A:644–652, July 1989

It was proposed previously that in patients with Dupuytren's disease, early onset, bilateral involvement, a positive family history, and involvement of other areas are prognostic for a more aggressive course and a greater tendency for disease recurrence. A recently completed multicenter trial found that the rate of recurrence or extension is 78% when all 4 factors are present and only 17% when all 4 factors are absent. A classification for histologic staging of Dupuytren's disease was developed.

During an 8-year study period, 9 women and 54 men aged 32–82 years with Dupuytren's disease, underwent selective fasciectomy as a primary procedure on 77 hands. Based on evolutionary clinical criteria, 1 hand had early disease characterized by the presence of nodules in the absence of retraction, 66 hands had active disease characterized by increasing retraction, and 10 hands had advanced disease characterized by a long-standing condition that had not worsened during recent months. Based on microscopic analysis of surgical specimens, a histologic classification of Dupuytren's lesions into 3 types was defined. Type I denotes a proliferative stage characterized by high cellularity and mitosis; type II, a fibrocellular stage characterized by high cellularity but no mitosis; and type III, a fibrotic stage characterized by dense fibrous material containing no reticulin fibers. By these criteria, 13 specimens were histologic type I; 42, type II; and 22, type III.

All patients were reexamined within an average of 5 years after operation. Of 13 hands classified histologically as type I, 2 were free of disease, 9 had disease recurrence, and 2 had extension without recurrence. Of 42 type II hands, 9 were free of disease, 17 had recurrence, and 16 had extension. Of 22 type III hands, 11 were free of disease, 4 had recurrence, and 7 had extension. Total disease activity rates were 85% for type I hands, 70% for type II hands, and for type III hands. There was a significant relationship between histologic stage at operation and recurrence of Dupuytren's disease but not between histologic stage and disease extension.

Histologic staging may have prognostic value for predicting recurrence. No correlation was found between clinical staging and histologic type.

▶ Recurrence or extension of Dupuytren's disease after surgical excision is not infrequent. The authors have proposed a practical histologic classification that seems to have a prognostic value with respect to recurrence rate although the risk of extension was not correlated with the histologic type. The classification presented will aid the surgeon in predicting recurrence of disease.—A.J. Weiland, M.D.

Extensor Carpi Ulnaris and Flexor Carpi Ulnaris Tenodesis of the Unstable Distal Ulna
Breen TF, Jupiter JB (Univ of Massachusetts, Worcester; Massachusetts Gen Hosp, Boston)
J Hand Surg [Am] 14A:612–617, July 1989   5–16

Subluxation of the distal ulna often causes considerable pain and disability. Many reconstructive procedures have been proposed for treating chronic instability of the distal ulna. One such procedure was evaluated in 8 patients with painful dorsal subluxation of the distal ulna.

Three patients had had Darrach procedures, and 5 had severe degenerative arthritis of the distal radioulnar joint before the study. All 8 patients underwent tenodeses of the extensor carpi ulnaris and flexor carpi ulnaris (Figs 5–5 through 5–7); 5 also underwent Darrach procedure done extraperiosteally for degenerative articular disease of the distal radioulnar joint.

After tenodesis, all patients had stable ulnae with a mean motion of 67 degrees of supination and 86 degrees of pronation. This was a mean increase of 32 degrees of supination and 43 degrees of pronation. Follow-up averaged 28 months.

In patients with chronic dorsal subluxation of the distal ulna, tenodesis using a weave of a proximally based slip of extensor carpi ulnaris and a distally based slip of flexor carpi ulnaris in combination with a Darrach

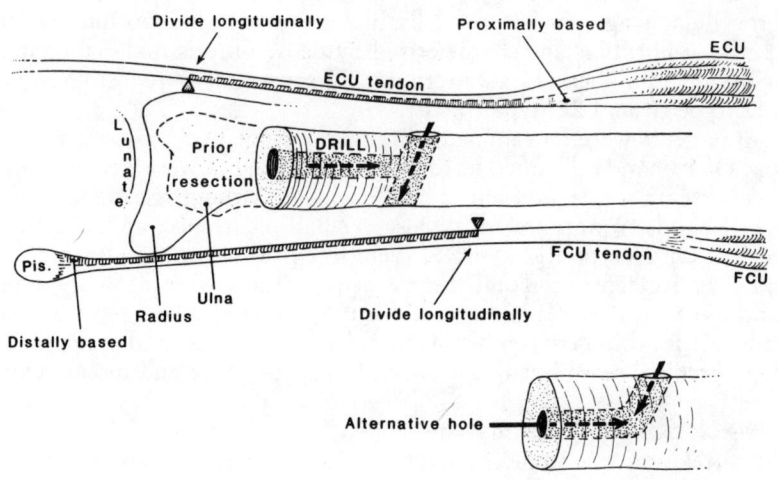

Fig 5-5.—Extensor carpi ulnaris *(ECU)* slip. (Courtesy of Breen TF, Jupiter JB: *J Hand Surg [Am]* 14A:612-617, July 1989.)

procedure is a reliable salvage procedure. The technique is appropriate after failed Darrach procedures, and it may be used in conjunction with distal ulnar resection when end-stage degenerative arthritis of the unstable distal radioulnar joint is encountered.

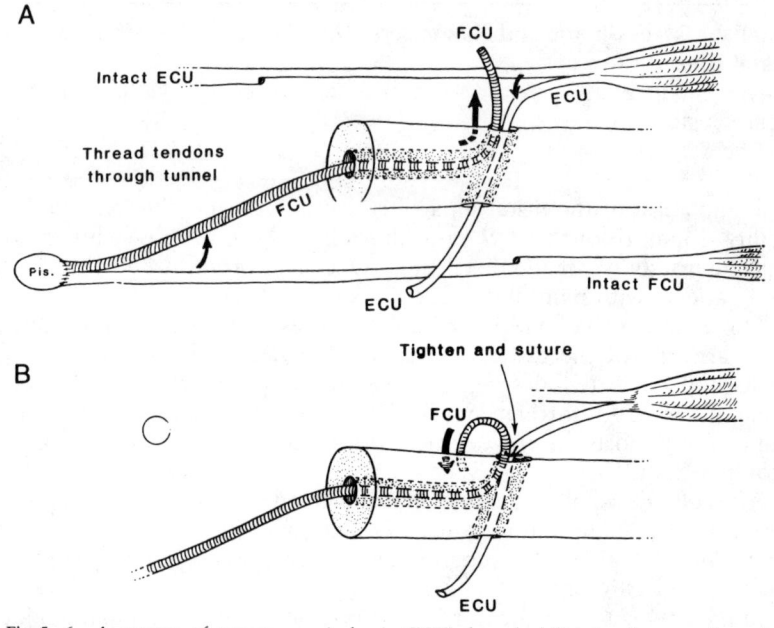

Fig 5-6.—**A,** passage of extensor carpi ulnaris *(ECU)* through drill holes; **B,** start of tenodesis weave. *FCU,* flexor carpi ulnaris. (Courtesy of Breen TF, Jupiter JB: *J Hand Surg [Am]* 14A:612—617, July 1989.)

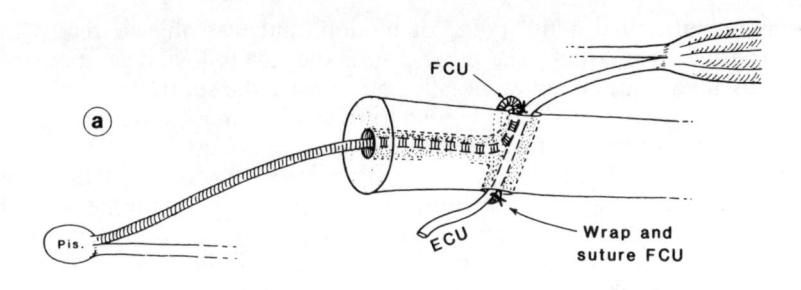

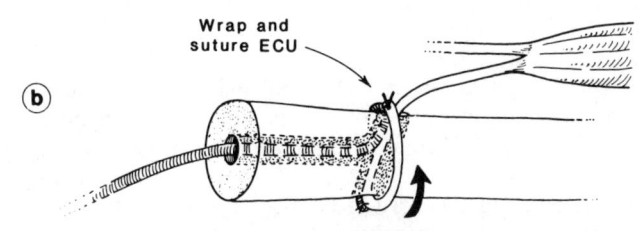

Fig 5–7.—Weave and suturing of extensor carpi ulnaris *(ECU)* and flexor carpi ulnaris *(FCU)*. (Courtesy of Breen TF, Jupiter JB: *J Hand Surg [Am]* 14A:612–617, July 1989.)

▶ A salvage procedure for stabilization of the distal ulna in 8 patients using both the extensor carpi ulnaris and flexor carpi ulnaris tendons is described. In the past, the solution to this difficult problem has not been satisfactory as evidenced by the many procedures that have been described in the literature. The results achieved in this study are encouraging; however, longer follow-up will be needed.— A.J. Weiland, M.D.

Wrist Pain and Distal Growth Plate Closure of the Radius in Gymnasts
Albanese SA, Palmer AK, Kerr DR, Carpenter CW, Lisi D, Levinsohn EM (State Univ of New York, Syracuse and Binghamton)
J Pediatr Orthop 9:23–28, January–February 1989   5–17

The skeletal system appears to respond to the stresses of intense athletic training by adaptive structural changes. However, the occurrence of stress fractures related to athletic activities suggests that the skeletal system's ability to respond to chronic stress is limited. Furthermore, there is evidence that intense athletic training by children may damage the growth plates in these skeletally immature individuals.

A group of 3 girls aged 12 to 14 years experienced wrist pain. All the girls had participated actively in competitive gymnastics before experiencing wrist pain, but none had had acute gymnastic injuries. Radiographic findings were suggestive of premature growth plate closure, which had resulted in shortening of the radius and alterations in the normal distal radioulnar articulation. A single patient underwent a successful ulnar-shortening osteotomy and plate fixation. At followup, she was asymptomatic, had a full range of motion, and was able to return to competitive gymnastics. The other 2 girls did not follow suggestions of activity modification and eventually had to leave the sport.

Chronic overuse in skeletally immature children may cause wrist pain associated with premature fusion of the distal radial growth plate. Some clinical evidence suggests that a growth plate's structure and function may be altered by repetitive subfracture loading. To maintain the normal anatomical relationship between the distal portions of the radius and ulna, both bones need to grow at the same rate during a given period. The findings in these 3 patients suggest that closure of the distal ulnar growth plate should precede that of the distal radial growth plate. A reversal in the sequence of the closure of the growth plates probably contributed to the alteration of the ulnar variance.

▶ Increased emphasis on competitive athletics has encouraged intense athletic training of children, especially gymnasts. The authors have demonstrated findings consistent with premature closure of the distal radial epiphysis in 3 patients, none of whom had a history of an acute injury. This resulted in radial shortening and alteration of the normal distal radial ulnar joint anatomy. It is hoped that with the information provided in this article, wrist pain in the highly competitive preadolescent gymnast will not be passed off as "sprain" but evaluated for possible growth plate abnormality.—A.J. Weiland, M.D.

Osteotomy of the Metacarpals and Phalanges Stabilized by AO Plates and Screws
Lucas GL, Pfeiffer CM (Wichita Clinic, Wichita, Kan; Kantonsspital, Basel, Switzerland)
Ann Chir Main 8:30–38, 1989   5–18

Malunion after fractures of the hand may cause severe limitation of finger function and weakness in grip. Corrective osteotomy has not often been performed because of a perceived risk of the deformity being made worse. Thirty-six cases in which osteotomies in phalanges or metacarpals were stabilized with AO plates and screws were reviewed, and the results were satisfactory in most cases.

The majority (64%) of the fractures had been treated in plaster after the original injury. Twenty-two percent had no immobilization, whereas 14% had various forms of internal fixation. Angular or rotary malunion or both was the indication for the osteotomy. Stabilization was accomplished with 1 of 4 types of AO plates and screws. The patients were followed up for an average of 12.5 months.

Results were judged to be very good in 23 cases, good in 8, and poor in 5, yielding an overall satisfactory rate of 86%. Two of the 5 failures were thought to have been poor candidates for the procedure (table). Fixation devices were removed in 66% of patients by the time of the last follow-up. Bony union occurred in all of the cases, and 86% of the patients had little or no joint stiffness. Results indicate that transverse meta-

Patient Summary and Results

Patient	Age	Malunion site	Osteotomy site	Type deformity	Other surgery	Result
LD	41	Prox. phalanx I	Same	Angular/Rotation	0	Very good
MB	27	"	"	Angular	0	Very good
MK	22	"	"	"	0	Very good
JB	23	Metacarpal II	"	Rotation	0	Very good
GL	18	"	"	Angular/Rotation	0	Very good
JD	18	"	"	Angular	0	Good
FM	34	"	"	Rotation	0	Very good
GG	43	"	"	"	0	Very good
MT	54	Middle phalanx III	Same	Angular	0	Good
GR	36	Prox. phalanx III	"	Rotation	0	Very good
KS	23	Metacarpal III	"	Angular/Rotation	0	Very good
GW	19	"	"	Rotation	0	Very good
JG	30	"	"	Angular	0	Very good
AB	37	"	"	Rotation	0	Good
HR	40	Prox. phalanx IV	"	"	0	Very good
EM	54	Metacarpal IV	"	Angular	0	Very good
AL	28	"	"	"	0	Very good
ON	25	"	"	Rotation	0	Good
MA	35	"	"	Angular	0	Very good
CA	29	Prox. phalanx V	Metacarpal	Rotation	Tenolysis/Silastic sheet	Poor
RF	20	"	Same	"	0	Poor
AT	58	"	"	"	0	Poor
PK	27	"	"	"	0	Very good
AZ	65	"	"	"	0	Very good
HS	24	"	"	"	0	Very good
FV	15	"	"	Angular/Rotation	0	Poor
JO	34	Metacarpal V	"	Angular	0	Poor
MA	24	"	"	"	0	Very good
BK	27	"	"	"	0	Very good
JW	20	"	"	"	0	Very good
FG	38	"	"	"	0	Very good
EJ	16	"	"	"	0	Very good
JD	18	"	"	"	0	Very good
AL*	28	"	"	"	0	Good
MA*	35	"	"	"	0	Good
CA*	29	"	"	"	0	Good

*Patients AL, MA, and CA had osteotomies of 2 different bones in the same hand at the same surgical procedure and are listed twice.
(Courtesy of Lucas GL, Pfeiffer CM: *Ann Chir Main* 8:30–38, 1989.)

carpal and phalangeal osteotomy can be a successful procedure for correction of angular or rotary deformity, or both.

▶ A malunion of metacarpal and phalangeal fractures can result in significant functional disability to the injured hand. The authors described the technique of using AO plate and screws to correct angular and rotational deformities. The advantage of this technique is that, with rigid fixation, active and passive range of motion can be started immediately after surgery. There is, however, a significant disadvantage in using this technique in that 66% of the patients described in this series needed removal of the internal fixation devices. I agree with the authors that internal fixation provides an optimal way of fixing osteotomies; however, I disagree with their statement that osteotomies always should be performed at the site of deformity. In certain instances, phalangeal malunions with rotational deformity are best treated with metacarpal osteotomy.—A.J. Weiland, M.D.

6 The Spine

Introduction

Spinal disorders continue to grow as a source of intensive clinical and research interest. More residents are seeking fellowship training, and the size of societies devoted to spinal disease are growing in size and stature. Much of this interest stems from the increasing complexity and sophistication of spinal surgery. Rigid fixation devices permit an attack on more complex spinal deformities and surgical failures, as does the aggressive use of anterior approaches. We now have good information from laboratory studies that confirm the clinical hypothesis that increased union follows the use of these appliances (McAfee: *Spine* 1990). However, the same studies show stress shielding does occur, the long-term impact of which is uncertain. Clinical experience such as that reported by Whiteside demonstrates the higher than usual complication rate, particularly during the learning phase. At the same time, newer surgical constructs continue to move us away from the use of traditional bone graft sources. For example, the use of hydroxyapatite is advocated in one article reviewed here; many other examples could have been chosen.

Correction of deformity and the magnitude of operations to deal with it are growing in complexity, but small is still thought to be better when decompression of disk herniation is attempted. Percutaneous diskectomy is used increasingly. Will this approach rise and fall like chymopapain, or will its place become established clearly? Only time will tell.

Spinal stenosis remains a topic of continued and growing interest. Who needs surgical treatment? Who can have decompression only? Who requires decompression with fusion? These questions are still open to debate. As part of dealing with the often elderly patient, the coincident management of osteoporosis is of increasing importance.

Despite the justifiable "hype" attached to spinal surgery, the reality is that this is a small part of the overall issue. Although the articles I chose for review have some intriguing basic science, notably absent are good clinical trials of conservative care. It is hoped that the growth of interest in spinal surgery will spill over to nonoperative care and prevention.

John W. Frymoyer, M.D.

Reference

1. McAfee PC, et al: *Spine* 14:919, 1989.

Cervical Fractures and Fusion Techniques

The Quadrangular Fragment Fracture: Roentgenographic Features and Treatment Protocol
Favero KJ, Van Peteghem PK (Shaughnessy Hosp–Univ of British Columbia, Vancouver)
Clin Orthop 239:40–46, February 1989   6–1

The quadrangular fragment fracture (QFF), thought to result from flexion with simultaneous axial loading, is difficult to manage. It does not respond well to posterior fusion and is characterized by a fracture line that creates an anterior quadrangular fragment, significant posterior sub-

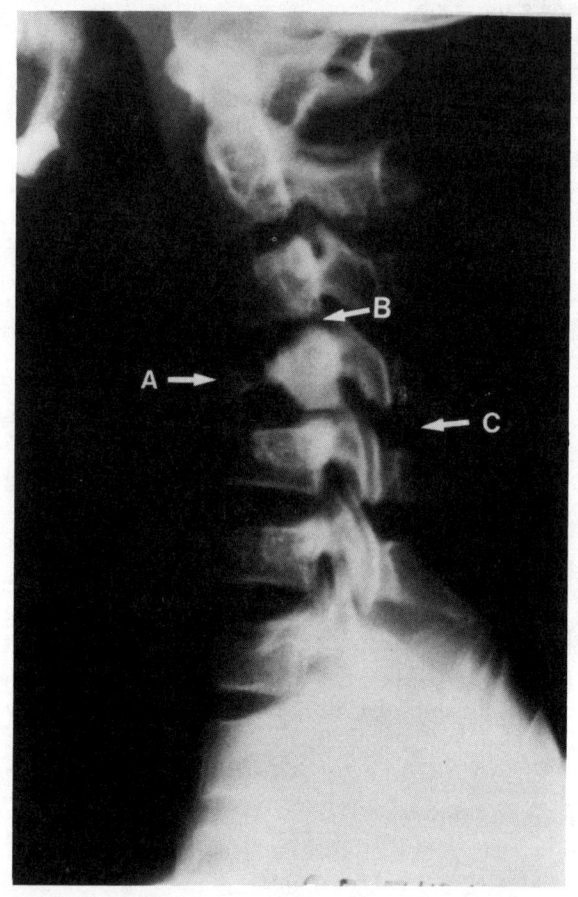

Fig 6–1.—A lateral roentgenogram showing a typical QFF with the 4 characteristic lesions: a quadrangular fragment *(A)*, posterior subluxation and kyphosis *(B)*, and the increased interspinous space indicative of disruption of the posterior elements *(C)*. (Courtesy of Favero KJ, Van Peteghem PK: *Clin Orthop* 239:40–46, February 1989.)

```
                    ┌─────────────────────┐
                    │   skull traction    │
                    │ 26-30 pounds over   │
                    │ an extension bolster│
                    └──────────┬──────────┘
                               │
                               ▼
   ┌──────────────────────┐        ┌────────┐   yes  ┌──────────────┐
   │ anterior inter-body  │        │        │───────▶│ traction for │
   │ strut from level above│──────▶│ stable │        │   6 weeks    │
   │ to level below injury │        │        │        └──────────────┘
   └──────────────────────┘        └────┬───┘
                                         │ no
                                         ▼
                              ┌─────────────────────┐
                              │   mobilization in   │
                              │ halo-thoracic brace │
                              └─────────────────────┘
```

Treatment B

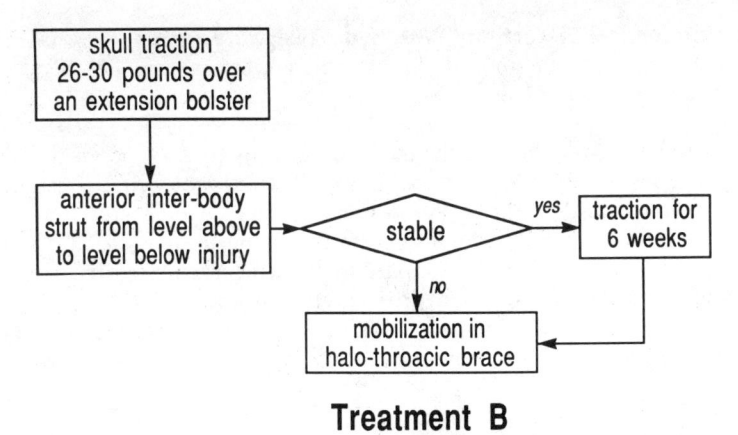

Fig 6-2.—Treatment B algorithm. Treatment B was developed when treatment A produced poor results in the first 23 patients with QFF. Treatment B was used in the final 15 patients. (Courtesy of Favero KJ, Van Peteghem PK: *Clin Orthop* 239:40-46, February 1989.)

luxation, some angular kyphosis, and an increased interspinous space with facet subluxation caused by disruption of the soft tissues (Fig 6-1).

Medical records and roentgenograms of 38 patients with confirmed QFF were reviewed. The patients' average age was 23 years; 29 patients were male. Fifteen patients had been ejected from motor vehicles at the time of an accident, and 11 were injured when diving. Twenty-five of the patients had associated head injuries; only 7 had escaped neurologic injury. Complete quadriplegia occurred in those patients with more than 5 mm of posterior displacement. Location of the QFF was C4-C5 in 9 patients, C5-C6 in 23, C6-C7 in 4, and C7-T1 in 1 patient.

The first 23 patients underwent treatment A, consisting of closed or open reduction with wire fixation with or without external fixation. Treatment B (Fig 6-2), a new protocol, was applied to the second group of 15 patients. Twelve patients in the treatment A group had a poor result with significant residual posterior subluxation at the fracture site. Although all fractures eventually healed with bony fusion, all patients had significant residual kyphosis resulting in neck pain. Thirteen patients who received treatment B had a satisfactory union at 4 weeks, and none needed reoperation or had significant neck pain.

Treatment B clearly is the modality of choice for QFF fractures. This method prevents further displacement, allows early mobilization, results in accurate reduction, and prevents pain at the fracture site.

▶ This well-documented series of patients with a relatively rare cervical fracture details the mechanisms of injury and radiographic findings. The greater value is in the comparison of treatments A and B, again demonstrating that spinal fusion is essential to successful outcomes in unstable injuries. In this retrospective and uncontrolled analysis, the goal was best achieved with anterior strut graft stabilization.—J.W. Frymoyer, M.D.

Anterior Cervical Discectomy With Hydroxylapatite Fusion

Senter HJ, Kortyna R, Kemp WR (Western Pennsylvania Hosp, Pittsburgh)
Neurosurgery 25:39–43, July 1989   6–2

Controversy over the benefits of fusion during anterior cervical diskectomy is considerable. Specific criticisms of autologous iliac crest interbody fusion include pain at the donor site, risk of iliac crest infection, meralgia paresthetica, eventual absorption of the bone plug, and failure to fuse. The outcomes were compared between patients treated with autologous iliac crest fusion or hydroxyapatite fusion.

During the first 2½-year study period, 75 patients underwent anterior cervical diskectomy and autologous interbody fusion with iliac crest. The

Comparison of Results in Groups 1 and 2

Number of Patients	Number of Cervical Levels Treated	Complications — Kind	n	%	Angulation >30% with Midline Pain — n	%
Group 1[a]						
33	1	None			0	
31	2	Slipped bone plug with second operation	2		0	
		Meralgia paresthetica	3	23	0	
		Chronic hip pain	1			
		Radiculopathy at a new level with second operation	1			
11	3	Iliac crest infection	1	18	1	9
		Radiculopathy at a new level with second operation	1			
75			9	12[b]		
Group 2[c]						
53	1	Partial slippage or fracture[d]	3	6	0	
		Slippage requiring second operation[d]	0		0	
27	2	Partial slippage or fracture[d]	1	7	0	
		Slippage requiring second operation[d]	1	7	0	
3	3	None				
1	4[e]	None				
84			5	6		

[a]Treated by anterior cervical diskectomy and fusion.
[b]Rate of second operations, 5%.
[c]Treated by anterior cervical diskectomy and hydroxyapatite fusion.
[d]Treated with 12 weeks of wearing a cervical collar, rather than 6 weeks.
[e]Performed as 2 separate 2-level procedures.
(Courtesy of Senter HJ, Kortyna R, Kemp WR: Neurosurgery 25:39–43, July 1989.)

operating microscope was used for all procedures, and the Smith-Robinson technique for interbody fusion was used exclusively. Indications for operation included radioculopathy in 61 patients, of whom 21 had spondylytic osteophytic spurs. Fourteen patients had myelopathy with or without radioculopathy, and 35 had soft disk herniation. Clinical follow-up ranged from 4 to 6 years.

During the second 2.5-year study period, 84 patients underwent anterior cervical diskectomy and fusion with synthetic, dense, nonresorptive hydroxyapatite spacers. Indications for operation included radiculopathy in 72 patients, of whom 50 had soft disk herniations and 22 had spondylytic osteophytic spurs. Twelve patients had myelopathy. Clinical follow-up ranged from 6 months to 3 years.

All patients with radiculopathy who had iliac crest fusions obtained relief at the appropriate level (table). However, in 2 patients radiculopathy recurred within 6 months at adjacent levels and both patients needed new fusion procedures. Infection developed at the iliac crest donor site in 1

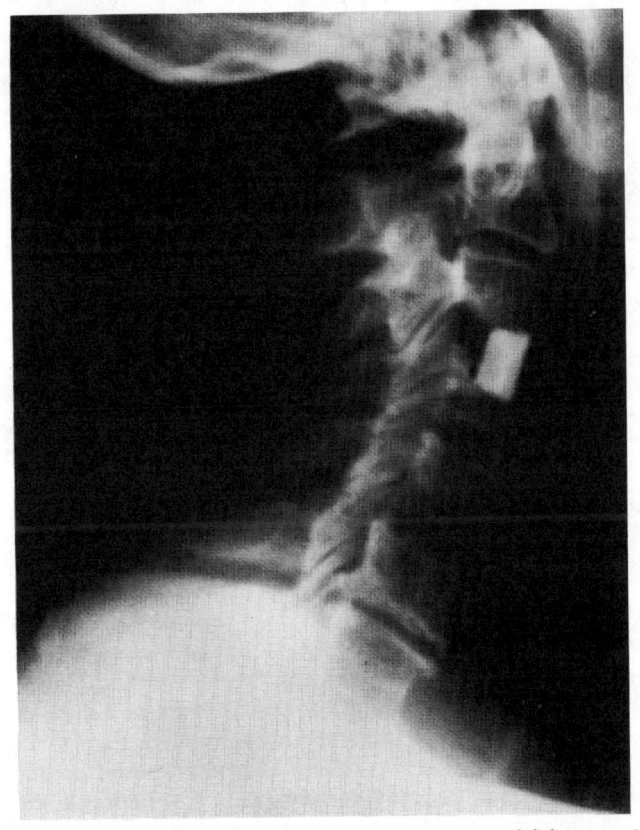

Fig 6–3.—Roentgenogram of cervical spine 3 years after anterior cervical diskectomy with hydroxyapatite fusion and partial vertebrectomy at C3–4 in a patient with myelopathy. (Courtesy of Senter HJ, Kortyna R, Kemp WR: *Neurosurgery* 25:39–43, July 1989.)

patient, and meralgia paresthetica developed in 3. Chronic hip pain developed in 1 patient after graft removal. Ten of the 14 patients with myelopathy were improved after operation. All patients with radiculopathy who received the hydroxyapatite bone plugs also obtained relief at the appropriate level. Although 3 hydroxyapatite bone plugs slipped and 2 fractured, only 1 patient needed a second operation. Nine (75%) of the patients with myelopathy had improvement (Fig 6–3).

Hydroxyapatite is biocompatible, is nonresorptive, and bonds strongly to adjacent bone without fibrous encapsulation within 6–8 weeks. The compound is equal or superior to iliac crest for anterior cervical fusion, and its use is recommended highly.

▶ Basic laboratory research and an increased understanding of the biochemistry of bone formation are leading to clinical applications of these newer insights. The experience presented here suggests adequate stabilization is obtained, but the clinical follow-up is short. The obvious and basic question is whether the construct will withstand the test of time. Six of the 84 patients already have failed by radiographic criteria. A review of the postoperative radiographs leaves open the question of whether any of the "grafts" have united or are still simply behaving as spacers. Although the basic premise that donor graft sites are a source of problem is correct, I remain unconvinced the technique yet deserves widespread application.—J.W. Frymoyer, M.D.

Spinal Stenosis—Causes and Treatment

Developmental Spinal Canal Stenosis and Somatotype
Nightingale S (Queen Elizabeth Hosp, Birmingham, England)
J Neurol Neurosurg Psychiatry 52:887–890, July 1989   6–3

The pathogenesis of developmental spinal canal stenosis has not been studied extensively. The reason may be that canal size is related to overall skeletal size, but most clinicians find that the canals of large people are not unusually large nor are the canals of small people stenotic. If canal dimensions are not related to overall skeletal size, they might be associated with a particular body shape or somatotype. The hypothesis that somatotype and developmental cervical spine canal stenosis may be associated was investigated.

Ninety-one persons had the following measurements taken using standard anthropometric techniques: standing and sitting heights; foot, tibia, upper arm, and lower arm lengths; bicondylar femur and humerus diameters; bi-iliocristal and biacromial diameters; head and chest circumferences; and weight. Cervical spine radiographs were then taken with a constant focus-image distance of 2 m. The anteroposterior diameter of the cervical spinal canal was measured at the C6 vertebral level from the midpoint of the posterior surface of the vertebral body to the nearest part of the line formed by the junction of the laminae. After correction for magnification, mean anteroposterior diameters of the sixth vertebral canal for men and women were 14.8 and 14.3 mm, respectively. Several individual anthropometric variables were associated with cervical canal size. The most significant correlation was between canal size and upper arm length, which was still significant after control for the effect of sex and when men were considered alone. Height, foot length, tibia length, forearm length, and the widths of the knee and elbow also were correlated with canal size; controlling for sex or considering men alone, however, abolished those associations.

Only 22% of the variation in developmental canal size can be related to somatotype. Cervical developmental stenosis is part of a generalized skeletal misproportion. Prenatal and postnatal processes that determine the adult skeletal proportions affect the relationship of cervical size to the long bones of the body and to body length.

▶ This article addresses a basic question: "Is spinal stenosis part of a generalized skeletal misproportion?" The authors quite meticulously have measured a series of anthropometric variables and found some correlation of canal size to upper arm length. The article does not really answer the question, but leaves it open for debate. Perhaps results would have been different it they had the benefit of more accurate measures of developmental stenosis, such as magnetic resonance imaging.—J.W. Frymoyer, M.D.

Fluorotic Cervical Myelopathy
Naidu MRC, Raja Reddy D, Reddy PK, Sastry Kolluri VR (Nizam's Inst of Med Sciences; Osmania Gen Hosp, Hyderabad; Natl Inst of Mental Health and Neurosciences, Bangalore, India)
Fr J Orthop Surg 3:204–207, June 1989   6–4

In India, fluorosis affects half a million persons. Manual laborers are especially vulnerable because of the large quantities of water drunk in tropical regions and the acceleration of the process by muscle activity. Nearly all the retained fluoride is fixed in the skeleton, especially in cancellous bone. The skeletal concentration is dependent on how much and for how long fluoride is ingested. The cervical spine, because of its mobility, often is affected (Fig 6–4). The role of surgical intervention is not widely recognized.

Forty patients, 36 of them men, were operated on for cervical myelopathy and other manifestations of fluorosis (table). Computed tomography

Clinical Signs

Radiculo-myelopathy :	40
Indefinite sensory level :	10
Cervical stiffness :	36
Joint stiffness :	30

(Courtesy of Naidu MRC, Raja Reddy D, Reddy PK, et al: Fr J Orthop Surg 3:204–207, June 1989.)

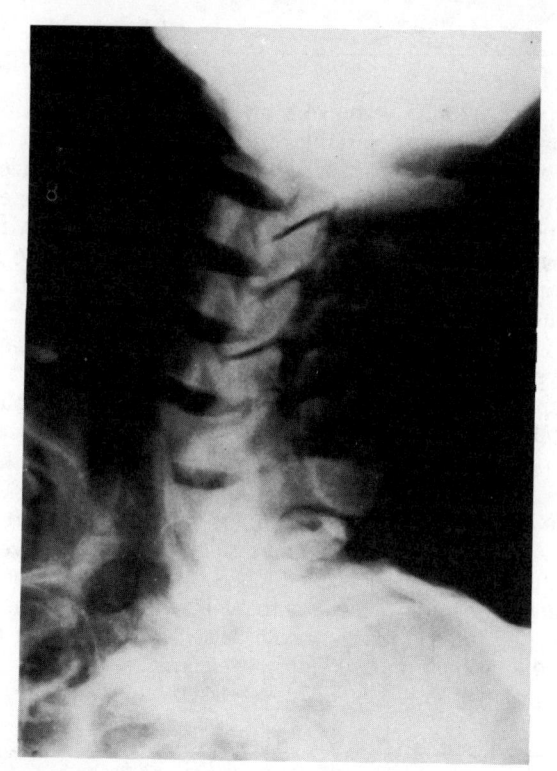

Fig 6–4.—Lateral radiograph of the cervical spine showing bone sclerosis and calcification of the ligaments. (Courtesy of Naidu MRC, Raja Reddy D, Reddy PK, et al: *Fr J Orthop Surg* 3:204–207, June 1989.)

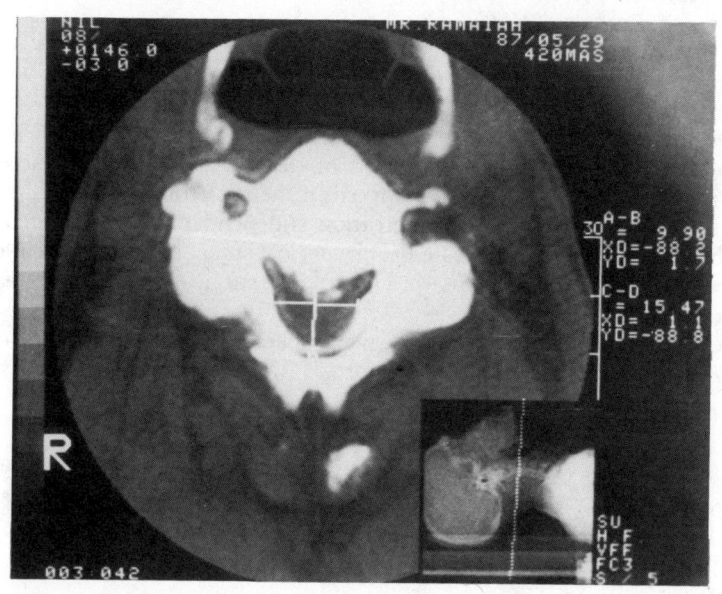

Fig 6–5.—Computed tomography scan appearances showing osteophytic stenosis of the cervical spinal canal. (Courtesy of Naidu MRC, Raja Reddy D, Reddy PK, et al: *Fr J Orthop Surg* 3:204–207, June 1989.)

revealed ligamental calcification, increased bone density, and osteophytes (Fig 6-5). Spinal cord compression was limited to the cervical region, and respiratory function was adequate. Patients first had laminectomy over at least 4 vertebrae, with avoidance of excessive neck flexion, and then physiotherapy.

Three deaths occurred soon after operation, 1 from myocardial infarction and 2 from respiratory paralysis. Neurologic recovery was satisfactory in 32 patients. All 12 patients who were observed for 1-3 years were able to do reduced work and to care for themselves.

The results of cervical surgery in selected patients are encouraging. Success requires excellent anesthesia and respiratory care. Defluorination of patients' drinking water is necessary to stop progression of myelopathy.

▶ An extensive experience with cervical myelopathy is presented, secondary to environmental fluoride ingestion. The value of this article is threefold: (1) despite this condition being uncommon in the United States, surgeons will encounter this condition more often, much in the same way we now are seeing and having to deal with OPLL; (2) the experience is large and suggests the outcomes are not uniquely different from those of problems encountered with cervical myelopathies caused by other conditions; and (3) the advice for halting the progression of myelopathy makes me wonder whether we will begin to see myelopathies secondary to patients receiving fluorides for osteoporosis.— J.W. Frymoyer, M.D.

Cervical Kyphosis and Myelopathy: Treatment by Anterior Corpectomy and Strut-Grafting
Zdeblick TA, Bohlman HH (Case Western Reserve Univ)
J Bone Joint Surg [Am] 71-A:170-182, February 1989   6-5

Kyphotic deformity of the cervical spine with compression of the spinal cord can cause cervical myelopathy, which can result in severe disability secondary to quadriparesis. Whatever the cause of the kyphosis, the resulting deformity is difficult to correct surgically.

During an 8-year study period 11 men and 3 women aged 21-73 years (mean, 46 years) with cervical kyphosis and myelopathy underwent anterior decompression and arthrodesis. The lesions preceding the development of kyphosis were spondylosis in 8 patients, traumatic injury in 5, and a benign intradural tumor in 1 (Fig 6-6). Severe kyphosis and myelopathy had developed after laminectomy of 3, 4, or 5 cervical vertebrae, or an average of 2.25 vertebral bodies, with subsequent average fusion of 3.25 levels.

Eight patients had fibular grafts that spanned an average of 4.10 levels (Fig 6-7). Six patients had iliac grafts that spanned an average of 2.70 levels. Four of the 5 patients with traumatic lesions had anterior decompression and arthrodesis combined with posterior arthrodesis, which was performed during the same anesthesia period. However, in 3 of these 4

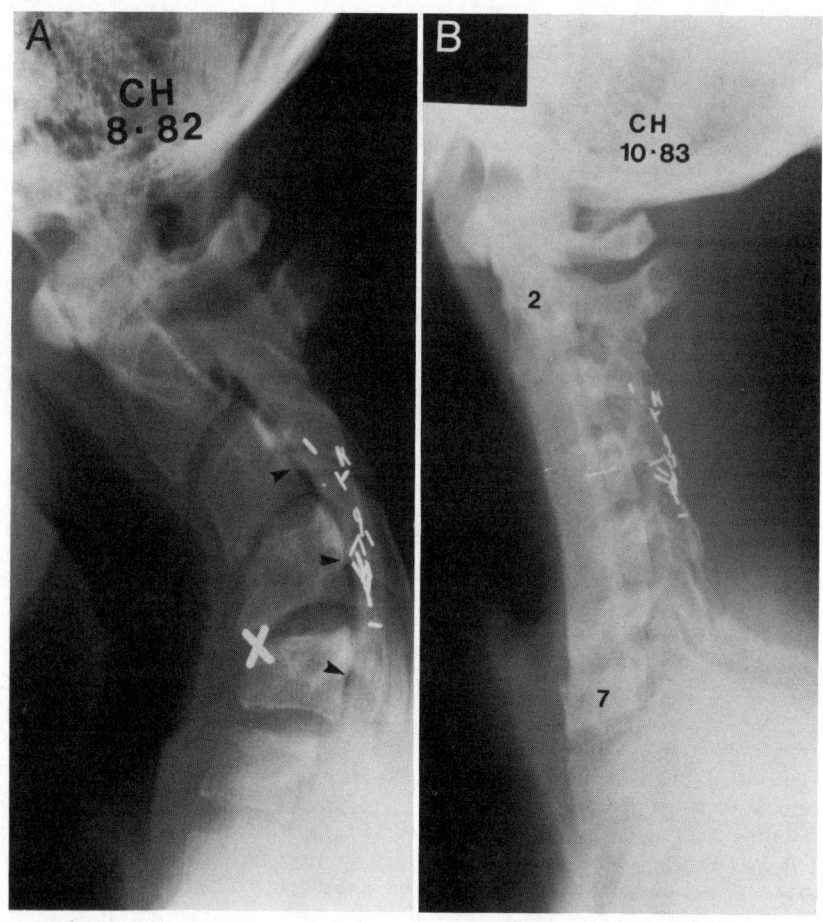

Fig 6–6.—A young man had progressive quadriparesis and pain in the neck caused by an arteriovenous malformation at the third cervical level. This was treated with laminectomy from the third to the sixth cervical vertebra, myelotomy, excision of the tumor, and drainage of a syrinx. After surgery, the patient remained quadriparetic (grade-3 motor strength). A progressive kyphosis developed 4 years later, as did quadriplegia. The kyphosis measured 43 degrees. **A,** myelography demonstrated several points of anterior compression of the cord *(arrows)* at the level of the kyphosis. **B,** a multilevel decompression was performed through an anterior approach. To do this, subtotal corpectomies were carried out from the third to the sixth cervical level. Traction was applied to reduce the kyphosis, and a fibular strut graft was inserted to provide stability. After 34 months, fusion was solid with minimum residual kyphosis. Motor strength had returned to grade 3. (Courtesy of Zdeblick TA, Bohlman HH: J Bone Joint Surg [Am] 71-A:170–182, February 1989.)

patients the anterior grafts because dislodged in the immediately postoperative period; 2 of these grafts subsequently were revised to restore stability. Two patients died within a year of operation, but both had solid fusions and stable recovery of neural function before death. The other 12 were followed for an average of 2.6 years, during which all fusions remained solid. Nine patients had complete recovery of neural function and 4 had partial recovery. One patient continued to be completely quadriplegic.

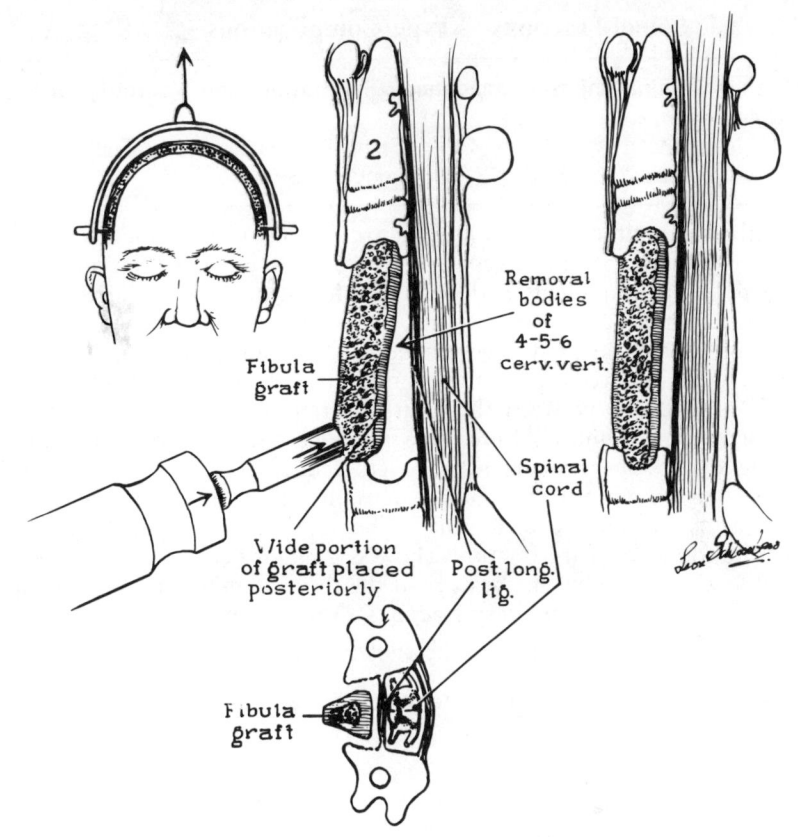

Fig 6–7.—The steps of the procedure that are performed after anterior corpectomy and decompression. Skeletal traction is increased to reduce the kyphosis. Extension of the neck also may be needed. Seating holes are made in the end plates of the superior and inferior intact vertebral bodies with a burr. The ends of the graft are then rounded, and the graft is impacted into place. When the traction is released, the graft is locked into place. (Courtesy of Zdeblick TA, Bohlman HH: *J Bone Joint Surg [Am]* 71-A:170–182, February 1989.)

In patients with severe cervical kyphosis and myelopathy, adequate anterior decompression of the spinal cord, correction of the kyphosis, and anterior arthrodesis using a strut graft can accomplish fusion, which will allow recovery of the myelopathy. However, the surgical procedures are technically demanding.

▶ How best to treat myelopathy of the cervical spine is open to debate. When postural deformity is absent, the good results can be achieved with posterior decompression or, in selected cases, the use of laminoplasty. When a significant deformity is present other strategies may be necessary. In particular, the authors have shown that the difficult problem of cervical kyphosis with myelopathy may be managed with anterior decompression over multiple levels with fusion. Their admonition is well taken; these are technically demanding procedures.—J.W. Frymoyer, M.D.

Thoracic Spinal Fractures—Type/Complications

Multilevel Spinal Injuries: Incidence, Distribution, and Neurological Patterns
Gupta A, El Masri WS (Midland Ctr for Spinal Injuries, Oswestry, England)
J Bone Joint Surg [Br] 71-B:692–695, August 1989   6–6

Although multilevel spinal injuries are not uncommon, the neurologic patterns of injury and recovery have not been well studied. During a 26-year-period, 935 patients had treatment for acute spinal injuries, 91 of whom had multilevel spinal injuries.

Injuries were classified as contiguous when more than 3 adjacent vertebrae were involved and as noncontinuous if there was at least 1 uninjured articulation between the injured vertebrae. By these criteria, 71 multilevel spinal injuries were noncontiguous and 20 were multiple but contiguous lesions. Primary lesions were defined as those responsible for a patient's symptoms or neurologic signs on admission; secondary lesions were defined as those contributing to the patient's neurologic deficit. The distribution of primary fractures showed a major peak at the lower cervical level and another major peak at the thoracolumbar level (Fig 6–8). The distribution of secondary fractures showed 2 major peaks at upper cervical and cervicothoracic levels, and 2 minor peaks at middorsal and sacral levels.

A definite pattern of injury in terms of the relationship between the pri-

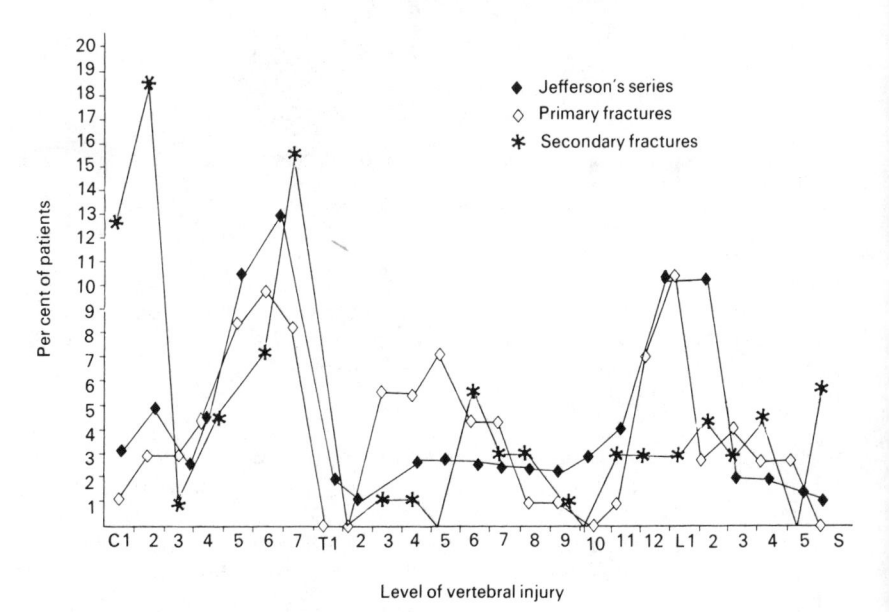

Fig 6–8.—Distribution of primary and secondary lesions in 91 patients with multiple noncontiguous fractures compared with Jefferson's series of 2,006 spinal fractures. (Courtesy of Gupta A, El Masri WS: J Bone Joint Surg [Br] 71-B:692–695, August 1989.)

Neurologic Patterns in Patients With Multilevel Spinal Injury at
the Time of Admission and at Final Review

Group	Number		Frankel grade				
			A	B	C	D	E
I	91	Admission	41	13	9	14	14
		Result	41	2	4	20	24
II	20	Admission	10	3	3	3	1
		Result	10	1	1	5	3
III	71	Admission	31	10	6	11	13
		Result	31	1	3	15	21
IV	61	Admission	24	8	6	10	13
		Result	24	1	2	14	20
V	10	Admission	7	2	0	1	0
		Result	7	0	1	1	1

(Courtesy of Gupta A, El Masri WS: *J Bone Joint Surg [Br]* 71-B:692–695, August 1989.)

mary and secondary level could not be identified in 52% of the patients, but 7 patterns of injury were defined for the remaining 42%. In 55% of the patients, multilevel spinal injuries had caused only incomplete neurologic lesions, possibly because the impact force was dissipated over several segments. At the final follow-up evaluation, 56% of these patients had neurologic improvement. Multilevel noncontiguous lesions at more than 2 levels had the worst prognosis, as 70% of these patients had complete paraplegia (table).

The 9.7% incidence of multilevel spinal injury in this study population underscores the importance of early recognition of this type of injury, as nondiagnosed secondary spinal lesions may have serious neurologic consequences.

▶ If a meticulous search is made, multiple spinal fractures are more common than usually suspected, when there is high energy trauma. Two somewhat different perspectives emerge from these articles, 1 suggesting the lesser, and usually overlooked, fracture is usually stable, the other suggesting nondiagnosed secondary spinal lesions may have serious neurologic consequences. The important lesson is to look for multiple fractures, which seem to occur in almost 10% of patients, particularly when a patient is unconscious.—J.W. Frymoyer, M.D.

Multiple-Level Noncontiguous Spinal Fractures
Powell JN, Waddell JP, Tucker WS, Transfeldt EE (St Michael's Hosp, Toronto; Univ of Toronto)
J Trauma 29:1146–1151, August 1989

278 / Orthopedics

Summary of Multiple-Level Noncontiguous Spinal Injury Cases

Patient No.	Age (years)/Sex	Mechanism	ISS	Site of Injury	Stability	Neurologic	Treatment	Outcome
1	30/F	MVA	34	T7 burst fracture, T12 compression fracture	Unstable, stable	Intact	Brace	United
2	30/M	MVA	41	C6-C7 fracture-dislocation, T10 burst fracture	Unstable, unstable	Incomplete T10 cord lesion	Anterior fusion, posterior fusion	Root deficit C7 postoperative
3	42/M	Fall from a height	24	T7 compression fracture, L1 burst fracture	Stable, unstable	L1 incomplete paraplegia	Brace Posterior instrumentation	Partial neurological recovery with union of the fractures
4	52/F	Fall off ladder	22	C2 hangman's fracture, T8 burst fracture	Unstable, unstable	T8 root lesion	Brace	Fractures united
5	72/M	Injured by falling tree	20	C5-C6 spinous process and laminar fractures, T2 dislocation, T2 fracture-dislocation	Stable, unstable	T2 partial paraplegia	Laminectomy ×2, brace	Eventual improvement to dependent ambulation
6	29/M	MVA	17	C2 lateral mass Fracture sacral alar	Stable, stable	L5 root lesion	Brace, ORIF pelvis	Union of fracture
7	22/F	Diving accident	75	Type II, odontoid fracture, C7 fractured lamina spinous process	Unstable, stable	Complete high cervical cord	Ventilatory support	Died

8	54/F	Fell down 2 flights of stairs	34	C1 Jefferson fracture, T7 burst fracture	Stable, unstable	T4 paraplegia	Collar Bed rest	Died of Gram-negative sepsis
9	22/M	MVA	19	C6-C7 fracture-dislocation, T4-T5 compression fracture	Unstable, stable	Intact	Anterior fusion, brace	Union of fusion and fracture
10	18/M	MVA	22	Type II odontoid C3-C4 subluxation	Unstable, unstable	Intact	Posterior fusion, anterior fusion	Union but chronic pain syndrome
11	56/M	MVA	18	C5 spinous process fracture, C6 lamina fracture, C7 facet fracture	Unstable,	L5 root lesion	Brace and bed rest	Union of the fracture, partial recovery L5 nerve root
12	45/M	MVA	50	Sacral body T10 paraplegia (no skeletal injury)	stable Stable	T10 paraplegia	Bed rest until pelvis stabilized and then mobilized	Early satisfactory, lost to followup
13	28/F	MVA	18	C7 compression fracture, T4 burst fracture	Stable, unstable	Intact	Bed rest and brace	Union of fractures
14	21/M	Fall from a height	17	T11 compression fracture, L3 burst fracture	Stable, unstable	Intact	Brace	Union of fracture, significant spinal stenosis, asymptomatic at present

(Courtesy of Powell JN, Waddell JP, Tucker WS, et al: *J Trauma* 29:1146–1151, August 1989.)

Double-level noncontiguous spinal injury may be more common than previously reported. The records of 212 patients with spinal injury were reviewed retrospectively to determine the incidence, associated findings, and treatment of multiple-level noncontiguous spinal fractures.

Fourteen patients (6.6%) aged 18–72 years (mean, 37) had multiple-level noncontiguous spinal injury (table). Motor vehicle accidents and falls from a height were the most common cause of injury. All patients had Injury Severity Scores of 16 or greater, with an average of 29. Neurologic injury was present in 9 patients; 3 patients had complete cord lesions at C1, T4, or T10; 3 had partial cord lesions at T2, T10, or L1; 1 patient had a cauda equina, and 2 had single root involvement at T8 or L5. Usually the pattern of skeletal injury was 1 unstable and 1 stable injury. Only 1 patient had a potentially unstable injury that was diagnosed late. Treatment was individualized and depended on the pattern of injury. Generally, the presence of a second level of spinal injury did not affect the indications for surgery. Treatment outcome was largely associated with the presence or absence of neurologic injury.

Double-level noncontiguous spinal injury is relatively more common than is generally appreciated. All patients with high-energy injury must be suspected of having spinal fracture until proven otherwise. A complete radiologic survey of the spine must be included in the emergency room evaluation when clinical assessment is impaired. Treatment must be individualized using the same guidelines as for treating the isolated injury.

Fibrinolysis and Spinal Injury: Relationship to Post-Traumatic Deep Vein Thrombosis
Petäjä J, Myllynen P, Rokkanen P, Nokelainen M (Helsinki Univ Hosp)
Acta Chir Scand 155:241–246, April–May 1989   6–8

Venous thrombosis occurs in 70% to 100% of patients with acute spinal cord injury as a result of several factors such as immobility, muscle paralysis, and trauma, but the hemostatic changes are not well understood. Therefore, 9 paralyzed patients with acute spinal injury and 12 unparalyzed control patients immobilized for cervical spine fracture were examined taking fibrinolytic measurements at rest, after venous occlusion, and during 10 days' monitoring.

Venous thrombosis, detected by the fibrinogen ^{125}I test, occurred in 78% of the paralyzed patients and 8% of controls 5–10 days after injury. Tissue plasminogen activator levels were similar in both paralyzed patients and controls. However, levels of tissue plasminogen activator activity were significantly lower in paralyzed patients than in controls after venous occlusion. On admission the levels of tissue plasminogen activator inhibitor were somewhat higher in paralyzed patients, and venous occlusion intensified this difference. On day 6 after injury, paralyzed patients had significant increases in von Willebrand factor antigen, fibrinogen, and, on day 10, factor VIII procoagulant activity as well.

Thrombogenesis in patients with acute spinal cord injury is preceded by reduced fibrinolytic capacity. Impairment of fibrinolysis probably contributes to thrombogenesis, but thus far fibrinolytic measurements are unable to predict which patients will have venous thrombosis.

▶ Deep venous thrombosis (DVT) and pulmonary emboli (PE) are a major problem after spinal cord injury. Many of us naively assume this relates to the hemodynamics of the peripheral vessels, akin to the increased risk of DVT and PE in patients at prolonged bedrest. Although this study is preliminary and incomplete, it raises the question of altered clotting mechanisms as either causative or contributory. Although the authors readily admit they do not know how to use this information predictively, even the possibility opens the door for future therapeutic trials aimed at prevention.—J.W. Frymoyer, M.D.

Cause of Death for Patients With Spinal Cord Injuries
DeVivo MJ, Kartus PL, Stover SL, Rutt RD, Find PR (Univ of Alabama, Birmingham)
Arch Intern Med 149:1761–1766, August 1989

The life expectancies of patients with spinal cord injuries remain substantially low. To define ways of preventing or managing potentially fatal complications after these injuries, the leading causes of death within the first 7 years after spinal cord injury were evaluated in 5,131 patients. These patients were admitted to 1 of 7 federally designated regional spinal cord injury care systems and survived for at least 24 hours after injury.

By the end of follow-up, 459 patients (9%) had died. The leading cause of death was pneumonia, followed by unintentional injuries and suicides (table). The highest ratios of actual to expected deaths (standard mortality ratios [SMRs]) were for septicemia, pulmonary embolism, and pneumonia. Pneumonia was the leading cause of death among quadriplegic patients and patients at least 55 years of age, whereas unintentional injuries and suicides were common among paraplegic patients and patients younger than age 55. Except for cancer and unintentional injuries and suicides, SMRs were highest during the first month after injury for all causes. Pneumonia was the leading cause of death during the first 6 months after injury; unintentional injuries and suicides were the leading cause of death more than 6 months after injury. Urinary tract infection and severe pressure sores often were cited as contributory causes of death.

Conclusive evidence was found that mortalities for spinal cord injury patients have declined dramatically since World War II, but many cause-specific mortalities remain substantially above normal. Septicemia appears to be a leading cause of death for these patients. Life expectancies may be improved with patient education, particularly in the areas of proper skin care and bladder management, and regular home visits by skilled personnel to provide early diagnosis and problem management.

Cause of Death for 459 Deceased Patients
With Spinal Cord Injuries

Cause of Death	Actual Deaths	Expected Deaths	SMR	SMR, 95% Limits
Septicemia (038)	38	0.27	140.7	96.0-185.4
Cancer (140-239)	29	17.00	1.7	1.1-2.3
Ischemic heart disease (410-413)	30	21.87	1.4	0.9-1.9
Other heart disease (420-429)	37	2.48	14.9	10.1-19.7
Cerebrovascular disease (430-438)	20	5.23	3.8	2.1-5.5
Diseases of arteries (440-448)	8	1.40	5.7	1.7-9.7
Venous thrombosis and embolism (450-453)	28	0.62	45.2	28.5-61.9
Influenza and pneumonia (470-486)	79	1.75	45.1	35.1-55.1
Other respiratory disease (490-519)	15	2.34	6.4	3.2-9.6
Diseases of digestive system (531-533, 550-553, 560, 571)	17	3.01	5.6	2.9-8.3
Diseases of urinary system (580-599)	12	0.94	12.8	5.6-20.0
Symptoms and ill-defined conditions (780-796)	36	1.80	20.0	13.5-26.5
Unintentional injuries and suicides (E800-E959)	59	17.92	3.3	2.5-4.1
Residual (all others)	18	13.10	1.4	0.7-2.0
Unknown	33	...	...	...

SMR, standardized mortality ratio; *International Classification of Diseases Adapted*, ed 8; codes are in parentheses.
(Courtesy of DeVivo MJ, Kartus PL, Stover SL, et al: *Arch Intern Med* 149:1761–1766, August 1989.)

▶ The risks and causes of death in the acute phase after spinal cord injury seem quite well understood. The value of this article is its presentation of the later cause in a huge group of patients. The 10% mortality is striking, but most of the causes would be expected. What particularly caught my attention is the suicides that occur, particularly in younger paraplegics, 6 months or more after injury. Although not totally surprising, the article again emphasizes the need for careful follow-up and monitoring of these people who not only are severely injured physically but have had major and ongoing psychological trauma.—J.W. Frymoyer, M.D.

Epidemiology of Vertebral Fractures in Women
Melton LJ III, Kan SH, Frye MA, Wahner HW, O'Fallon WM, Riggs BL (Mayo Clinic and Found, Rochester, Minn)
Am J Epidemiol 129:1000–1011, 1989   6–10

Vertebral fracture prevalence was assessed in an age-stratified random sample of 200 women aged 50 years and older. Three different approaches were used to define vertebral fractures. In the first approach, the

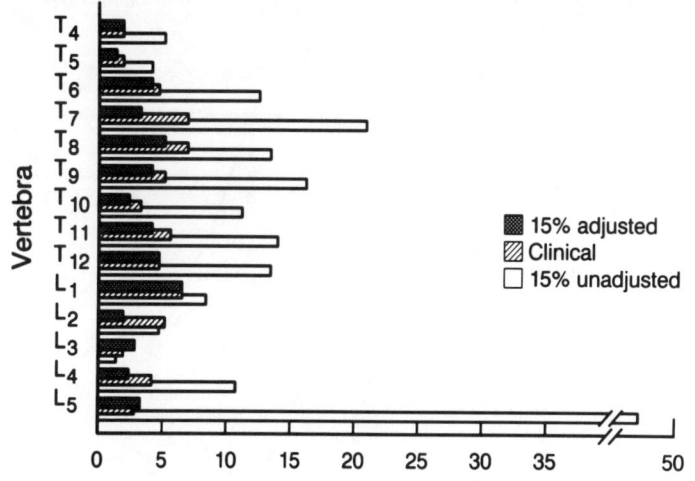

Fig 6–9.—Distribution of vertebral fractures by various criteria among Rochester, Minnesota, women aged 50 years and older, by vertebra. *Horizontal scale* is marked in 5% intervals. (Courtesy of Melton LJ III, Kan SH, Frye MA, et al: *Am J Epidemiol* 129:1000–1011, 1989.)

roentgenograms of all patients were read by a physician unaware of a patient's age or medical history. The second approach involved empirical criteria using a 15% reduction in vertebral body height to define a new fracture. In the third method, fractures were reassessed using the measured vertebral heights and the algorithm from the 15% criteria after adjustment for normal variations in vertebral shape and size.

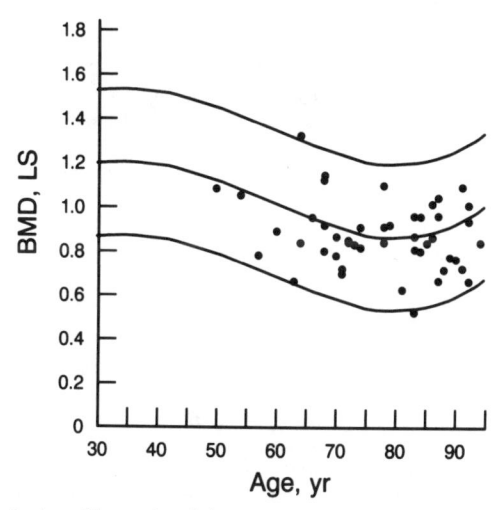

Fig 6–10.—Distribution of bone mineral density *(BMD)* of lumbar spine *(LS)* by age, among Rochester, Minnesota, women. The relation is best described by a cubic model: $\mu = 0.517835 + 0.492212 \times 10^{-1} \times \text{age} - 0.105822 \times 10^{-2} \times \text{age}^2 + 0.625726 \times 10^{-5} \times \text{age}^3$; $\sigma = 0.158749$, $R^2 = 0.33$. Values for women aged 50 years and older with 1 or more vertebral fractures are indicated by *circles*. (Courtesy of Melton LJ III, Kan SH, Frye MA, et al: *Am J Epidemiol* 129:1000–1011, 1989.)

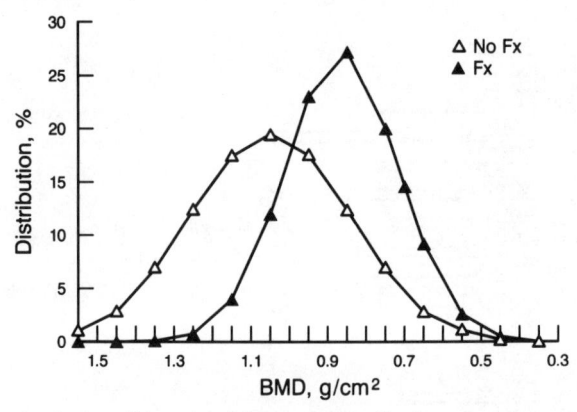

Fig 6–11.—Distribution of bone mineral density *(BMD)* of lumbar spine, by age, among Rochester, Minnesota women aged 50 years and older with *(Fx)* or without *(no Fx)* 1 or more vertebral fractures. (Courtesy of Melton LJ III, Kan SH, Frye MA, et al: *Am J Epidemiol* 129:1000–1011, 1989.)

Regardless of which of the approaches was used, distribution of fractures by vertebra showed concentrations in the midthoracic area and in the region of transition from thoracic to lumbar vertebrae (Fig 6–9). Using the second method, 166 (83%) women were classified as having at least 1 vertebral fracture. With the third method, 56 (28%) women had fractures. The prevalence of vertebral fractures increased with age, and reached an estimated 78% among women aged 90 years and older. When traumatic vertebral fractures were excluded this incidence was 51.7%. Bone mineral density as described in a cubic model decreased with age (Fig 6–10). Bone mass in women with vertebral fractures was not dra-

Estimated Prevalence of Atraumatic Vertebral Fractures by Bone Mineral Density of Lumbar Spine Among Rochester, Minnesota, Women Aged 50 Years and Older on January 1, 1980

Bone mineral density (g/cm²)	Expected no. with fractures	Estimated population	Prevalence (%)
≥1.30	4.8	229.5	2.1
1.20–1.29	22.7	498.9	4.6
1.10–1.19	82.4	1,031.7	8.0
1.00–1.09	199.0	1,563.1	12.7
0.90–0.99	322.4	1,734.8	18.6
0.80–0.89	350.3	1,401.5	25.0
0.70–0.79	255.3	815.0	31.3
0.60–0.69	124.8	337.1	37.0
<0.60	51.3	121.4	42.3
Total	1,413	7,733	

(Courtesy of Melton LJ III, Kan SH, Frye MA, et al: *Am J Epidemiol* 129:1000–1011, 1989.)

matically lower than other women of similar age, and the bone mineral density distributions overlapped considerably in both groups (Fig 6–11). From the total population (1,413) the total number of women with 1 or more vertebral fractures was estimated using the smoothed age-specific prevalence rates, and bone density-specific vertebral fracture prevalence rates were estimated (table). As bone density decreased, vertebral fracture prevalence increased, reaching levels of 40% among 6% of women aged 50 years and older who had spinal bone mineral density less than 0.7 g/cm^2. The mean number per patient among women with a vertebral fracture increased from 1 in women with bone density levels 1.1 g/cm^2 or greater to more than 3 per person in women with bone density less than 0.8 g/cm^2.

A close relation between spinal bone mass and vertebral fracture prevalence was observed; because spinal bone mass is decreased with age, fracture risk also is increased with age. Bone mineral density, however, as assessed by dual photon absorptiometry in the lumbar spine, does not entirely account for the age-related increase in fracture prevalence.

▶ I continue to be intrigued by osteoporotic compression fractures and, in particular, the newer diagnostic techniques to predict who is at risk, as well as the more general question of how major a problem this is becoming with our aging population. The conclusions are fairly obvious and not unexpected. However, the article does leave unanswered how much we can rely on dual photon absorptiometry for any 1 patient.—J.W. Frymoyer, M.D.

Dural Laceration Occurring With Burst Fractures and Associated Laminar Fractures
Cammisa FP Jr, Eismont FJ, Green BA (Univ of Miami–Jackson Mem Hosp Med Ctr, Miami)
J Bone Joint Surg [Am] 71-A:1044–1052, August 1989   6–11

The incidence of dural laceration in burst thoracic or lumbar fractures with associated laminar fractures has not been well documented. The relationship between burst vertebral fracture and coexisting laminar fracture was examined in 47 men and 13 women, aged 14–70 years, who underwent operation for a burst thoracic or lumbar fracture between July 1984 and February 1988. All patients were operated on within 2 weeks of injury through a posterior approach and treated with posterior spinal instrumentation.

Thirty of the 60 patients did not have associated laminar fractures, and no dural lacerations were identified at operation. This finding was statistically significant and indicated that posterior dural lacerations occurred only when a laminar fracture was present.

The other 30 patients had burst fractures with associated laminar fractures. Five of the fractures were in the thoracic spine, and 25 were in the lumbar spine. Sixteen (53%) of the 30 patients had preoperative neurologic deficits; the other 14 were not neurologically impaired. Eleven

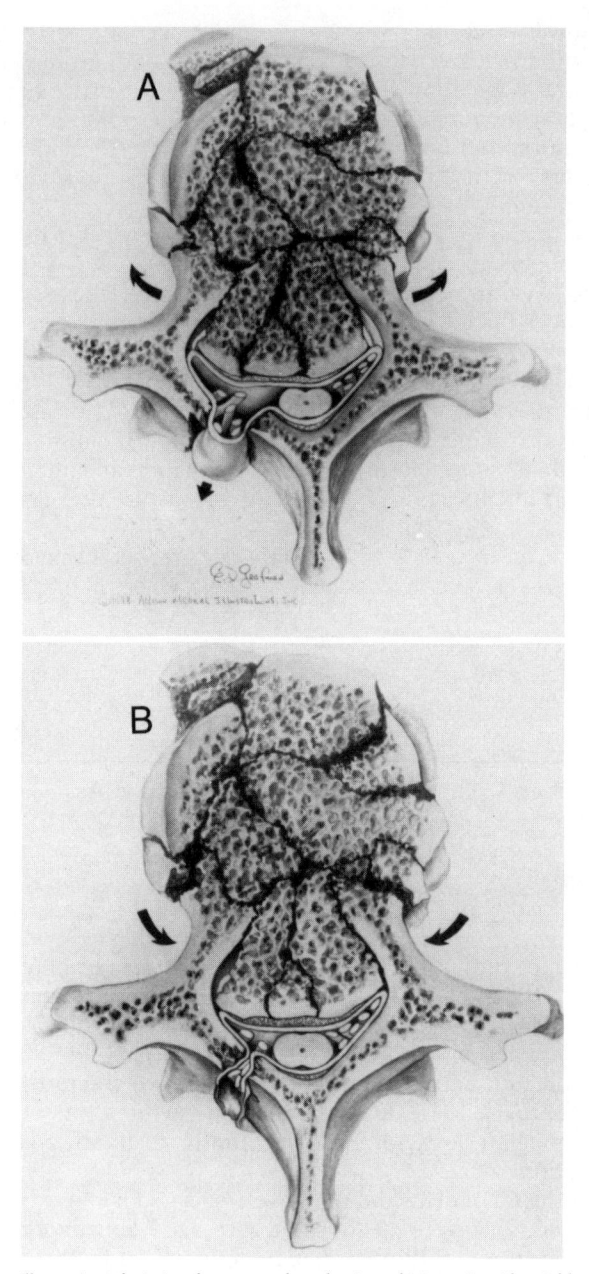

Fig 6–12.—Illustrations depicting the proposed mechanism of injury. **A,** with axial loading, the pedicles are spread laterally, the lamina fractures, and bone is retropulsed from the vertebral body, which may result in protrusion of the dura between the laminar fracture fragments. **B,** as the axial load is dissipated, the laminar fragments recoil, possibly entrapping the dura and nerve rootlets. (Courtesy of Cammisa FP Jr, Eismont FJ, Green BA: *J Bone Joint Surg [Am]* 71-A:1044–1052, August 1989.)

(69%) of the 16 patients with neurologic deficit had dural laceration in association with lumbar fractures. In 4 of those 11 patients, neural elements were entrapped between fragments from the laminar fracture (Fig 6-12).

Univariate and multivariate statistical analysis revealed no significant association between dural laceration and a patient's age, sex, or radiographic findings, including interpedicular distance, compression of the vertebral body, grade of compromise of the spinal canal, or the type of laminar fraction. However, the association between dural laceration and neurologic deficit was statistically significant.

A preoperative neurologic deficit in a patient with a burst vertebral fracture and an associated laminar fracture is a highly sensitive and specific predictor of dural laceration. This fracture pattern is also predictive of a finding of trapped neural elements at operation.

▶ This is a useful clinical study because it gives a clear set of clinical guidelines of who is at risk for a burst fracture, an associated laminar fracture, and a preoperative neurologic defect. More important, this pattern predicts trapped neural elements, which may provide 1 reversible cause of neural injury.—J.W. Frymoyer, M.D.

Basic Diagnosis in Low Back Pain

Fibrous Structure in the Intervertebral Disk: Correlation of MR Appearance With Anatomic Sections
Yu S, Haughton VM, Lynch KL, Ho K-C, Sether LA (Med College of Wisconsin, Milwaukee)
AJNR 10:1105-1110, September-October 1989   6-12

To correlate the magnetic resonance (MR) appearance of the intervertebral disk with its fibrous structure, the lumbar intervertebral disks in 10 cadavers were examined with MR, CT, cryomicrotome anatomical sections, and, in selected disks, with histologic and dried sections.

After MR imaging, specimens were frozen at −70C for 3 days, and a block of tissue including the entire lumbar spine was removed, which then was embedded in carboxymethylcellulose solution in a Styrofoam box. The frozen block was imaged using a GE 9800 CT scanner. A block of tissue was cryosectioned and photographed. The 6-μm sections were stained with hemotoxylin-eosin. The MR images were correlated with their corresponding CT, cryomicrotomic, histologic, and dried sections. Immature, transitional, and normal adult lumbar disks had different fibrous patterns. In newborns, the only fibrous tissue seen was in the laminated fibers in the disk periphery. Immature disks at age 2 years showed an increase in fibrous tissue in the midportion of the nucleus. At age 10 years, fibers in the lumbar nucleus pulposus could be seen, at age 19 years, disks had a solid, opaque, fibrous-appearing nucleus pulposus and lacked a sharp demarcation between nucleus and anulus. In adult disks (Fig 6-13), nuclei were opaque and fibrous. Pigmented regions were con-

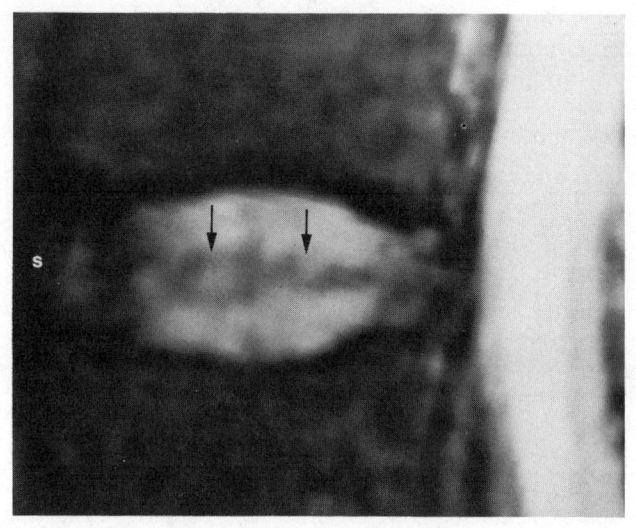

Fig 6–13.—L4–L5 intervertebral disk of 54-year-old patient. Magnetic resonance image (2,500/80) demonstrates fibrous band *(arrows)* and Sharpey's fibers *(S)* as regions of low signal intensity. (Courtesy of Yu S, Haughton VM, Lynch KL, et al: *AJNR* 10:1105–1110, September–October 1989.)

spicuous. Sometimes a plate of tissue in the equator of the disk, slightly darker yellow than the rest of the disk, was evident. Histologic examination revealed that the plate in the equator consisted of collagen with some elastic and reticular fibers. On MR images, regions of compact fibrous tissue showed lower signal intensity than the mucoid regions in the rest of the disk.

This study clarified the sources of high- and low-signal intensities within disks and elucidated the development of fibrous tissue in lumbar

Sharpey's fibers
Hyaline cartilage
Fibrous plate
Anulus fibrosus

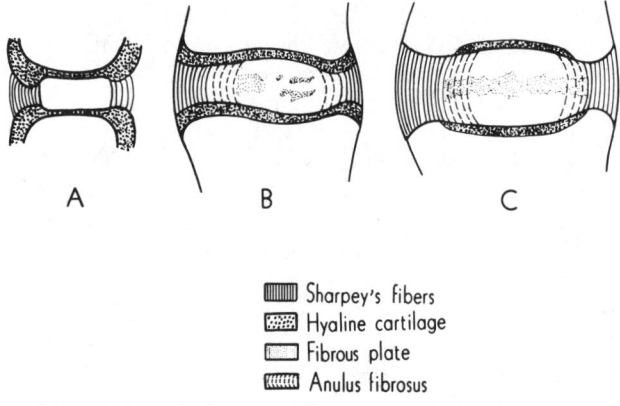

Fig 6–14.—Schematic shows development of fibrous tissue in lumbar disks. In newborn (**A**), the fibrous tissue is evident only in Sharpey's fibers. In 10-year-old (**B**), vertically oriented fibers appear on ventral or dorsal aspect of the nucleus. Clumped fibers are visible in the ground substance of nucleus pulposus. In adult (**C**), there is a fibrous plate in equator of disk. (Courtesy of Yu S, Haughton VM, Lynch KL, et al: *AJNR* 10:1105–1110, September–October 1989.)

disks (Fig 6-14). The band of fibrous tissue in the equator of the disks previously has been called, inexactly the "intranuclear cleft."

▶ We now are getting down to the "nitty-gritty" of what the various images seen on MRi mean in pathophysiologic terms. This article defines some of the attributes of fibrous tissue as a function of aging, specifically, the issue of the "intranuclear cleft." For those of you who like to outshine your radiologic confreres, this article gives you the opportunity for "one-upmanship."—J.W. Frymoyer, M.D.

Comparison of MR and Diskography in Detecting Radial Tears of the Anulus: A Postmortem Study
Yu S, Haughton VM, Sether LA, Wagner M (Med College of Wisconsin, Milwaukee)
AJNR 10:1077-1081, September-October 1989   6-13

Previous studies of structural changes in the lumbar anulus fibrosus have suggested that a radial tear of the anulus may be a primary cause of disk degeneration. Although a radial tear of the anulus can be detected with diskography or magnetic resonance (MR) imaging, the sensitivity of MR imaging in demonstrating such tears has not yet been determined. A comparison was made of the sensitivity of diskography and of MR imaging in demonstrating radial tears of the anulus fibrosus.

Spines were obtained from 6 fixed and 2 fresh cadavers, including a newborn, a 2-year-old, and 6 adults aged 54-87 years. The spines had been removed from the bodies before diskography, MR imaging, and cryomicrotomy anatomical sectioning were performed.

On the basis of diskographic appearance, disks were classified into 4 categories as described by Adams and Kieffer. A disk was called type 1 if contrast medium collected in a regular ovoid-shaped nucleus pulposus, type 2 if contrast medium showed an irregular ovoid shape, type 3 if contrast medium collected in 2 or more lobular-shaped collections, and type 4 if contrast medium escaped from the nucleus into the spinal epidural

Comparison of Cryomicrotomy, Diskography, and MR Imaging for the Detection of Anular Tears

Diskogram		Cryomicrotome		MR	
		Intact Anulus	Radial Tears	Intact Anulus	Radial Tears
Intact anulus	(n = 21)	21	0	21	0
Radial tear	(n = 15)	2	13	5	10
Total		36	23	13	26	10

(Courtesy of Yu S, Haughton VM, Sether LA, et al: AJNR 10:1077-1081, September-October 1989.)

space through a tear in the anulus. In all, 36 intervertebral disks were studied.

Radial tears were confirmed by diskography in 15 of the 36 intervertebral disks. Ten of the 15 radial tears were correctly identified on T_2-weighted MR images as high-signal intensity regions; 13 tears had diminished signal intensity. Therefore, the sensitivity of MR for detecting radial tears when compared with diskography was 67% (table). Magnetic resonance imaging can be used to demonstrate radial tears in the anulus fibrosus, but it is less precise than diskography.

▶ The debates go on about the clinical significance of anular radial tears and the sensitivity and specificity of the MRI versus diskographic imaging in detecting these tears. Putting aside the first issue, this postmortem study shows (alas!) diskography is the better of the 2. Obviously it does not answer the first and more crucial issue: what exactly is the significance of these tears?—J.W. Frymoyer, M.D.

Connective Tissue Changes of the Multifidus Muscle in Patients With Lumbar Disc Herniation: An Immunohistologic Study of Collagen Types I and III and Fibronectin
Lehto M, Hurme M, Alaranta H, Einola S, Falck B, Järvinen M, Kalimo H, Mattila M, Paljärvi L (Univ of Turku; Univ of Tampere; Univ of Kuopio, Finland)
Spine 14:302–309, March 1989   6–14

Nerve root lesions caused by herniation may cause denervation of paraspinal muscles and structural alterations of contractile and connective muscle tissue. The distribution of different types of collagen in muscle can be determined with indirect immunofluorescence using type-specific anticollagen antibodies. Type I collagen is found mainly in the epimysium, which surrounds the whole muscle; to a lesser extent in perimysium, which surrounds muscle fiber bundles; and in endomysium, which surrounds individual muscle fibers. Type III collagen is prominently present in the perimysium and to a lesser extent in the epimysium and endomysium. Fibronectin is present in skeletal muscle in the sarcolemma surrounding individual muscle fibers and in the perimysium. Changes in the distribution of collagen type I, collagen type III, and fibronectin were studied in multifidus muscle biopsy specimens obtained from 21 women and 25 men younger than 55 years who were operated on for nerve root compression caused by lumbar disk herniation. Multifidus muscle biopsy specimens from the cadavers of 2 women and 7 men who had no known back problems were studied as controls.

In multifidus muscle biopsy specimens obtained from the cadaver controls, type I collagen was present in both the endomysium and the perimysium. Type III collagen antibodies had more affinity to perimysial structures. Fibronectin was present in both the endomysium and the perimysium together with type III collagen. Control muscles showed no or only a slight thickening of endomysial and perimysial structures. In most patient muscle biopsy specimens, the distribution of types I and III collagen and fibronectin was similar to that of the controls. However, in some patient muscle biopsy specimens, there was evidence of an abnormal staining pattern and thickening of connective tissue structures, endomysium, and perimysium. Specifically, fibrosis of the perimysium, and to a lesser extent of the endomysium, involved all type I and type III collagen and fibronectin. A correlation was found between the severity of connective tissue structural changes to muscle atrophy and the patient's degree of disability after 1 year of postoperative follow-up. These findings suggest that marked muscle fibrosis may hamper recovery during postoperative follow-up in patients who have undergone operation on a herniated lumbar intervertebral disk.

▶ For those of you who have basic science at heart, this article nicely details the histologic changes that occur after posterior lumbar surgery. For those of you who want only the clinical message, my encapsulation of this article is (a) in planning a postoperative rehabilitation program, deconditioning and denervated muscles are issues that have to be managed before a patient can be exposed to mechanical loading; and (b) incisional length and protection of the paravertebral muscle's posterior primary ramus innervation is important, whenever possible.—J.W. Frymoyer, M.D.

Pathogenesis of Square Bodies in Ankylosing Spondylitis
Aufdermaur M (Cantonal Gen Hosp, Lucerne, Switzerland)
Ann Rheum Dis 48:628–631, August 1989   6–15

The pathogenesis of squaring of the vertebral bodies was evaluated in a fully recorded case of ankylosing spondylitis.

Man, 20, had ankylosing spondylitis. Radiographs showed spondylitis with destruction, rebuilding, and squaring of the vertebral bodies (Fig 6–15). The patient committed suicide at 25 years of age. Autopsy showed an acute and chronic spondylitis with destruction and simultaneous rebuilding of the cortex and the spongiosa of the vertebral bodies (Fig 6–16). The cortex of the vertebral bodies was missing in many areas, being replaced by scars and granulation tissue with lymphocytes and monocytes as well as woven bone with osteoclastic bone reabsorption and osteoblasts with new bone formation. Bone formation appeared to increase in proportion to decreasing inflammation. Sections with recently constructed cortex showed features of a transition from woven to lamellar bone with irregularly shaped osteons having superficial seems of osteoids.

The development of square bodies in ankylosing spondylitis is based on a combination of destructive osteitis and repair.

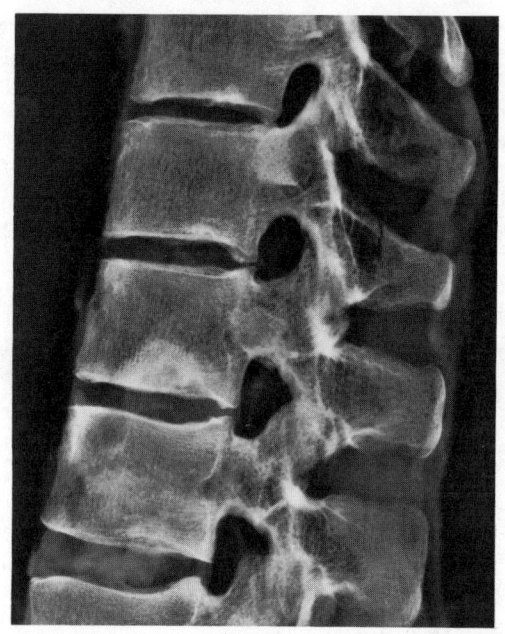

Fig 6–15.—Roentgenogram from T10 to L2. Erosions and simultaneous bone formation are seen at the anterior vertebral margins, resulting in squaring of the vertebral bodies. Localized radiolucencies occur with slight marginal bone sclerosis. The intervertebral disk spaces are maintained. Disk prolapses are seen into the vertebral bodies T10 to T12. (Courtesy of Aufdermaur M: *Ann Rheum Dis* 48:628–631, August 1989.)

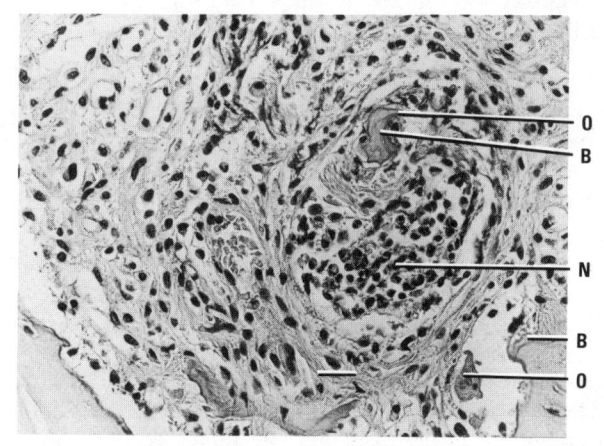

Fig 6–16.—Acute and chronic spondylitis and osteoclastic bone destruction. Hematoxylin and eosin. *Bar*, 30 µm. *O*, osteoclast; *B*, bone fragment; *N*, spot of polynuclear neutrophilic leukocytes. (Courtesy of Aufdermaur M: *Ann Rheum Dis* 48:628–631, August 1989.)

▶ A tidbit for those of you who want to know why some vertebral bodies are square.—J.W. Frymoyer, M.D.

Cross Leg Pain and Trunk List
Khuffash B, Porter RW (Doncaster Royal Infirmary, South Yorkshire, England)
Spine 14:602–603, June 1989   6–16

Gravity-induced trunk list and cross leg pain are signs of lumbar disk protrusion. The prevalence and prognostic significance of these 2 symptoms were studied in 113 patients who had root tension signs from a lumbar disk lesion. The mean age of the patient was 33 years (range, 23–49 years).

Twelve patients had both cross leg pain and trunk list, 21 had cross leg pain and no list, 20 had a list and no cross leg pain, and 60 had neither list nor cross leg pain. Surgery was required in 58%, 48%, 30%, and 10% of these patients, respectively. Among the 17 patients with cross leg pain requiring surgery, 11 had disk sequestration; 3 had disk protrusion, and 1 patient had a protrusion with an intact outer anulus.

A high incidence of disk sequestration or extrusion is found in surgically treated patients with cross leg pain. Because of this association, the presence of cross leg pain is probably a contraindication to chymopapain injections. Surgeons should be aware of the possibility of a migrated disk fragment during surgery in patients with cross leg pain.

▶ The specificity of cross straight leg raising has been known for many years; this article confirms that perspective and shows a significant association with a free disk fragment. The authors suggest a cross straight leg raising should serve as a relative contraindication to chymopapain. A better conclusion in today's surgical approach would have been that the test may serve as a relative contraindication to percutaneous diskectomy.—J.W. Frymoyer, M.D.

The Role of Thermography in the Evaluation of Lumbosacral Radiculopathy
So YT, Aminoff MJ, Olney RK (Univ of California, San Francisco)
Neurology 39:1154–1158, September 1989   6–17

Although there are many published studies on the use of thermography in the evaluation of low back pain, only 1 used a controlled study design. The diagnostic accuracy of thermography in the diagnosis of lumbosacral radiculopathy was evaluated in 30 patients aged 27–76 years with suspected lumbosacral radiculopathy and 27 asymptomatic controls aged 23–66 years. Twenty-one of the 30 patients had clinical signs of radiculopathy. After an initial clinical examination, each study participant underwent thermography, conventional electromyography, and nerve conduction studies. Thermography was done first to avoid the potential effects of nerve stimulation on skin temperature. Thermograms were interpreted without knowledge of clinical or electrodiagnostic findings. Abnormal thermographic studies were defined as an interside temperature difference exceeding 3 standard deviations above the normal mean.

Of 21 patients with clinical signs of radiculopathy, 17 (81%) had abnormal thermographic studies and 15 (71%) had abnormal electrodiagnostic studies. Four patients with abnormal thermograms had normal electrodiagnostic studies, and 2 patients with normal thermograms had abnormal electrodiagnostic studies. The more symptomatic limb was colder in 12 patients, was warmer in 3 patients, and did not differ from the contralateral limb in 6 patients. Thus, it was impossible to identify the side of the root lesion on the basis of thermographic evidence. Furthermore, thermographic abnormalities did not seem to follow a dermatomal distribution.

Serious questions are raised about the localizing value of thermography, as neither the side of the root lesion nor the level of root involvement could be identified on the basis of thermographic evidence in this study.

▶ The thermography debate goes on, and on, and on. I have never understood why thermography was necessary for patients with obvious radiculopathies; the clinical symptoms and signs are highly predictive. Alternatively, if a patient has "subtle" signs, why would you want to prove it or operate unless it was to satisfy your friendly neighborhood attorney? Although that position sounds cynical, I have been impressed by the heat of the debate and the absence of much in the way of true science (1). This article will not be popular with the thermography advocates, and we can be assured there are and will be articles to counter it.—J.W. Frymoyer, M.D.

Reference

1. Frymoyer JW, Haugh LD: *Orthopedics* 9:699, 1986.

Vertebral Infections

Pyogenic Vertebral Osteomyelitis of the Posterior Elements
Ehara S, Khurana JS, Kattapuram SV (Massachusetts Gen Hosp, Boston; Harvard Med School)
Skeletal Radiol 18:175–178, 1989   6–18

When pyogenic osteomyelitis of the vertebra involves the posterior elements alone, it is difficult to differentiate from neoplastic processes and the arthritides. Part of the difficulty is the nonspecific early signs and symptoms or their concealment by preceding infection, such as the diabetes mellitus noted in 2 of 3 patients observed. None of the patients had surgery or injection therapy or an open wound. In these 3 patients and 3 others reported previously there was articular destruction.

Man, 63, was referred because of a firm mass in the left posterior part of the neck. The history included diabetes. Plain films yielded no useful information, but a CT scan revealed destructive changes in the articular facet and lamina. The white blood cell count was 15,200, and the erythrocyte sedimentation rate was 103 mm. A loculated mass with low density was detected by another scan at the caudal part of the destructive process in the facet. After open biopsy, culture of the purulent fluid grew *Staphylococcus aureus*. Treatment with nafcillin and vancomycin administered intravenously was successful.

Diabetes mellitus may precede pyogenic vertebral osteomyelitis. Involvement of the facet joint helps in differentiation from neoplasm. However, erosive arthritides, multicentric reticulohistiocytosis, and scleroderma are other possible causes of facet arthritis. Facet involvement may be caused by primary hematogenous osteomyelitis of the facet with extension into the facet joint.

▶ This article caught my attention because, in 20 years, I have seen but 2 patients with infectious processes involving posterior elements, both of which were postsurgical. The authors again emphasize the factors that place patients generally at risk for any spinal infection. Involvement of the facet seems to be a particularly useful radiographic sign and raises the intriguing possibility these rare infections arise as a hematogenous pyarthrosis. Given the commonality of facet degeneration, one wonders why we don't see more of these infections.—J.W. Frymoyer, M.D.

Sacroiliac Joints

Movements of the Sacroiliac Joints: A Roentgen Stereophotogrammetric Analysis
Sturesson B, Selvik G, Udén A (Malmö Gen Hosp, Lund Univ, Lund, Sweden)
Spine 14:162–165, February 1989   6–19

Previous postmortem studies have demonstrated the load displacement behavior in the sacroiliac joint. To measure movements of the sacroiliac joint under different loads and compare the movements of symptomatic and asymptomatic sacroiliac joints, 21 women aged 19 to 45 years and 4 men aged 18 to 45 years with sacroiliac joint disorders were studied. All had stereophotogrammetric examination and percutaneous insertion of tantalum balls under local anesthesia with fluoroscopic guidance. Seven patients had bilateral symptoms.

Exposures were made in 5 positions: supine, prone with hyperextension of the left leg, prone with hyperextension of the right leg, standing, and sitting with straight knees. The sacrum was defined as the fixed segment, with movement defined as rotation around and translation along the axis (Fig 6–17).

There was a constant pattern of motion with different loads, particularly around the transverse axis. However, rotations were small, with the maximal mobility observed between end points in extension and flexion in each joint ranging from 1.6 degrees to 3.9 degrees (mean, 2.5 degrees). Translations ranged from 0.1 to 1.6 mm (mean, 0.7 mm). There was no difference in rotation or translation between symptomatic and asymptomatic joints and no decrease in total mobility of the sacroiliac joint with age.

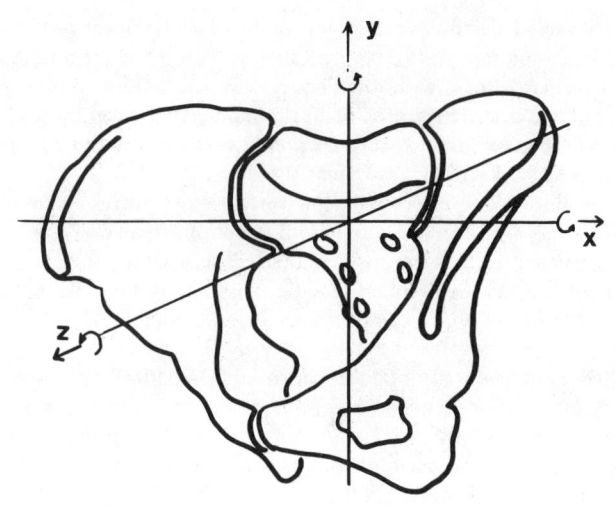

Fig 6–17.—Pelvis with rotational axes. (Courtesy of Sturesson B, Selvik G, Udén A: *Spine* 14:162–165, February 1989.)

The identical movements of symptomatic and asymptomatic sacroiliac joints demonstrate that analyses of the mobility under physiologic loads is not useful for diagnosing a joint dysfunction in patients with sacroiliac joint syndrome.

▶ The sacroiliac joint is making a comeback! This extraordinary study involved a highly sophisticated and accurate method for measuring minute motions in the living human being. Contrary to some clinical studies, this research again confirms the minimal movement possible, as well as the absent correlation of pain with movement. Although the sacroiliac joint may be the source of overlooked symptoms, it seems unlikely pain comes from abnormal movement, except in a small number of patients with posttraumatic or postsurgical destabilization.—J.W. Frymoyer, M.D.

Surgical Techniques and Results

Assessment of the Outcome of Low Back Surgery
Waddell G, Reilly S, Torsney B, Allan DB, Morris EW, Di Paola MP, Bircher M, Finlayson D (Western Infirmary, Glasgow; Univ of Glasgow, Scotland)
J Bone Joint Surg [Br] 70-B:723–727, November 1988   6–20

The wide variation in reported success rates for low back operations has been attributed to patient selection, surgical technique, or methods of assessing the outcome. To analyze the relationship between various methods of assessing outcome after such surgery, 185 white, native-born British patients aged 20 to 60 years were studied before and after various types of surgery for low back pain and sciatica. Forty-nine patients had chemonucleolysis, 91 had first operations for disk prolapse, 20 had spinal fusions for low back pain, and 25 had repeat spinal operations.

Identical preoperative and postoperative assessment by an independent observer included pain, disability, physical impairment, psychological distress, and illness behavior. At follow-up outcome was assessed independently by the patient and the observer and from the work record, which was analyzed for return to work, type of employment, and duration of sick leave before and after operation. There was 96% follow-up at 2 years.

Overall, the patient's assessment was more favorable than either the observer's assessment or the return to work record. Both patient and observer based their assessment mainly on postoperative status, rather than on the actual change produced by the operation. The observer was influenced most by postoperative pain, disability, and physical impairment, but the patient was influenced most by residual physical impairment, type of surgery, and proportional change in disability.

The degree of psychological distress and illness behavior did not affect the patient's assessment. Return to work was influenced most by postoperative disability and the nature of the patient's occupation. Thus the patient's and observer's assessments and return to work record were all arrived at from different aspects of the low back disorder.

The findings that postoperative pain scores and physical impairment were the strongest influences on outcome assessments made it possible to develop a simple method for rating the outcome of back surgery. The use of this formula agreed well with the total clinical assessment in nearly every case.

▶ Waddell continues to study carefully the issues of low back pain, spinal surgery, and clinical outcomes from a broad perspective. The article points out how we, as surgeons, may have perspectives of success different from those of our patients. Equally important, it challenges the traditional wisdom that psychological dysfunction is incompatible with good surgical results. This perspective has been present for some time, with a scientific basis, but was lost because of the relative obscurity of the article (1). In his prospective study, Weber compared the outcomes of patients with abnormal results of the Minnesota Multiphasic Personality Inventory treated conservatively and operatively versus people who were ostensibly psychologically normal. Those with psychological dysfunction did better with surgery, which also flies in the face of predictive scoring systems such as that devised by Spengler and associates (2). I am increasingly becoming convinced the critical determinants are compensation, disability behavior, and the patient's occupation: a perspective further strengthened by this article.—J.W. Frymoyer, M.D.

References

1. Weber H: *J Oslo City Hosp* 28:89, 1978.
2. Spengler DM, et al: *Spine* 5:356, 1980.

Quantitative Measurement of Disc Space Area Before and After Chemonucleolysis and Nucleotomy

Gördes W, Feuchtgruber G, Fritz W (Orthopädische Abteilung des Krankenhauses der Barmherzigen Brüder, Munich)
Int Orthop 13:89–93, 1989

Changes in the intervertebral disk space height have been noted after chemonucleolysis and nucleotomy. To determine how chemonucleolysis and nucleotomy affect the volume of disk space during a period of time, measurements of the area of the intervertebral disk space shown in radiographs were made, for 400 days or more, in 16 patients who underwent chemonucleolysis and in 20 patients after nucleotomy.

The anterior and posterior disk space heights were measured together with the anteroposterior diameter of the intervertebral disk (Fig 6–18). In the superimpositioning method, a fixed point was established once for each intervertebral body for the entire radiographic series of the patient. Only areas that differed from volumes in just a single dimension but showed good correlation were measured as compared with measurement of intervertebral disk space heights alone.

Narrowing of the interveretebral disk space was evident up to 50 days after both chemonucleolysis and nucleotomy. Thereafter, a comparison between these 2 treatments showed highly significant differences. With chemonucleolysis, the relative area remained constant up to 180 days and

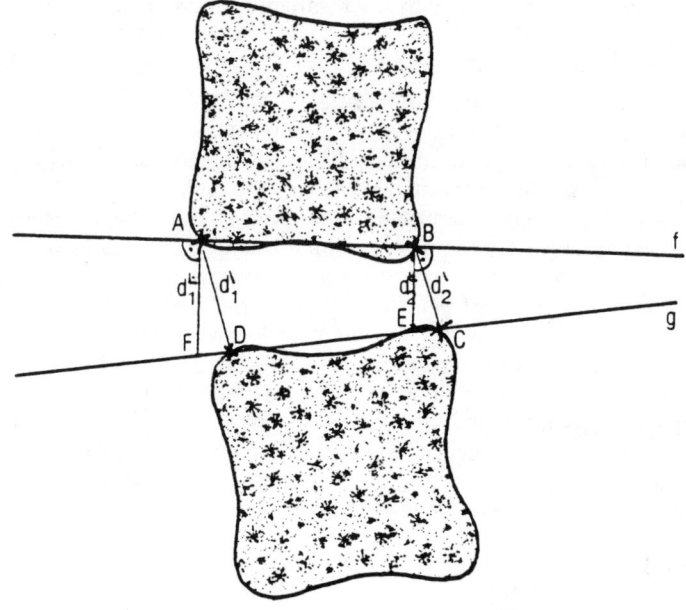

Fig 6–18.—Measuring parameters for establishing the area: *ABCD*. (Courtesy of Gördes W, Feuchtgruber G, Fritz W: *Int Orthop* 13:89–93, 1989.)

gradually increased, by as much as 2.5%, up to day 355. In contrast, an unequivocal reduction in area was noted after nucleotomy.

Chemonucleolysis produces a gain in disk substance by the enzymatic effect of chymopapain, probably indicating restoration with replacement tissue and the reestablishment of proteoglycan synthesis. Nucleotomy is associated with a loss of substance as well as loss of proteoglycan synthesis, resulting in irreversible narrowing of the disk space.

▶ Long-term radiographic studies have shown disk space narrowing is an inevitable consequence of lumbar disk excision (1). Clinical observation has suggested disk space height was regained after chymopapain. This article rigorously confirms the earlier clinical "impressions" and fits with animal experiments, which show biomechanical and biochemical "recovery" after chemonucleolysis (2). What is less clear and important is whether this regained disk space height has any relevance to clinical outcomes. Comparative long-term studies of chymopapain and surgical disk excision have shown little difference in clinical outcome (3). Despite chymopapain no longer being favored, newer enzymatic agents will again raise these questions.—J.W. Frymoyer, M.D.

References

1. Frymoyer JW, et al: *Spine* 4:435, 1979.
2. Spencer DL, et al: *Spine* 10:555, 1985.
3. Weinstein J, et al: *J Bone Joint Surg [Am]* 68A:43, 1986.

Does Percutaneous Nucleotomy With Discoscopy Replace Conventional Discectomy? Eight Years of Experience and Results in Treatment of Herniated Lumbar Disc
Schreiber A, Suezawa Y, Leu H (Univ of Zurich)
Clin Orthop 238:35–42, January 1989   6–22

The goal of percutaneous nucleotomy is to reduce the volume of the involved lumbar disk by partial removal of the nucleus pulposus while leaving all structures important to segmental stability intact. Since 1982 additional intradiskal optical control has been achieved with an adapted arthroscopic kit, which allows more accurate and effective removal of the nucleus pulposus under direct view.

During an 8-year period, 68 men and 41 women aged 19–71 years underwent percutaneous nucleotomy in the treatment of lumbar disk herniation. Follow-up ranged from 3 to 93 months, (mean follow-up, 33 months). For stabilization, 6 patients also underwent percutaneous cancellous bone grafting of the intercorporeal space after radical percutaneous nucleotomy through the same cannula.

Of the 109 patients, 22 had excellent, 45 had good, 12 had fair, and 30 had poor results. The overall success rate was 72.5%. Twenty-nine patients subsequently underwent classic open surgery. Nineteen patients had residual disk herniation detectable with CT and myelography. Three patients had herniation relapse more than 3 months after operation. Procedural complications were few. Two patients had nervous system injuries involving the lumbar plexus, but the injuries were resolved spontaneously in both. The sigmoid artery in another patient was damaged. Follow-up data on the patients who also had percutaneous bone grafting are not yet available.

In terms of the number of reoperations needed in this study population, percutaneous nucleotomy in the treatment of lumbar disk herniation seems only moderately successful. However, that the procedure is much less traumatic than conventional diskectomy is a definite advantage.

▶ This article is only one of many that could have been selected for review on the topic of percutaneous diskectomy. Why removal of a small amount of disk tissue will cause symptom relief remains enigmatic to me. The article also raises significant questions about what causes the pain in lumbar disk herniation. What emerges from this article is quite similar to most others: the results of percutaneous diskectomy are less predictable than those of conventional techniques, and in experienced hands neurologic and arterial injuries can occur. The uniqueness of the article is the combination of arthroscopy and percutaneous diskectomy, as well as the possible future application to percutaneous bone grafting.—J.W. Frymoyer, M.D.

Cauda Equina Syndrome After Surgical Treatment of Lumbar Spinal Stenosis With Application of Free Autogenous Fat Graft: A Report of Two Cases
Mayer PJ, Jacobsen FS (West Virginia Univ, Morgantown)
J Bone Joint Surg [Am] 71-A:1090–1093, August 1989   6–23

The formation of a fibrous epidural scar is a common cause of failure in patients undergoing surgical treatment of the back. Both fat grafts and absorbable gelatin sponge have been used to create an interpositional membrane to reduce the likelihood of scar formation. Compression by a free fat graft has been reported in only a few patients.

Woman, 56, with mild non-insulin-dependent diabetes mellitus stated that, for 1 year, she had had pain in the left buttock that radiated down the posterolateral aspect of the left lower limb to the ankle. Bilateral laminectomy of the fourth lumbar vertebra, bilateral foraminotomies of the third and fourth lumbar vertebrae, and bilateral lateral arthrodesis of the fourth and fifth lumbar vertebrae were performed. The third and fourth lumbar nerve roots were explored and decompressed bilaterally. A large, free autogenous fat graft about 2 cm thick, which filled the 3 × 4.5-cm site of the laminectomy, was placed over the exposed dura. After surgery, the patient had immediate relief of pain. Three days later, however, extension of the left toes was weak. On day 4, after the catheter was removed, the patient was unable to void spontaneously. On day 7, she had reduced sensation and dysesthesias in the left perianal region. Computed tomography revealed compression of the dura by the overlying fat graft. Reoperation was performed 7 days after the first procedure. The original graft was removed, and a new, thinner fat graft was used. Her second postoperative course was uneventful. She had a gradual improvement of sphincter control, muscle power, and sensation.

Because of the danger of nerve compression, surgeons should avoid using a fat graft that is too large. The graft should be between 0.5 and 1 cm thick to protect the dura sufficiently and allow for some graft shrinkage without fibrous tissue formation. The height of the graft should not exceed that of the cephalad and the caudad spinous processes of the remaining posterior elements. This precaution might shield the graft from the direct compressive forces of the overlying soft tissues.

▶ This complication has been reported before, and these 2 cases simply reaffirm that too large a fat graft can cause a major postoperative problem requiring urgent evaluation and relief.—J.W. Frymoyer, M.D.

The Role of External Spinal Skeletal Fixation in the Assessment of Low-Back Disorders
Esses SI, Botsford DJ, Kostuik JP (Univ of Toronto; Toronto Gen–Mt Sinai Hosps)
Spine 14:594–600, June 1989   6–24

Various tests are used to predict pain relief after arthrodesis of the lumbar and lumbosacral spine. The usefulness of temporary external spinal skeletal fixation (ESSF) in predicting the outcome of surgical fusion was investigated in 35 patients with chronic low-back pain nonresponsive to previous conservative or surgical treatment. The predictive usefulness of ESSF was compared with use of plain radiographs, diskograms, and facet blocks.

Technique.—While the patients were under general anesthesia, Schanz screws were inserted under image intensifier control. These screws were connected either by using the frame designed by Magerl or by building a quadrilateral frame using the AO external fixation set (Fig 6–19). The patients were discharged a day later and encouraged to perform daily activities. After 6–14 days, the patients were readmitted and the nuts on the cross-linking bars were loosened or the connecting rods were removed, so that immobilization of the instrumented levels no longer existed. Unknowingly, the patients were not in a placebo trial. The Schanz screws were removed 2 days later.

Of the 35 patients who underwent ESSF, 2 were immobilized at 1 spinal motion unit, 21 at 2 levels, 11 at 3 levels, and 1 at 4 levels. After temporary ESSF, complete pain relief was achieved in 15 patients and significant pain relief in 12. In 1 patient, 1 sacral screw loosened, requiring removal of the ESSF device. In the placebo trial, low-back pain recurred in 22 patients after the frame was loosened. After fusion was achieved as

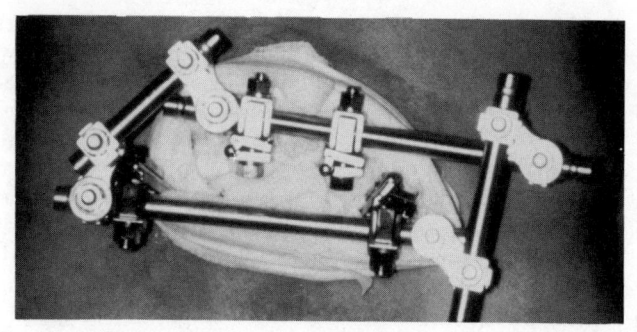

Fig 6–19.—External fixation using AO frame. (Courtesy of Esses SI, Botsford DJ, Kostuik JP: *Spine* 14:594–600, June 1989.)

the result of definitive surgery, 6 of 23 evaluable patients reported complete relief of back pain and 11 noted significant relief. Statistical analysis showed a strong association between the pain relief from external fixation and the positive outcome of subsequent fusion. None of the other tests was predictive of the subsequent surgical outcome.

The superiority of temporary ESSF in predicting surgical outcome was shown as compared with plain radiographs, diskograms, and facet blocks.

▶ This article represents an independent verification of the study presented earlier by Olerud and colleagues in 1986 (1). The logic is obvious and an extension of the historic use of braces to predict the outcome of spinal fusion, by preoperatively relieving symptoms through temporary stabilization. What has been less clear to me has been whether the invasiveness of the diagnostic test was almost as bad as simply doing the fusion. Since this article was published, new information from Esses and Kostuik's laboratory (2) suggests this preliminary optimism may not be standing up with additional clinical experience. Until the issue is resolved, I believe this technique, interesting as it may be, is still experimental.—J.W. Frymoyer, M.D.

References

1. Olerud S, et al: *Clin Orthop* 203:76, 1986.
2. Kostuik J: Personal communication, 1990.

Preoperative and Postoperative Instability in Lumbar Spinal Stenosis
Johnsson K-E, Redlund-Johnell I, Udén A, Willner S (Malmo Gen Hosp, Malmo, Sweden)
Spine 14:591–593, June 1989

Previous studies have shown a correlation between postoperative instability and unsatisfactory results of laminectomy for lumbar spinal stenosis. To assess the importance of some preoperative parameters and the extent of the laminectomy in postoperative outcome, data were reviewed on 40 men and 21 women aged 38 to 80 years who underwent laminectomy for spinal stenosis in a 14-year period. Postoperative follow-up ranged from 12 to 156 months. Four patients previously had undergone operation for lumbar disk protrusion. None of the patients had fusion, and epidural fat grafts were used in all cases.

Follow-up examinations included serial radiologic studies of the lumbar spine in the anteroposterior and lateral views. Fifty-one patients also had myelography. Preoperative and postoperative vertebral slipping was measured on plain films without provocation. Films also were evaluated for degenerative spondylolisthesis.

Thirty-six patients (59%) had good or excellent results, and 25 had poor results. Age at operation did not affect outcome. Ten of 40 men and 16 of 21 women (43% of total group) had postoperative slipping; 8 of the 26 had good results. Twenty-eight of 35 patients with no postoperative slipping (80%) had good results. Slipping was most pronounced at the L4–L5 level.

Myelography showed that spinal extension, on average, had a greater effect on stenosis in patients with poor results. Patients with postoperative slipping had greater preoperative sagittal mobility than those who had no postoperative slipping. Postoperative slipping occurred in 16 (53%) of 30 patients with degenerative spondylolisthesis and in 10 (32%) of 31 patients with degenerative stenosis.

Preoperative instability as seen on diagnostic myelography seems to be a poor prognostic sign. Radical decompression without stabilization increases the risk of postoperative slipping and a poor outcome. Postoperative slipping worsens the prognosis. Women are at greater risk of poor postoperative results than men.

▶ This meticulous follow-up gives additional information about who should have fusion at the time of decompression. It is not surprising that the predictors are preoperative instability and radical decompression. Many of us (1) have thought women also were at greater risk, and this article confirms that viewpoint. It does not, on a case-by-case basis, tell us absolute indications, but rather provides clinically useful guidelines.—J.W. Frymoyer, M.D.

Reference

    1. Goldner JL: *Spine* 6:293, 1981.

Segmental ("Floating") Lumbar Spine Fusions
Brodsky AE, Hendricks RL, Khalil MA, Darden BV, Brotzman TT (Texas Inst for Spinal Disorders; Baylor College of Medicine, Houston)
Spine 14:447–450, April 1989   6–26

Traditional teaching in orthopedic surgery holds that fusion for L4–L5 discopathy or instability should include the lumbosacral joint. This

Table 1.—Primary Diagnosis in 184 Cases

	No. of cases	Percent
Discopathy		
Herniated disc	115	62.5
Internal disc disruption	9	5.0
Extruded disc	1	0.5
Spinal stenosis		
Spondylotic spinal stenosis	28	15.2
Pseudospondylolisthetic spinal stenosis	8	4.3
Spondylolisthesis	6	3.3
Mechanical insufficiency	17	9.2
Post-laminectomy	9	
Post-chymopapain	4	
No previous surgery	4	
Total	184	

(Courtesy of Brodsky AE, Hendricks RL, Khalil MA, et al: *Spine* 14:447–450, April 1989.)

dictum is based on the assumption that fusion at L4–L5 will place increased mechanical stresses on the L5–S1 joint below. The validity of this theory never has been supported in published studies.

During a 32-year period, 206 segmental lumbar fusions were performed in which the L5–S1 joint was excluded. A total of 184 patients were available for follow-up. The primary diagnosis in 125 patients (68%) was discopathy, 115 of whom had a herniated disk, 9 had internal disk disruption, and 1 had an extruded disk. The remaining patients had spinal stenosis, spondylolisthesis, and mechanical insufficiency (Table 1). Only patients with a lumbosacral spinal unit relatively free of pathologic changes were considered for segmental fusion. Follow-up ranged from 6 months to 32.5 years, averaging 4.6 years.

Of 125 patients with primary discopathy, 105 (84%) were rated as having excellent or good results at follow-up (Table 2). Similar success rates were obtained in patients with spinal stenosis, spondylolisthesis, and mechanical insufficiency.

Preoperative and postoperative radiographs were available for 94 pa-

Table 2.—Clinical Results by Diagnosis ("Excellent" and "Good" Results)

	No. patients		Percent
Primary discopathy	105	(of 125)	84
Spinal stenosis	25	(of 28)	89
Spondylolisthesis	5	(of 6)	83
Pseudospondylolisthesis	4	(of 8)	50
Mechanical insufficiency	15	(of 17)	88

(Courtesy of Brodsky AE, Hendricks RL, Kahlil MA, et al: *Spine* 14:447–450, April 1989.)

Table 3.—Postoperative Radiologic Changes in 94 Patients

	Level above fusion		Level below fusion	
	Patients	Percent	Patients	Percent
Sclerosis	10	10.6	4	4.3
Osteophytes	22	23.4	23	24.5
Disc space narrowing	60	64	56	59.6
Symptomatic	2	2	9	9.6

(Courtesy of Brodsky AE, Hendricks RL, Khalil MA, et al: *Spine* 14:447–450, April 1989.)

tients. Postoperative changes in the disks above and below the floating fusion included occasional sclerosis and osteophytes and some disk space narrowing, but postoperative radiologic changes were not correlated with clinical symptoms (Table 3).

Twenty-five of the 184 patients needed additional operation, including 15 who had subsequent disk herniation. Five of these 15 new herniations occurred at the lumbosacral level. Operation consisted of diskectomy and extension of the fusion to incorporate the sacrum. Thus, the incidence of discopathy below a segmental fusion in this study population was 2.7%.

Inclusion of the lumbosacral disk in a lumbar fusion is unnecessary, provided the lumbosacral joint is in reasonably good condition.

▶ This is neither a controlled nor prospective study, but it gives 1 man's long-term experience with floating fusion. Traditional wisdom always taught that fusions should be extended to the lumbosacral joint, because the mechanical forces otherwise would lead to inevitable symptomatic degeneration. That this is not the case is shown here: only 2.7% of his patients needed further operation for new pathology. Less clear is how we determine the lumbosacral joint is in "reasonably good condition." For example, should a person with any magnetic resonance imaging abnormality at that joint have incorporation into the fusion, or should we use discography, a controversial subject of itself?—J.W. Frymoyer, M.D.

The Wiltse Pedicle Screw Fixation System: Early Clinical Results

Horowitch A, Peek RD, Thomas JC Jr, Widell EH Jr, DiMartino PP, Spencer CW III, Weinstein J, Wiltse LL (California Spine Surgery Med Group Inc, Long Beach; Mem Med Ctr of Long Beach; Univ of Iowa)
Spine 14:461–467, April 1989   6–27

Pedicle screws have been used in a number of spine fixation systems designed to achieve reduction and stabilization. Early clinical results of the Wiltse system in 99 patients undergoing posterolateral fusion were reviewed. The patients' average age was 52 years; average follow-up was 20 months. Prior spine surgery had been performed in 76 of the patients.

Common diagnoses included degenerative disk disease, pseudarthrosis, instability, stenosis, degenerative spondylolisthesis, and scoliosis.

Surgery approaches were midline or paraspinal. A Steffee gearshift was used in inserting pedicle screws of proper diameter and length. Fluoroscopic guidance aided those maneuvers. In many multilevel fusions, a vertebral level was skipped and no pedicle screw was inserted. When reduction was necessary, specialized pedicle screws with extension rods were used. Postoperative immobilization was not needed. Flexion and extension lateral radiographs assessed the success of fusion.

Of 82 patients evaluable at 1 year, 56 (68%) had radiographic union. The only significant variable affecting union was prior surgery. Although all 18 patients with no previous surgery had successful union, only 38 (59%) with prior surgery had successful union. The success rate also was lowered by smoking and by fusion of multiple levels. Two patients had permanent neurologic damage. Less serious complications included infection and hardward failure. One patient died after cardiopulmonary arrest in the immediate postoperative period and another died 10 months after surgery of underlying sarcoma.

The advantage of pedicle screws is their solid fixation to vertebral bodies from a posterior approach. With the Wiltse system, risks to neurologic structures are minimized because variable screw lengths and diameters are available. The overall union rate, however, is disappointing. Better results may be obtained with recent modifications of hardware design.

▶ The indications for pedicle screw fixation still are evolving. This series gives a realistic appraisal of a state of the art. Most important, the major indication was the management of previous failures (76%) rather than primary operations. Only 68% had radiographic union, probably because of this high percentage of second operations. Like other studies, the rate was decreased as a result of smoking and multilevel fusion. It is reassuring to see a 100% successful fusion rate in primary operations. The neurologic complications were 2%, lower than Whitecloud's experience reported below.—J.W. Frymoyer, M.D.

Complications With the Variable Spinal Plating System
Whitecloud TS III, Butler JC, Cohen JL, Candelora PD (Tulane Univ)
Spine 14:472–476, April 1989 6–28

Solid arthrodesis of the lumbar spine is difficult to achieve, and various devices have been developed to provide internal stability while the arthrodesis is accomplished. The variable spinal plating (VSP) system, which consists of bone plates with beveled screw slots that can be contoured to conform to the sagittal curves of the spine, was used in 40 patients who underwent fixation during an 18-month period because of complex spinal instability.

Twenty-one patients had not undergone previous spinal surgery and 19 had averaged at least 2 previous operations. Among the patients with no previous surgery 7 had spondylolisthesis, 11 had fractures of the thora-

Results With the Variable Spinal Plating System

	Overall	Without previous surgery	With previous surgery
Excellent	13	8	5
Good	12	—	5
Fair	7	1	6
Poor	8	5	3

(Courtesy of Whitecloud TS III, Butler JC, Cohen JL, et al: *Spine* 14:472–476, April 1989.)

columbar or lumbar spine, 2 had internal disk derangement, and 1 had spinal stenosis that required extensive decompression. The minimal follow-up was 14 months.

Overall, results in 25 patients (62.5%) were rated good or excellent, 7 were rated fair, and 8 were rated poor. Eight of the 21 patients with no previous surgery had excellent results, 7 had good results, 1 had a fair result, and 5 had poor results (table). Four of the 5 poor results occurred with thoracolumbar fractures that probably should have been treated with anterior grafting of the fractured body.

The overall complication rate was 46%, with the rate being 29% in patients with no previous surgery and 63% in those with previous operations. Six patients had increased postoperative nerve root irritation, which resolved spontaneously within 3 months in 4 cases. Improper placement of screws was responsible in the other 2 cases and the screws were removed. Two patients had deep wound infections and 1 had a superficial wound infection. There has been no plate breakage, but screw breakage has occurred in 7 patients.

Transpedicle internal fixation for problematic lumbar spinal fusion is technically demanding and still associated with a high complication rate. It is expected that the complication rate will drop somewhat as orthopedic surgeons become more expierenced in the use of VSP techniques.

▶ This is a diverse group of patients treated with the variable spinal plating system. However, the impressive figure is the 46% complication rate, which rose to 63% among patients who had previous surgery. Of 40 patients, 6 (15%) had neurologic complications and 2 (5%) had deep wound infections. Screw breakage occurred in 17.5%, which again demands us that pedicle screws, despite the obvious benefit to stabilization, extract a price, particularly early in one's surgical experience.—J.W. Frymoyer, M.D.

Adult Idiopathic Scoliosis Treated With Luque or Harrington Rods and Sublaminar Wiring
Winter RB, Lonstein JE (Minnesota Spine Center, Minneapolis)
J Bone Joint Surg [Am] 71-A:1308–1313 October 1989

Posterior spinal arthrodesis with Harrington instrumentation used to be the operation of choice in the treatment of adult idiopathic scoliosis. However, the rate of pseudarthrosis after this procedure was high. The concept of segmental posterior spinal instrumentation with sublaminar wiring was introduced by Luque in 1976. Since then, these 2 techniques have been combined for treating idiopathic scoliosis in adolescents.

The results of spinal arthrodesis with sublaminar wires, attached to either double L-shaped Luque rods or to a Harrington distraction rod, were assessed in 47 adults aged 23–61 years with idiopathic scoliosis seen during a 4-year period (Fig. 6–20). The average follow-up was 3 years. All underwent a combined procedure. Three patients were lost to follow-up. A single Harrington rod and sublaminar wires were used in 31 patients, of whom 18 had posterior arthrodesis only and 13 had preliminary anterior arthrodesis followed by posterior arthrodesis. Double L-shaped Luque rods were used in the other 11 patients, of whom 6 had posterior arthrodesis only and 5 had preliminary anterior arthrodesis followed by posterior arthrodesis.

The preoperative curve for the entire group averaged 67 degrees. The curve was corrected at operation to an average of 37 degrees, and averaged 44 degrees at the latest follow-up. Thus, the average correction at discharge was 30 degrees, the average loss of correction over the follow-

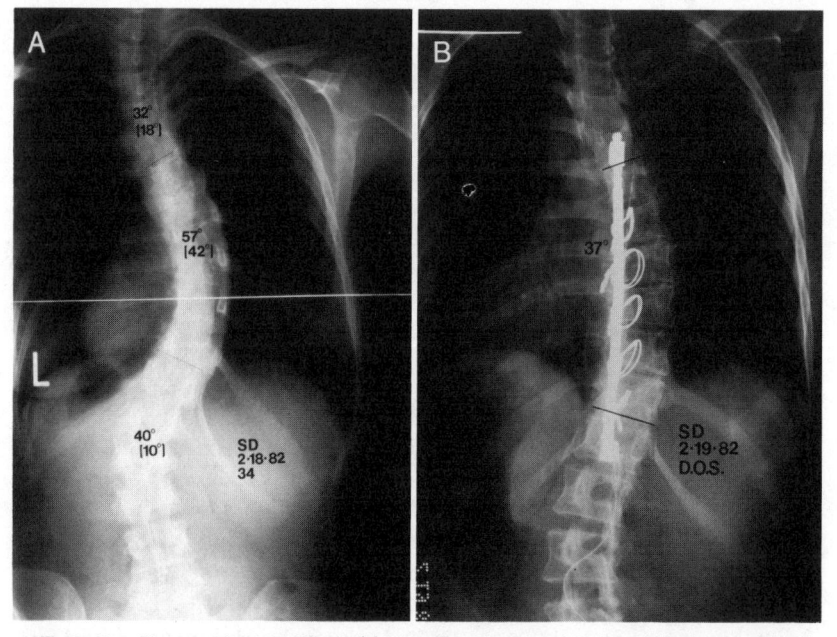

Fig 6–20.—Woman, 34 years, with painful major thoracic curve of 57 degrees that corrected to only 42 degrees on supine side-bending. There were flexible compensatory curves cephalad and caudad to the major curve. **A,** preoperative radiograph. **B,** radiograph made immediately after posterior arthrodesis from the fifth to the twelfth thoracic vertebra, accomplished with a square-ended Harrington distraction rod and 5 double loops of 16-gauge wire. The curve was corrected to 37 degrees. The patient wore an orthosis for 4 months postoperatively. *(Continued.)*

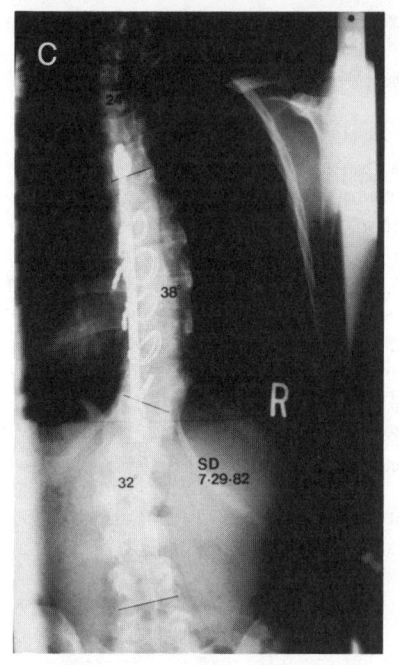

Fig 6–20, cont.—C, radiograph made 5 months after operation and 1 month after removal of the orthosis. The curve was stable and measured 38 degrees. Two years postoperatively, it measured 40 degrees. The patient had no complications and the preoperative pain was completely relieved. (Courtesy of Winter RB, Lonstein JE: *J Bone Joint Surg (Am)* 71A:1308–1313, October 1989.)

up period was 7 degrees, and the final correction averaged 34%. There was no statistically significant difference in the amount of final correction between the surgical subgroups.

Only 1 patient had a surgery-related neurologic deficit. This patient's wake-up test was positive, and the rod and wires were removed immediately. One patient had pneumonia, 1 had atelectasis, and 3 had urinary tract infections. There were no incidents of broken rods or wires. One patient needed removal of a painful rod tip. Three patients who had undergone posterior arthrodesis only had pseudarthrosis in the lumbar area. Thirty patients (71%) had no complications.

Segmental fixation with sublaminar wiring gives satisfactory results in the treatment of idiopathic scoliosis in adults, but only when performed by surgeons skilled in this technique.

▶ With all due respect to Drs. Winter and Lonstein, their published technique is already out of date. Since they initiated their series, newer fixation devices, particularly the Cotrel-Dubosett apparatus, has emerged as a favored technology. However, this article shows the results that can be achieved in the adult and forms one of a number of "baseline" outcome studies against which we should measure the newer devices. Equally important, it again reemphasizes that adult scoliosis is a clinical problem of significance and can be managed successfully by skilled surgeons using modern anesthetic techniques and appropriate monitoring of spinal cord function.— J.W. Frymoyer, M.D.

Anterior Zielke Instrumentation for Spinal Deformity in Adults
Kostuik JP, Carl A, Ferron S (Toronto Gen Hosp)
J Bone Joint Surg [Am] 71-A:898–912, July 1989　　　　　　　　　6–30

Spinal deformity was treated with anterior arthrodesis of the spine and Zielke instrumentation in 58 adult patients. The patients' average age was 37.4 years; 51 of the patients were women. Most (49) of the patients had idiopathic scoliosis. Other causes of deformity were paralytic scoliosis or hyperlordosis in 7 and congenital scoliosis in 2.

Fifty-one patients had disabling pain, usually aching at the apex of the curve. Medication or use of a spinal orthosis or both did not relieve their discomfort. Those patients who did not complain of pain had progression of the curve and a loss of height. Average follow-up for the 58 patients was 42 months.

Of the patients with idiopathic scoliosis, 30 had a single curve and 19 a double curve. The Zielke instrumentation was used to fix an average of 5 vertebral levels. Postoperatively, the curve in those patients improved 68%. In the remaining 9 patients, the curve improved 40%. Use of a derotator apparatus resulted in greater correction, and the derotator is now employed routinely, Preoperative traction was not used.

The 38 patients in whom the curve was convex to the left underwent a left thoracoabdominal approach. In 19 patients, the curve was convex to the right and a right thoracoabdominal approach was used. One patient needed a left paramedian exposure for a lower lumbar arthrodesis. On average, 5 vertebral levels were included in the instrumentation.

Only 4 of the 44 patients with idiopathic scoliosis and disabling pain continued to have pain. Single idiopathic curves improved the most, and the correction was not lost postoperatively. The average improvement for pelvic obliquity was 33%. Patients with paralytic deformities had complete relief from pain and a mean correction of the curve of 29 degrees. Good results also were obtained in patients with congenital scoliosis. Overall, intraoperative complications were minor.

▶ Aggressive surgical management of adult scoliosis can achieve good results in experienced surgeons' hands. In this group of 58 patients, the major indication was for pain; curve progression was a less common reason. The excellent results and minimal complications add to a growing belief that anterior spinal surgery is an excellent solution to the adult, more rigid curve.—J.W. Frymoyer, M.D.

Progression of Kyphosis in Tuberculosis of the Spine Treated by Anterior Arthrodesis
Rajasekaran S, Soundarapandian S (Madras Med College; Government Gen Hosp, Madras, India)
J Bone Joint Surg [Am] 71-A:1314–1323, October 1989　　　　　　6–31

Pretreatment Characteristics, Intraoperative Correction, and Final Result, According to Site of Lesion

	Site of Lesion			
	Thoracic (T1-T10)	Thoraco-lumbar (T11-L2)	Lower Lumbar (L3-S1)	Total
No. of patients	22	29	30	81
Vertebral involvement *(no. of vertebrae)*				
Narrrowing of disc space	0	2	2	4
One disc space	4	7	4	15
Two disc spaces	11	16	19	46
Three disc spaces	7	2	2	11
Four disc spaces or more	0	2	3	5
Total vertebral loss				
Narrowing of disc space	0	2	2	4
<1	12	18	15	45
1.1-2	9	4	11	24
2.1-3	1	1	1	3
>3	0	4	1	5
Pre-treatment kyphotic angle *(no. of patients)*				
0-10 degrees	2	4	20	26
11-20 degrees	5	7	4	16
21-30 degrees	3	11	4	18
31-40 degrees	7	4	1	12
>40 degrees	5	3	1	9
Intraoperative change in angle* *(no. of patients)*				
Correction >10 degrees	1	7	2	10
Correction <10 degrees	6	5	2	13
No change	10	12	24	46
Increase <10 degrees	4	3	2	9
Increase >10 degrees	1	2	0	3
Final result†				
Excellent	5	11	17	33
Good	5	6	4	15
Fair	6	4	5	15
Poor	6	8	4	18
Favorable results (excellent and good)	10/22 (45%)	17/29 (55%)	21/30 (70%)	48/81 (60%)

*The kyphotic angle as seen on the first postoperative radiograph compared with that seen on the preoperative radiograph.
†The kyphotic angle as seen on the 8-year follow-up radiograph compared with that seen on the preoperative radiograph.
(Courtesy of Rajasekaran S, Soundarapandian S: J Bone Joint Surg [Am] 71A:1314-1323, October 1989.)

Anterior spinal arthrodesis is used in spinal tuberculosis to prevent deformity from progressing, but few long-term studies on the fate of the graft have been done. Therefore, 81 patients (table) having had anterior arthrodesis during an 8-year-period were studied by comparing preoperative and postoperative radiographs. The results were graded as excellent

Fig 6-21.—Final results according to the length of the graft. The *broken line* indicates a favorable result, and the *solid line*, an unfavorable result. (Courtesy of Rajasekaran S, Soundarapandian S: *J Bone Joint Surg [Am]* 71-A:1314–1323, October 1989.)

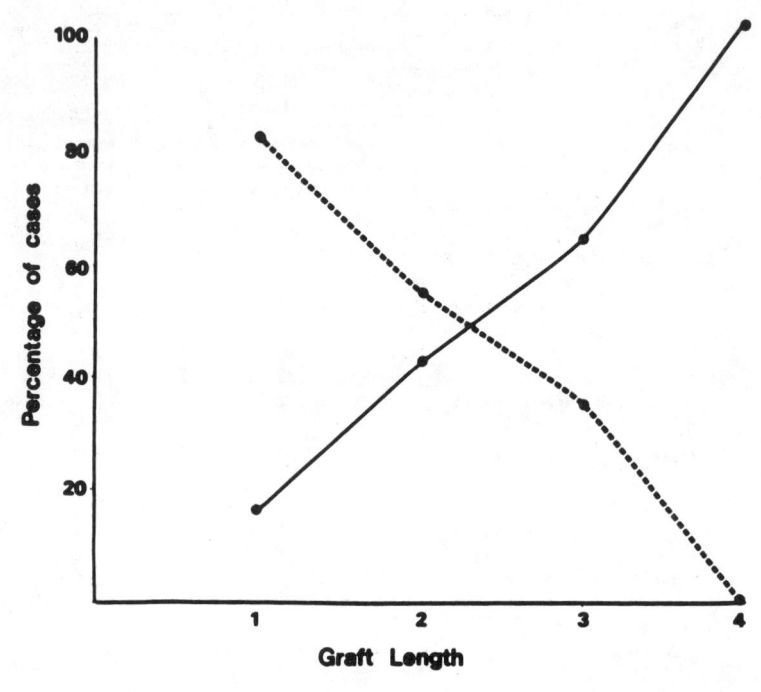

if the gibbus angle had been corrected, good if the angle had not progressed, fair if the angle had increased less than 20 degrees, and poor if the angle had increased more than 20 degrees.

Results were good or excellent in 59%. These patients had minimal bone deficit needing only a short graft. Results were fair in 19% and poor in 22%. An adverse result usually was associated with a graft that spanned more than 2 disk spaces (Fig 6–21).

Graft failure occurred in 59% of 81 patients. The reasons were graft slippage, which was the most common complication; graft fracture, often occurring during the first year and asymptomatic; graft absorption, which may indicate reactivation of disease; and graft subsidence, with failure of the graft to abut the end plates of the vertebrae.

A graft whose length exceeds 2 disk spaces should not be relied on fully to prevent vertebral collapse. Such patients may need non-weight-bearing for awhile, a brace until consolidation is complete, and posterior arthrodesis after a few weeks. All patients should be observed for graft failure, which requires posterior arthrodesis.

▶ Most of us see little tuberculosis. When we do, and elect a spinal stabilization, anterior strut grafting may not be enough, particularly when there is multilevel involvement. Such multilevel involvement is probably more common with adult spinal tuberculosis than has been appreciated. In a more general perspective, this article reinforces the growing belief that some spinal instabilities are best treated with combined anteroposterior procedures.—J.W. Frymoyer, M.D.

7 The Foot and Ankle

Introduction

This chapter is devoted to the significant contributions to better diagnosis and treatment of disorders of the foot and ankle made during the past year. More than 500 articles published in the English literature dealt directly with the foot and ankle. Twenty-five of these articles have been highlighted in this portion of the YEAR BOOK.

Several topics in this year's literature are particularly important. The biomechanics of the first cuneiform metatarsal joint has been better elucidated. This joint has been understood poorly in the past. Understanding the tarsometatarsal joint in normal and pathologic conditions may change our approach to hallux valgus surgery. Also, interest in ankle arthroscopy continues to expand, and other uses are being explored. The articles, however, emphasize that the procedure is fraught with potential complications, and its indications remain limited. The treatment of fractures of the foot and ankle has been refined further. Biodegradable pins have been shown to be useful and may have a greater role in the future. There is no doubt that injuries of the syndesmosis between the tibia and fibula must be stabilized. However, the approach to this remains controversial and many surgeons have different protocols for deciding how to stabilize this area, whether and when any implant is removed, and when weight bearing is begun.

Problems of the foot and ankle compose approximately 20% of a general orthopedist's practice. The awareness of foot and ankle problems is increasing, and it is gratifying that interest in orthopedic foot and ankle fellowships has increased significantly. Foot and ankle surgery is now in the mainstream of orthopedics, and the orthopedic knowledge and teaching of foot and ankle problems have increased significantly. The following 25 articles highlight the literature of the past year. They should lead to improvements in care. Each of the selections should be read in its entirety by those interested in the orthopedic management of foot and ankle disorders.

Kenneth A. Johnson, M.D.

Problems of the Forefoot

Bone Reaction to Silicone Metatarsophalangeal Joint-1 Hemiprosthesis
Verhaar J, Vermeulen A, Bulstra S, Walenkamp G (Univ Hosp, Maastricht, The Netherlands)
Clin Orthop 245:228–232, August 1989   7–1

Earlier assessments of inflammatory reactions to silicone small-joint implants emphasized the benign nature of such reactions. However, accumulating evidence suggests that these reactions are more aggressive than was previously thought. The radiographic and histologic aspects of inflammatory reactions in patients who underwent silicone hemiarthroplasties of the first metatarsophalangeal joint were assessed.

During a 5-year study period, 43 patients aged 17–60 years with hallux rigidus underwent implantation of 58 silicone hemiprostheses in the great toe. The mean length of follow-up was 59 months. Four patients with a mean age of 45 years needed revision operations because of persistent pain and signs of synovitis. The mean interval between prosthesis implantation and removal was 2 years.

Fifteen of the 58 implants showed substantial deformation on follow-up radiographs, and 1 implant appeared to be broken. Thirty-four implants had evidence of osteolysis around the base of the stem of the prosthesis in the proximal phalanx. Osteolysis was rated moderate in 15 feet and considerable in 18 feet (Fig 7–1). Only 14 of the 58 feet were free of

Fig 7–1.—Roentgenogram of the first metatarsophalangeal joint with a silicone prosthesis after 3.5 years in situ. The proximal phalanx shows multiple cysts at the base of the stem of the prosthesis. Cysts are seen in the head of the first metatarsal. (Courtesy of Verhaar J, Vermeulen A, Bulstra S, et al: *Clin Orthop* 245:228–232, August 1989.)

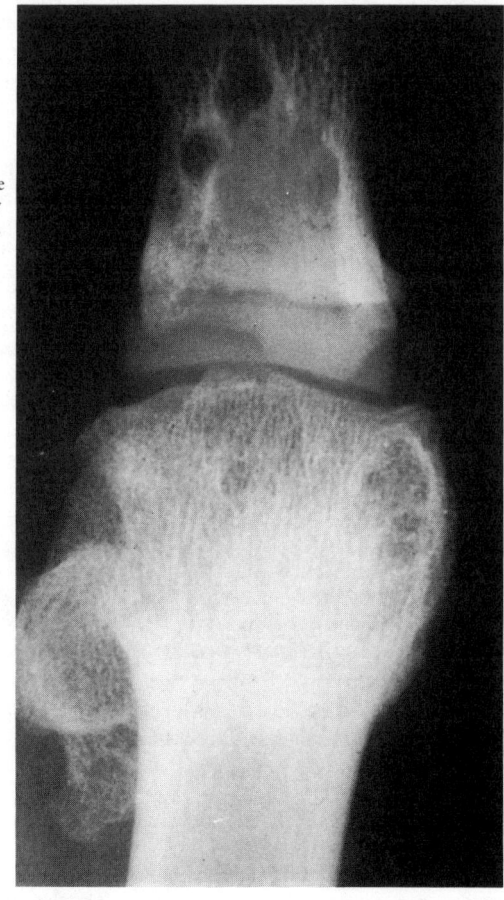

cysts. Two feet had 1 cyst each in the first metatarsal head and 40 feet had several cysts. The cysts ranged in size from 1 to 4 mm.

Wear had progressively decreased the length of the proximal phalanx over time and altered the shapes of the prostheses. The shape of the first metatarsal head had changed in 40 feet, with 28 deformations rated as slight and 12 as more serious. Histologic examination of the surgical samples removed at revision showed that the cysts were filled with an avascular cellular stroma containing histiocytes and multinucleated giant cells opsonizing silicone particles from the wear debris of the prosthesis. Replacement of the first metatarsophalangeal joint with a silicone implant in young, active patients is not recommended.

▶ Every year, additional studies document the high rate of complications with silicone implant arthroplasty (1). The majority of the patients in this study had significant osteolysis. It's difficult to recommend the use of silastic hemi-implant arthroplasty based on information such as this. In my experience, such osteolysis also occurs about the stems of the hinged Silastic implant also.— K.A. Johnson, M.D.

Reference

1. Lemon RA, et al: *Foot Ankle* 4:262, 1984.

First Tarsometatarsal Joint: Anatomical Biomechanical Study
Wanivenhaus A, Pretterklieber M (Univ of Vienna)
Foot Ankle 9:153–157, February 1989   7–2

The form, function, and malfunction of the first tarsometatarsal (TMT) joint have not been well studied. However, the first TMT joint is an important communication point between the longitudinal and transverse arch and has much clinical significance. An anatomical study used 100 feet from 53 cadavers.

The study material consisted of 66 feet from women and 34 feet from men. The patients ranged in age from 20 to 92 years with an average age of 68 years at the time of death. Dorsoplantar and lateral x-ray films were obtained for each specimen. Maximal approximation of the first and second metatarsals was attempted by manual compression. Kirschner wires were used to achieve fixation in the compressed state. After another x-ray film was made, the first metatarsal joint was exposed while preserving all ligamentous structures. Kirschner wires were placed so as to enable the measurement of movement around the first TMT joint's axis.

Only 11 of the 100 feet could be abducted or adducted in the first TMT joint. The average abduction in these 11 joints was 4.4 degrees, and the average adduction was 5 degrees. Study of the x-ray films revealed that lateral compression of the first and second metatarsals reduced the metatarsal angle in 40 feet. However, in only 26 cases could this reduction be attributed to movement in the first TMT joint. Furthermore, the first TMT joint showed no dorsiplantar flexion, and internal and external rotation were negligible.

The clinical implication of the finding that abduction and adduction in the first TMT joint are mostly lacking is that any operation involving the first TMT joint will have little or no success in terms of a correction. The anatomical findings support previously published clinical studies which found that permanent correction of the metatarsal angle could never be achieved with the widely used McBride procedure. Thus, these findings challenge the value of the McBride transfer in metatarsus primus varus.

▶ The first TMT joint has attracted much interest recently. These authors demonstrate that this joint normally has very little motion. This article and several others have elucidated the biomechanics and function of this joint (1). With metatarsus primus varus and hallux valgus, this motion probably is increased over the normal stable conditions shown by these authors. The concept of the "hypermobile first ray" with hallux valgus is probably a clinical entity that necessitates stabilization at the first TMT joint in some cases of hallux valgus.—K.A. Johnson, M.D.

Reference

1. Ouzounian TJ, Shereff MJ: *Foot Ankle* 10:140, December, 1989.

Proximal Closing Wedge Osteotomy and Adductor Tenotomy for Treatment of Hallux Valgus
Resch S, Stenström A, Egund N (Univ Hosp, Lund, Sweden)
Foot Ankle 9:272–280, June 1989   7–3

Proximal closing wedge osteotomy of the first metatarsal combined with adductor tenotomy and bunionectomy was used in the treatment of moderate to severe hallux valgus in 27 feet of 25 patients. Operative results were reviewed; the follow-up period was 37 months (range, 25–51 months).

Twenty patients (22 feet) were completely satisfied with the effect of the operation (Fig 7–2). All of the 5 patients who were not completely satisfied had metatarsalgia because of dorsal displacement of the second metatarsal head. Postoperative radiographic measurements showed a narrowing of the forefoot rather than a large change in the intermetatarsal angle. The reduction in the hallux valgus angle was impressive. The average recovery period was 11 weeks. A major complication was development of pain under the second metatarsal head. Other complications included pin inflammation in 5 patients and incisional neuromas in 2 patients.

Proximal closing wedge osteotomy is a technically demanding operation. Although the results are generally satisfactory, the risk of complications, particularly dorsal displacement of the second metatarsal head resulting in metatarsalgia, should be taken into consideration when using this operation.

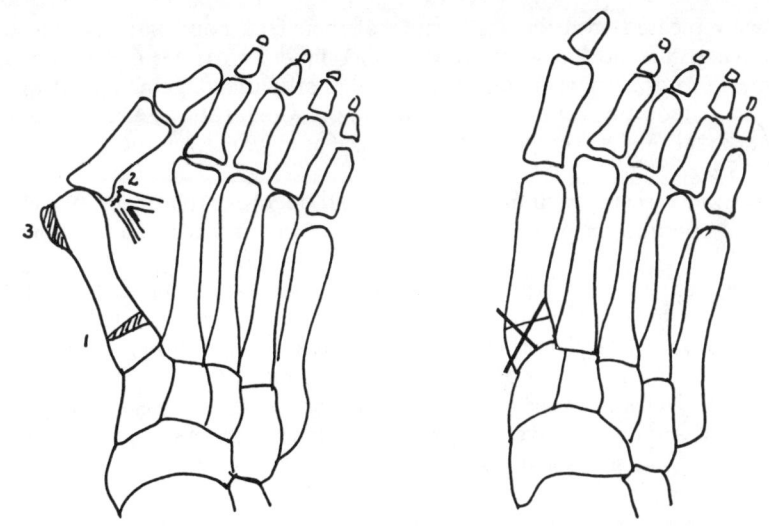

Fig 7-2.—Operative procedure: *1*, lateral wedge in the metaphysis of the metatarsal, fixation by K wire. *2*, always adductor tenotomy through a separate incision. *3*, in most cases, removal of the osteophytes at the metatarsal head. (Courtesy of Resch S, Stenström A, Egund N: *Foot Ankle* 9:272-280, June 1989.)

▶ This article substantiates why proximal first metatarsal wedge osteotomy has lost favor in the treatment of hallux valgus. These authors demonstrate the significant excessive transfer metatarsalgia in 20% of their patients with such an operative procedure. In addition, incisional neuromas developed in 8% of the patients. A proximal osteotomy for hallux valgus is not a trivial procedure, and methods to decrease this high rate of complications include basilar crescentic osteotomies and cuneiform metatarsal-I arthrodeses. It is most important to prevent shortening or elevation of the first metatarsal to avoid the transfer metatarsalgia.—K.A. Johnson, M.D.

Treatment of Hallux Valgus in Adolescents by the Chevron Osteotomy
Zimmer TJ, Johnson KA, Klassen RA (Mayo Graduate School of Medicine; Mayo Clinic and Mayo Found, Rochester, Minn)
Foot Ankle 9:190-193, February 1989   7-4

Many procedures are available for correction of hallux valgus in adolescents. Two males and 18 females aged 12 to 18 years (average, 15.6 years) underwent 35 chevron osteotomies of the first metatarsal for painful hallux valgus between 1978 and 1984. With 1 exception the patients had intermetatarsal angles of less than 15 degrees, and all had hallux valgus of 40 degrees or less. All had significant pain that limited activity. Fifteen patients had bilateral chevron operations.

The average follow-up was 64 months. Seventeen patients had no pain at follow-up, but 3 had some discomfort that limited activities. Seven patients still found some types of footwear uncomfortable. All patients but

2 were pleased with the appearance of their feet. Four patients had subjective recurrences associated with incomplete correction. The average time to radiographic union was 6 weeks; all patients gained solid union of the osteotomy, and none had malunion. Correction of the first intermetatarsal angle averaged 4.8 degrees. The average forefoot narrowing was 5.9 mm.

Few adolescents with hallux valgus need operative treatment, but when they do because of pain, the chevron osteotomy is a reasonable choice.

▶ Management of a bunion deformity in an adolescent patient remains controversial. As in older patients, pain remains the primary indication for correction of hallux valgus. Significant activity-limiting pain was present in all patients in this study, and a high rate of satisfaction was demonstrated using the Chevron procedure. As with all hallux valgus patients, conservative measures should be tried first and orthopedic surgeons should remain wary of operating on these patients.— K.A. Johnson, M.D.

Metatarsal Osteotomy Using a Double-Threaded Compression Screw: An Adjunct to Revision Forefoot Surgery
Sammarco GJ, Scioli MW (Univ of Cincinnati; Lubbock, Tex)
Foot Ankle 10:129–139, December 1989   7–5

A review was made of the early results of a lesser metatarsal osteotomy to repair metatarsal nonunions in patients in whom previous surgery failed. A double-threaded Herbert compression screw was used in 18 feet with 20 lesser metatarsal osteotomies and 6 nonunion repairs. Twelve of 16 patients also needed simultaneous correction of other conditions.

The rationale for using the double-threaded compression screw is that it can provide low-profile rigid compression of a wedge osteotomy or nonunion. The screw may be used in conjunction with bone grafting. Other advantages are that the screw eliminates the need for percutaneous pins, external fixators, electrical stimulation, and casts.

At follow-up, 11 of 15 feet had complete relief of plantar metatarsal pain, 3 feet had partial relief, and 1 foot was unrelieved. Nine patients returned to full activity. Five had improvement but had some limitations in standing or walking at presymptomatic levels. Of 8 preoperative callosities, 5 were resolved and 3 persisted with mild symptoms. Seven of 14 patients could wear higher heels for short periods, and 1 patient could wear any type of shoe. There was no infection or metatarsophalangeal joint degeneration. Subjectively, 11 of 14 patients with osteotomy believed that the surgery was satisfactory, 1 had some reservations, and 2 were disappointed. Screw fixation and bone grafting permitted union of 4 of 6 metatarsal nonunions, but complications made additional surgery necessary.

Internal fixation with a double-threaded screw had a success rate of 73% in this series. Treatment of metatarsal nonunion, however, remains a problem. Complications in of 6 metatarsals required further surgery.

▶ This article describes a new method of fixation of metatarsal osteotomies using the Herbert double-threaded bone screw. The authors insert the screw through the metatarsal head and state that the metatarsal head hole fills in with fibrocartilage. We must remember that metatarsal osteotomies are not trivial procedures and should be attempted only after failure of conservative therapy. Most surgeons prefer to fix lesser metatarsal osteotomies; however, this study reinforces that fixation can be fraught with complications.— K.A. Johnson, M.D.

Morton Neuroma: Sonographic Evaluation
Redd RA, Peters VJ, Emery SF, Branch HM, Rifkin MD (Brooke Army Med Ctr, San Antonio; Thomas Jefferson Univ; Wilford Hall US Air Force Med Ctr)
Radiology 171:415–417, May 1989   7–6

Before the advent of ultrasound (US), it was difficult to adequately image Morton neuroma, a focal mass of perineural fibrosis involving the plantar digital nerves of the foot. To evaluate the role of US in identifying, localizing, and quantifying these neuromas in the foot, 100 patients and 10 controls were examined with US. The mean patient age was 53 years. Forty-five patients subsequently had surgical resection and pathologic analysis of the interdigital masses. Patients also underwent clinical examination and plain radiography. Both coronal and sagittal images were obtained with US.

With ultrasound, 134 intermetatarsal masses were found. Twenty-six patients had multiple masses; 74 had solitary lesions. Surgical exploration revealed Morton neuromas. The typical sonographic appearance was that of an ovoid, hypoechoic mass with an orientation parallel to the long axis of the metatarsals. Most masses were between the second and third or the third and fourth metatarsals. When they reached a diameter of approximately 5 mm, patients usually had symptoms.

Imaging with US enhances the likelihood of successful surgical excision of Morton neuromas. Computed tomography and magnetic resonance imaging also could be used, but US may be more readily available and is less expensive.

▶ Interdigital neuroma remains a diagnosis based on symptoms only; thus, the absence of any specific laboratory or x-ray test contributes to its overdiagnosis. This article suggests that sonography may be useful for the diagnosis of Morton's neuroma and does an excellent job of reviewing the sonographic image of interdigital neuroma. It is not, however, a study that includes normal feet without interdigital neuromas. Further studies are indicated to see whether this technique has any clinical usefulness.— K.A. Johnson, M.D.

Prosthetic Replacement of the First Metatarsophalangeal Joint
Merkle PF, Sculco TP (Hosp for Special Surgery, New York)
Foot Ankle 9:267–271, June 1989   7–7

A semiconstrained prosthesis was designed as an alternative to Keller bunionectomy, Silastic implant replacement, and cheilectomy of the first metatarsophalangeal joint (MTPJ). The components are secured with polymethyl methacrylate and follow the contour of the normal joint and the first metatarsosesamoidal articulation. The flexor hallucis brevis and adductor hallucis are note disturbed.

Twelve patients underwent 15 MTPJ replacements with the implant. Nine patients (11 feet) were followed up for an average of 1 year, 9 months. Overall satisfaction was good to excellent in 4 patients. Aseptic loosening occurred in 6 (54.5%) of 11 patients. Deep sepsis developed in 1 patient with subsequent removal of the prostheses.

Cemented replacement arthroplasty of the first MTPJ is not a satisfactory procedure for the treatment of hallux rigidus. Further modification of the prosthesis and its fixation method currently is being considered. Until then, one of the standard operations—cheilectomy, arthrodesis, Silastic, or resection arthroplasty—should be used.

▶ This is yet another report of poor results after implant replacement of the first metatarsophalangeal joint. Their loosening rate was more than 50% with this semiconstrained component. These authors conclude that, until further data are obtained, the standard operations such as cheilectomy, arthrodesis, or resection arthroplasty should be used in the treatment of hallux rigidus.—K.A. Johnson, M.D.

Dorsiflexion Osteotomy in Freiberg's Disease
Kinnard P, Lirette R (Université Laval, Sainte-Foy, PQ)
Foot Ankle 9:226–231, April 1989   7–8

A number of surgical procedures are recommended when conservative treatment of Freiberg's disease fails, but little has been written about the dorsiflexion osteotomy technique. In a retrospective study of 10 patients who underwent this procedure, the 8 women and 2 men had failed to respond to conservative treatment for more than 2 years. Patients' ages ranged from 14 to 55 years. The procedure consisted of a large metatarsophalangeal arthrotomy (Fig 7–3) to expose the metatarsal head through a lateral or medial dorsal incision. After débridement, a closed dorsal wedge osteotomy was performed. Even in patients with extensive avascular necrosis of the metatarsal head, the procedure rotated the bone up sufficiently to remove the defect from the articular surface (Fig. 7–4). Patients were reviewed clinically and radiographically by an independent observer. Follow-up averaged 36.5 months.

All patients had excellent results with minimal loss of metatarsophalangeal motion. The average radiologic metatarsal shortening was 2.3 mm. There was no postoperative metatarsalgia. The dorsiflexion osteotomy is a satisfactory treatment for symptomatic Freiberg's disease. Re-

Chapter 7— The Foot and Ankle / **323**

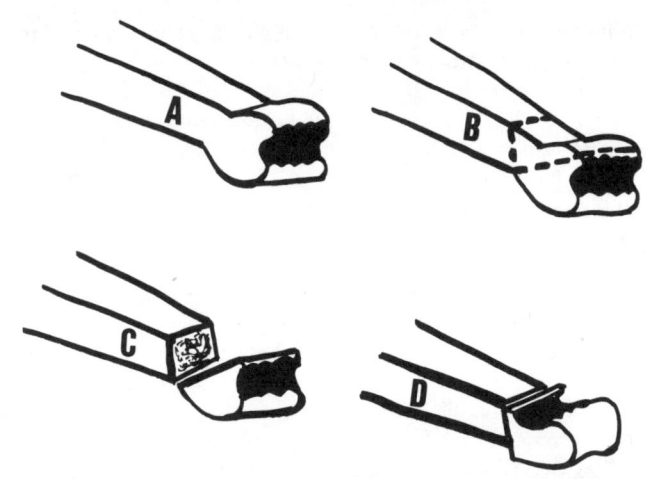

Fig 7–3.—Dorsiflexion osteotomy technique. (Courtesy of Kinnard P, Lirette R: *Foot Ankle* 9:226–231, April 1989.)

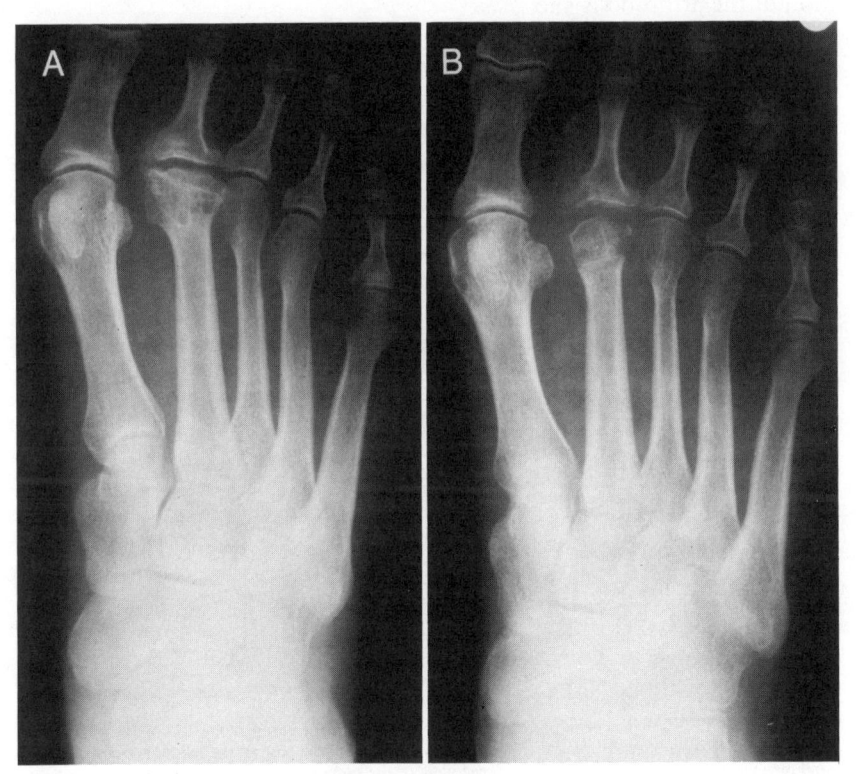

Fig 7–4.—A 57-year-old patient before *(A)* and 3 months after *(B)* surgery. (Courtesy of Kinnard P, Lirette R: *Foot Ankle* 9:226–231, April 1989.)

sults are reliable, and the procedure is not destructive, an attractive feature should further treatment be necessary.

▶ These authors studied the use of a dorsiflexion osteotomy for Freiberg's disease and illustrated the technique by which they obtained excellent results for all their patients. Metatarsal shortening was 2.3 mm, but transfer metatarsalgia was not a problem. It is a treatment of Freiberg's disease that deserves further consideration.—K.A. Johnson, M.D.

Modified Lapidus Procedure for Hallux Valgus
Sangeorzan BJ, Hansen ST Jr (Harborview Med Ctr; Univ of Washington, Seattle)
Foot Ankle 9:262–266, June 1989   7–9

Lapidus first described his surgical procedure for correcting hallux valgus complex in 1934. This procedure was adapted to treat hallux valgus with hypermobile first ray, which involves the use of rigid internal fixation of the arthrodesis site.

Procedure.—A longitudinal incision beginning in the first web space and extending proximally over the first tarsometatarsal joint is deepened distally, and a lateral longitudinal capsulotomy is done. The wound then is deepened proximally, and the tarsometatarsal joint is opened. The cartilage then is removed from the distal cuneiform and proximal metatarsal down to subchondral bone. Rigid internal fixation requires a planar surface for stability and the shape of the cuneiform-metatarsal varies; thus, some versatility is needed to remove as little bone as necessary to reposition the first metatarsal into a lateralized and slightly

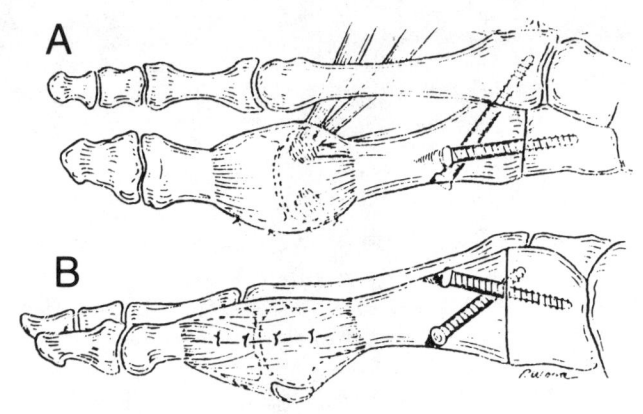

Fig 7–5.—**A,** a screw has been placed across the metatarsal articulation, compressing the planar surface. A second screw has been placed from the medial border of the base of the metatarsal into the second metatarsal as a derotation screw. **B,** lateral view of the same patient showing a closed elipse of soft tissue at the metatarsophalangeal joint capsule and the lateral view of the position of the proximal fixation screws. Note that a small notch has been made in the dorsal surface of the metatarsal to allow positioning of the fixation screw. (Courtesy of Sangeorzan BJ, Hansen ST Jr: *Foot Ankle* 9:262–266, June 1989.)

more plantar-flexed position (Fig 7–5). Sometimes a small plantar lateral wedge has to be removed. Resecting the whole joint is not necessary. A longitudinal medial capsulotomy over the metatarsophalangeal joint is done next. The metatarsal and hallus are reduced. Redundant medial capsule is excised. The metatarsocuneiform joint is held reduced, and provisional fixation is done. After the reduction is documented by radiography, a second screw is placed from the first metatarsal into the second cuneiform to ensure rotational stability of the cuneiform metatarsal fusion. With the metatarsal held in corrected position, the hallux valgus angle is corrected manually, and a capsular repair is done with absorbable sutures.

This procedure was successful in 75% of 33 feet operated on as a primary procedure. All 7 feet operated on for failed previous surgery were improved. The best results were obtained with multiple screw fixation, use of bone graft, and attention to plantar flexion of the first metatarsal.

▶ Arthrodesis of the cuneiform-metatarsal I articulation may be used to treat hallux valgus deformity. However, this article demonstrates that complications are significant when the surgical technique involves large surface joint resection before arthrodesis. Better results were obtained with secure fixation using AO screws and bone graft. Other techniques that avoid first ray shortening and destabilization may be preferable. This topic of the hypermobile first ray and the first metatarsocuneiform arthrodesis for hallux valgus probably will be receiving considerable attention in the near future.—K.A. Johnson, M.D.

Trauma and Sequelae

Effect of the Syndesmotic Screw on Ankle Motion
Needleman RL, Skrade DA, Stiehl JB (Med College of Wisconsin, Milwaukee)
Foot Ankle 10:17–24, August 1989   7–10

Syndesmotic screw fixation is used for the internal fixation of certain unstable ankle fractures. Whether it should be removed 6 weeks before weight bearing or left in place indefinitely remains controversial. To assess the effect of syndesmotic screw fixation on ankle motion, 8 unpaired osteoligamentous cadaver ankles were tested for ankle motion, talar tilt, ankle drawer, and tibiotalar motion rotation using an MTS biomechanical testing system. Each specimen was tested under 15-kg and 70-kg axial loads. The testing was repeated after the placement of a syndesmotic screw, a 4.5-mm cortical screw, in accordance with the AO technique.

After syndesmotic screw fixation of the ankle, there was a significant decrease in the tibiotalar external rotation and a significant decrease in the anterior and posterior drawer tests with the foot in plantar flexion. There was no difference in ankle flexion after syndesmotic screw fixation of the ankle.

Syndesmotic screw fixation significantly interferes with normal ankle motion. The syndesmotic screw should be removed before the return to full activity. Leaving it in place will contribute to abnormal ankle motion, which may result in local discomfort and possible fatigue fracture of the screw.

Stabilization of Ankle Syndesmosis Injuries With a Syndesmosis Screw
Kaye RA (Santa Clara Valley Med Ctr, San Jose, Calif)
Foot Ankle 9:290-293, June 1989

The treatment of displaced ankle fractures with associated syndesmosis disruptions is controversial. Some physicians favor the use of transfixation screws to stabilize the distal tibiofibular joint, whereas others prefer to limit the use of screws to patients in whom the syndesmosis cannot be stabilized by internal fixation of the fibular fracture or by ligament repair. A retrospective study was conducted to review the experience and outcome with the use of syndesmosis screws.

Between 1983 and 1987, 25 men and 6 women had syndesmosis screws placed during treatment of ankle fractures. Each patient had a fracture of the fibula above the tibial plafond with associated disruption of the distal tibiofibular syndesmosis. Eight patients had high fibular fractures of the Maisonneuve variety, and 10 patients had tears of the deep deltoid ligament. Synthes screw sizes ranged from 3.5 cortical to 6.5 cancellous. Most screws were placed transversely 1.5-3.5 cm above the joint line. The average time to weight bearing was 6.3 weeks, and the average time to plaster removal was 9 weeks. Most patients were mobilized before screw removal, but timing of screw removal varied by patient and physician choice.

Two thirds of the patients had some evidence of bony erosion around a screw before the screw was removed. No screw broke before removal. Seven patients had evidence of calcification within the interosseous membrane, which progressed to distal tibiofibular synostosis in 4 patients. However, the location of the calcification was associated most closely with the level of the fibular fracture rather than with the level of syndesmosis screw placement. After a follow-up ranging from 3 months to 3 years, final ankle range of motion averaged 9 degrees of dorsiflexion and 38 degrees of plantar flexion. Routine radiographs were not useful for assessment of the distal tibiofibular joint. Transfixation screws provide satisfactory stability of the syndesmosis to permit stable healing of the inteosseous membrane and distal ligaments after ankle fractures.

▶ There is much controversy about the timing of syndesmosis screw removal. The first article (Abstract 7-10) is a nice biomechanical study which shows that the syndesmosis screw significantly interferes with normal ankle motion. These authors recommended removal of the screw before return to full activity. The next study (Abstract 7-11) is a retrospective review of 30 patients that confirms the effectiveness of the syndesmosis screw in displaced ankle fractures with associated syndesmosis disruptions. The technique varied among surgeons, and most patients were mobilized before screw removal. They had no screw breakage, but did have lucent changes develop around some of the screws. Most surgeons currently recommend a cortical screw through 3 cortices inserted in a nonlag fashion. The screw should remain in place for at least 6 weeks and probably longer. It is reasonable to allow weight bearing before screw removal, and most surgeons accept the small risk of screw breakage or loosening over the risk of redisplacement of the syndesmosis.—K.A. Johnson, M.D.

Osteochondral Fractures of the Dome of the Talus
Anderson IF, Crichton KJ, Grattan-Smith T, Cooper RA, Brazier D (Royal North Shore Hosp of Sydney, St Leonards; North Sydney Orthopaedic and Sports Medicine Clinic, Crows Nest, Australia)
J Bone Joint Surg [Am] 71-A:1143–1152, September 1989   7–12

Osteochondral fractures of the dome of the talus traditionally have been difficult to diagnose. On plain ankle radiographs, stage I osteochondral fractures show no diagnostic changes and stage II lesions usually show only subtle changes. The advent of CT and magnetic resonance (MR) imaging has facilitated the diagnosis of these fractures.

During a 9-month period, 56 patients underwent MR imaging of the ankle. Thirty of the 56 patients had posttraumatic chronic disability of the ankle although plain radiographs revealed no abnormalities. Fourteen of those 30 patients were selected for further study. Ten other patients with a diagnosis of talar osteochondral fracture on the basis of plain radiographic evidence also were studied. The first 14 patients underwent scintigraphy of the ankle; all 24 patients also underwent CT.

Seventeen of the 30 patients with undiagnosed posttraumatic disability of the ankle had unexpected osteochondral fractures of the talar dome as confirmed by MR imaging and bone scanning. Three patients who had tibial plafond fractures only subsequently were excluded from the analysis. The remaining 14 patients had 15 fractures of the dome of the talus. One patient had both a medial and a lateral fracture, thought to be the first reported case of a double osteochondral talar dome fracture (Fig 7–6). The average delay to diagnosis in these patients had been 17.6 months. Staging of the fractures with CT corresponded to MR staging in 9 of the 14 patients. In the other 5 patients CT findings were normal. In 9 of 10 patients with confirmed osteochondral fractures, CT staging of the fractures corresponded to the staging based on radiographic findings. Diagnoses made with MR imaging agreed with radiographic findings in all 10 cases.

Because of the unexpectedly high incidence of osteochondral talar fractures detected by MR imaging in patients who remained symptomatic after apparently negative plain radiographs, a diagnostic protocol was prepared for future use in patients suspected clinically of having osteochondral talar head fractures (Fig 7–7). These patients should be assessed with scintigraphy; those who have positive scintiscans should be examined further with MR imaging. Magnetic resonance imaging offers no major benefits to patients whose plain radiographs provide evidence for diagnosis, and CT is adequate for staging fractures in those cases.

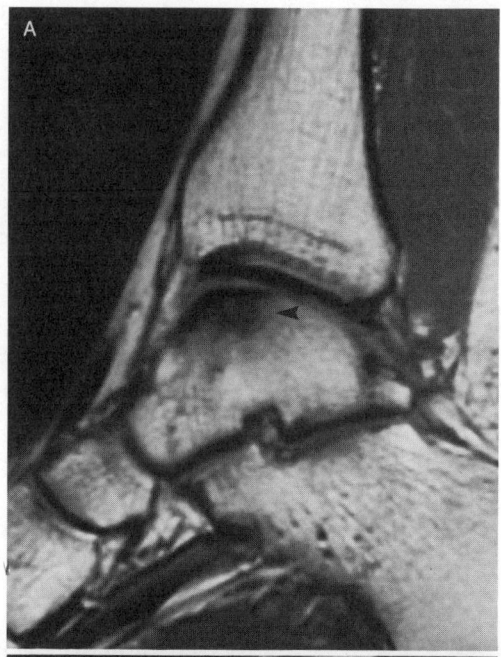

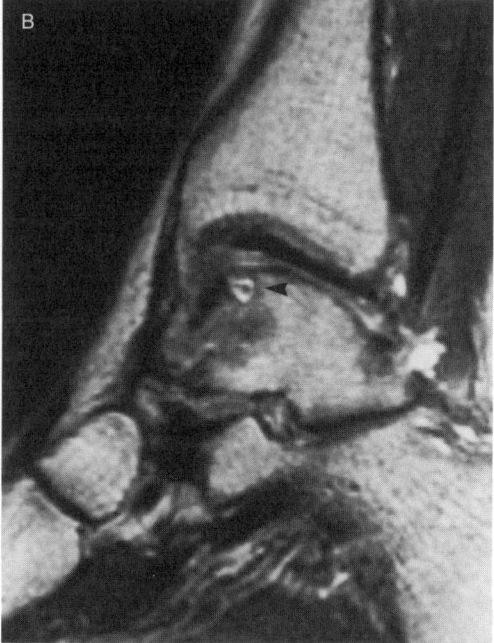

Fig 7–6.—Magnetic resonance images made 9 months after injury. Intermediate image (**A**) (pulse-repetition time, 2,000 ms; echo time, 20 ms) and T$_2$-weighted image (**B**) (pulse-repetition time, 2,000 ms; echo time, 70 ms) reveal a subchondral cyst in the anteromedial aspect of the talar dome *(arrowhead)*. (Courtesy of Anderson IF, Crichton KJ, Grattan-Smith T, et al: *J Bone Joint Surg [Am]* 71:A:1143–1152, September 1989.)

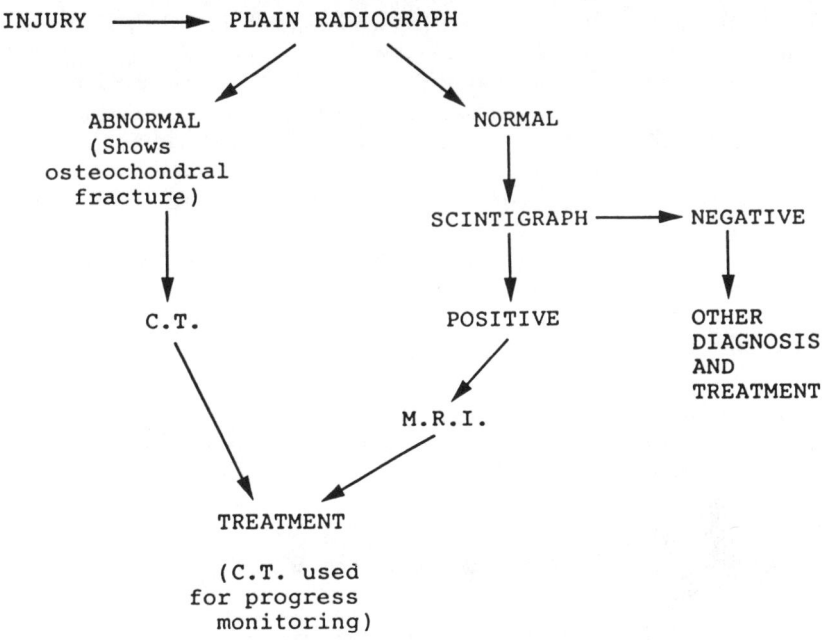

```
INJURY ──────▶ PLAIN RADIOGRAPH
                 ╱           ╲
         ABNORMAL           NORMAL
         (Shows                │
         osteochondral         │
         fracture)             ▼
            │         SCINTIGRAPH ──────▶ NEGATIVE
            │                │                │
            ▼                ▼                ▼
           C.T.           POSITIVE          OTHER
              ╲             ╱             DIAGNOSIS
               ╲           ╱                AND
                ╲         ╱              TREATMENT
                 M.R.I.
                 ╱    ╲
                ▼      
            TREATMENT

          (C.T. used
          for progress
          monitoring)
```

Fig 7-7.—Diagnostic protocol. The diagnosis of osteochondral fracture always should be considered for a patient who has a problem of the ankle that persists for more than 6 weeks after an inversion injury. Abbreviations: C.T., computed tomography; M.R.I., magnetic resonance imaging. (Courtesy of Anderson IF, Crichton KJ, Grattan-Smith T, et al: J Bone Joint Surg [Am] 71:A:1143–1152, September 1989.)

▶ The authors provide a useful algorithm for the diagnosis of these frequently missed lesions. Plain radiographs are often negative. In patients with persistent pain, bone scan and MR imaging scan may be helpful. The treatment remains controversial, although most chronic cases will need and benefit from surgery, whether it be open or arthroscopic.— K.A. Johnson, M.D.

Osteochondritis Dissecans of the Talus: Long-Term Results of Surgical Treatment
Angermann P, Jensen P (Central Hosp, Naestved, Denmark)
Foot Ankle 10:161–163, December 1989   7–13

Most authors recommend early surgical treatment of osteochondritis dissecans, but some advocate conservative treatment initially. Researchers investigated the long-term surgical results in 20 patients treated for osteochondritis dissecans of the talus 9 to 15 years after the procedure. Patients were reviewed both clinically and radiographically. Surgery had included multiple drilling of the lesion and excision of loose fragments.

Seventeen patients had satisfactory short-term results after surgery. Two of 3 patients with persistent symptoms later underwent talocrural fusion. At long-term follow-up more than half of the patients reported pain during activity, and 28% had noticeable ankle swelling. However, only a few had locking pain at rest. Two ankles examined clinically had reduced mobility, and 2 had swelling. Radiographic findings revealed only 1 patient with a reduction of the joint space of 1 mm on the treated side. Three patients had universal irregularity of the subchondral bone of the treated ankle but only local sclerosis. Only 2 ankles had no irregularity or sclerosis of the subchondral bone in the region of the lesion. Fourteen patients had osteophytes at the operated-on ankle, and 5 had osteophytes at the ankle that was not operated on.

Drilling combined with excision of destroyed fragments provides good short-term results in patients with osteochondritis dissecans of the talus, but results deteriorate with time. Nevertheless, the procedure is recommended for complete or displaced talar osteochondral lesions.

▶ With increased clinical awareness and improved diagnostic modalities, osteochondritis dissecans is being diagnosed more often. In this study all the surgery was done open through a medial malleolar osteotomy. In the patients with persistent symptoms and osteochondritis dissecans, surgery is recommended and provides good results. The exact timing and type of surgery—arthroscopic versus open—remain controversial.—K.A. Johnson, M.D.

Ankle Fractures Treated Using Biodegradable Internal Fixation
Böstman O, Hirvensalo E, Vainionpää S, Mäkelä A, Vihtonen K, Törmälä P, Rokkanen P (Helsinki Univ Central Hosp; Tampere Inst of Technology, Tampere, Finland)
Clin Orthop 238:195–203, January 1989   7–14

The introduction of biodegradable implants may abolish the need to remove the metallic fixation devices in fracture treatment. Absorbable implants were developed using self-reinforced lactide-glycolide copolymer and polyglycolide. These polymers biodegrade principally by hydrolysis, and the degradation time within the body is estimated at 60 to 100 days. A total of 102 patients with displaced unimalleolar or bimalleolar fractures of the ankle were managed using biodegradable internal fixation.

The internal fixation devices consist of cylindrical biodegradable implants 3.2 mm or 4.5 mm in diameter and 50 mm or 70 mm in length. After open reduction of the fracture, a channel is drilled from the tip of the malleolus into the cancellous bone through the fracture surfaces. A biodegradable rod of the same diameter is tapped into the drill channel. Fixation on the lateral side is reinforced by an absorbable figure-of-8 suture (Fig 7–8). Postoperatively, the ankle is immobilized with a plaster cast for 6 weeks.

An initial anatomical reduction was achieved in 93 patients (91%). Of these patients, 4 had slight secondary displacement of less than 2 mm. In 6 patients, a sinus was formed 2 to 4 months after operation and yielded remnants of the degradable implant. However, this complication did not influence the union of the fracture or functional recovery. At the 1-year

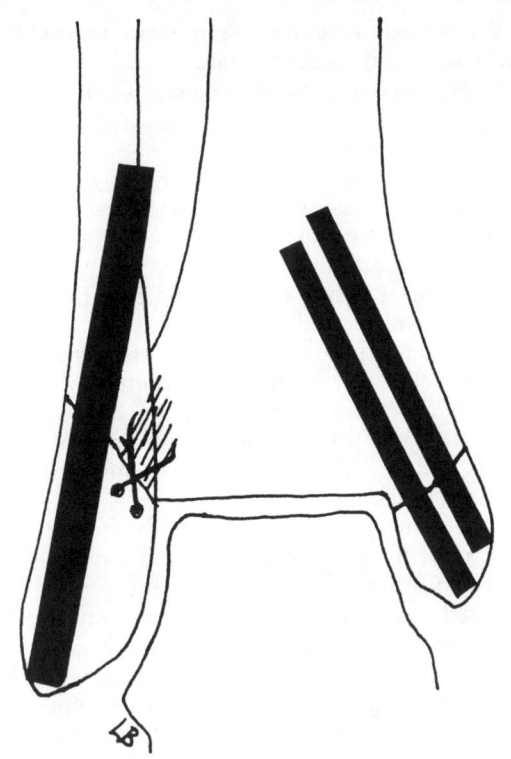

Fig 7–8.—A view of a bimalleolar fracture fixed using a 4.5-mm × 70-mm biodegradable rod in the lateral malleolus and two 3.2-mm × 50-mm rods in the medial malleolus. The lateral side is reinforced by a figure-of-8 suture through a hole in the distal fragment and behind the fibers of the distal tibiofibular syndesmosis. (Courtesy of Böstman O, Hirvensalo E, Vainionpää S, et al: *Clin Orthop* 238:195–203, January 1989.)

follow-up examination, no roentgenographic abnormalities were seen in 84 patients (82%). There was no change in participation in sports and other physical activities in 89 patients (87%).

These outcomes do not differ from those reported recently for comparable fractures treated by using the AO/ASIF instrumentation. These favorable results have encouraged the routine use of the biodegradable fixation method in the treatment of displaced unimalleolar and bimalleolar ankle fractures.

▶ These absorbable implants made of a lactide-glycolide copolymer and polyglycolide rods are commercially available, and their use is evolving for many clinical applications. This article demonstrates that they may have a useful role in foot and ankle surgery. Additional studies and those with longer follow-up will be necessary before these implants can be recommended routinely for ankle fractures. The 6% incidence of wound sinus formation is of concern, and this deserves further study.— K.A. Johnson, M.D.

Treatment of Open Ankle Fractures: Immediate Internal Fixation Versus Closed Immobilization and Delayed Fixation
Bray TJ, Endicott M, Capra SE (Univ of California, Sacramento)
Clin Orthop 240:47–52, March 1989   7–15

Two different approaches were used to treat 31 open ankle fractures over an 11-year period at a single institution. In 1973–1979, 15 patients, aged 17–85 years, had treatment initially with operative débridement and closed manipulative reduction. Minor wounds were allowed to close by secondary intention. Patients with Gustilo type III soft tissue wounds subsequently underwent delayed closure or skin grafting. Of the 15 patients in whom anatomical reduction could not be maintained by closed reduction, 7 underwent delayed internal fixation. In 1979–1984, 16 patients aged 18–77 years were treated with immediate open reduction and internal fixation. Delayed primary closure was performed at 5–7 days. After the wounds had healed, patients were encouraged to perform early range of motion exercises.

The average follow-up period was 90 months for patients treated during the early years of the study period and 33 months for those treated later. The mean final functional and pain scores were 78 for patients initially having closed reduction and 77 for those having immediate open reduction. Deep infections developed in 1 patient in each treatment group, which led to poor functional results. Ankles with fractures treated with immediate open reduction and internal fixation showed less impaired range of motion but a higher incidence of ankle swelling than did ankles with conservatively treated fractures. Patients treated with immediate open reduction and internal fixation needed significantly fewer days in the hospital than did those having had closed immobilization and delayed fixation.

Immediate open reduction and internal fixation of open ankle fractures enable earlier discharge from the hospital without increasing the risk of infection compared with closed reduction and delayed fixation.

▶ This retrospective review of 31 open fractures shows good results with immediate internal fixation. Early débridement, rigidity, and antibiotics remain a key to open fracture care. The authors demonstrate that, with good aggressive initial care, immediate open reduction can be performed without a higher complication rate than that with delayed fixation. Immediate open reduction shortened hospitalization time and hastened recovery. It should be emphasized that the key remains aggressive early débridement and proper wound management. The initial wounds were left open and were healed by secondary intention or were returned to the operating room for delayed closure or skin grafting.—K.A. Johnson, M.D.

Reconstruction for Lateral Ligament Injuries of the Ankle
Ahlgren O, Larsson S (Univ Hosp, Umeå, Sweden)
J Bone Joint Surg [Br] 71-B:300–303, March 1989   7–16

Chronic lateral instability of the ankle may lead to recurrent sprains and eventually to osteoarthritis. With the available procedures for restoration of efficient lateral stability, the ligaments usually heal, but with lengthening and consequent functional insufficiency. A new operation was designed for treatment of chronic lateral instability of the ankle.

Technique.—The operation involves the subperiosteal ligament release on the distal part of the lateral malleolus (Fig 7–9). The uncovered bone of the distal fibula is decorticated with an osteotome after which 4 channels for sutures are made into the bone, using a pricker and a hook (Fig 7–10). The released flap, including the insertions of both the anterior talofibular and calcaneofibular ligaments, is reattached to the malleolus, overlapping the proximal edge of the decorticated border by 3 mm to 5 mm (Fig 7–11). The skin is closed and the ankle immobilized in a below-knee plaster for 6 weeks. Full weight bearing is allowed after the first 2 weeks.

During a 7-year period, 50 males and 26 females aged 16 to 55 years in whom conservative treatment had failed to relieve symptoms or signs of chronic ankle instability underwent operation (83 ankles). The average time from primary injury to operation was 5.2 years. After a mean postoperative follow-up of 24 months, 82 ankles in 75 patients were available for reexamination. Full sagittal and inversion stability had been restored in 66 ankles. Inversion stability also had been fully restored in another 9 ankles, but slightly increased sagittal mobility remained. Only 1 ankle still had severe sagittal and inversion instability. However, this patient had had another severe ankle injury after operation. Of 51 patients,

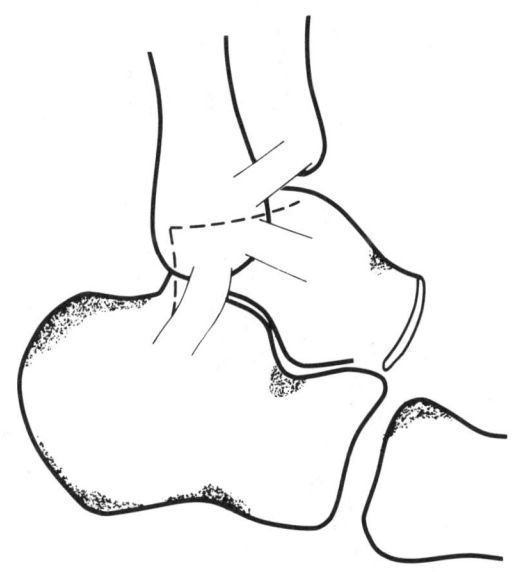

Fig 7–9.—Drawings (with Figs 7–10 and 7–11) of surgical technique. (Courtesy of Ahlgren O, Larsson S: *J Bone Joint Surg [Br]* 71-B:300–303, March 1989.)

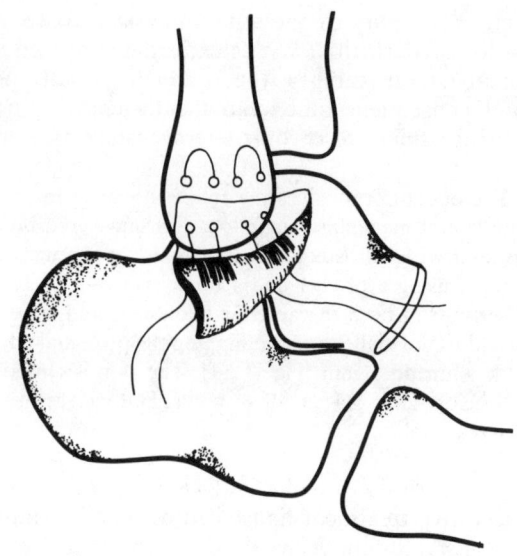

Fig 7–10.—(Courtesy of Ahlgren O, Larsson S: *J Bone Joint Surg [Br]* 71-B:300–303, March 1989.)

44 whose sporting activities had been restricted before operation reported no restriction at follow-up.

This simple reconstructive operation appears effectively to restore stability to ankles with chronic lateral instability.

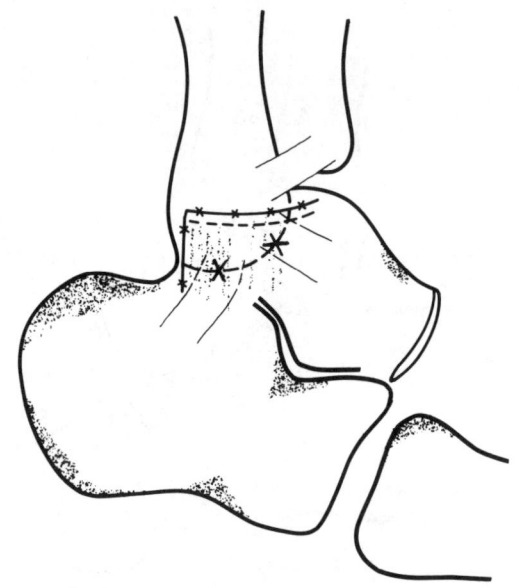

Fig 7–11.—(Courtesy of Ahlgren O, Larsson S: *J Bone Joint Surg [Br]* 71-B:300–303, March 1989.)

▶ Chronic lateral instability of the ankle can be quite debilitating, and several surgical methods exist in an attempt to treat this problem. These methods include tenodesis using the peroneus brevis tendons (Watson-Jones, Evans, Chrisman-Snook procedures), methods using a fascia lata graft such as the Elmslie procedure, and the Brostrom end-to-end repair of the ruptured ligaments. These authors describe a simple procedure that involves the subperiosteal release of the distal part of the lateral malleolus with advancement of this flap proximally. This simple procedure provides proprioception and additional support to the lateral aspect of the ankle.— K.A. Johnson, M.D.

Long-Term Follow-Up of Achilles Tendon Repair With an Absorbable Polymer Carbon Fiber Composite
Parsons JR, Weiss AB, Schenk RS, Alexander H, Pavlisko F (Univ of Medicine and Dentistry of New Jersey, Newark; Hosp for Joint Diseases, New York)
Foot Ankle 9:179–184, February 1989   7–17

There is still much controversy over the pathogenesis and treatment of the ruptured Achilles tendon. In 1981, a cooperative multicenter study was initiated to investigate the use of an absorbable polymer-carbon fiber composite ligament in the repair of the ruptured Achilles tendon. The implant acts as a scaffold for the regrowth of collagenous tissue.

During the 4-year study, 48 patients from 14 medical centers underwent 52 surgical repairs of a closed Achilles tendon rupture in which the composite implant was used; 1 patient had a bilateral rupture, and 3 patients needed reoperation. Most patients had complete Achilles tendon ruptures; all had severe functional deficits. A total of 27 patients were treated more than 4 weeks after injury; the average postinjury time to operation was 20.4 months. Postoperative follow-up evaluation was done at 3-month intervals during the first year and at 6-month intervals thereafter; 29 patients had at least a 1-year follow-up, 22 had at least an 18-month follow-up, 20 patients had at least a 2-year follow-up, and 5 patients had 4-year evaluations.

During the first postoperative year, all patients showed continuous functional improvement and lessening of pain. After 1 year of postoperative follow-up, patients with acutely repaired injuries showed a more dramatic improvement and tended to fare slightly better than those in whom repair had been delayed. Improvement leveled off throughout the second postoperative year. After an overall average of 2.1 years of postoperative follow-up, the outcome in 44 (86.2%) patients was rated excellent or good, even though many of these patients had had previous operations with severe debilitating injuries. Only 4 patients (13.8%) had fair results. At the 4-year follow-up, all 5 evaluated patients had excellent results.

The carbon-absorbable polymer implant appears to be useful in the treatment of the ruptured Achilles tendon as it restores immediate continuity in both the acute and chronic situation.

▶ Many controversies remain in the treatment of Achilles tendon rupture. These authors, in a cooperative multicenter study, demonstrate good results with no increased morbidity using a polymer-carbon fiber composite. This implant may be most useful where large gaps exist or when there is considerable fraying of the tendon ends. Further studies and longer follow-up will help determine the usefulness of this polymer-carbon fiber composite in the treatment of Achilles ruptures when compared with more conventional techniques utilizing autogenous grafts.— K.A. Johnson, M.D.

Sliding Fibular Graft Repair for Chronic Dislocation of the Peroneal Tendons
Micheli LJ, Waters PM, Sanders DP (Children's Hosp Med Ctr, Boston)
Am J Sports Med 17:68–71, January–February 1989

Chronic recurrent subluxation of teh peroneal tendons can disable young athletes. Conservative management is usually ineffective. Surgical reconstruction, including periosteal reattachment, groove deepening, tenoplasty procedures, and bone block procedures, has yielded some good results. A new procedure involves a sliding fibular bone graft that provides rigid stability against recurrent dislocation, yet preserves and deepens the fibro-osseous canal for tendon gliding.

Procedure.—A curvilinear skin incision is made along the lateral ankle just posterior to the standard lateral approach to the lateral malleolus, and the lateral

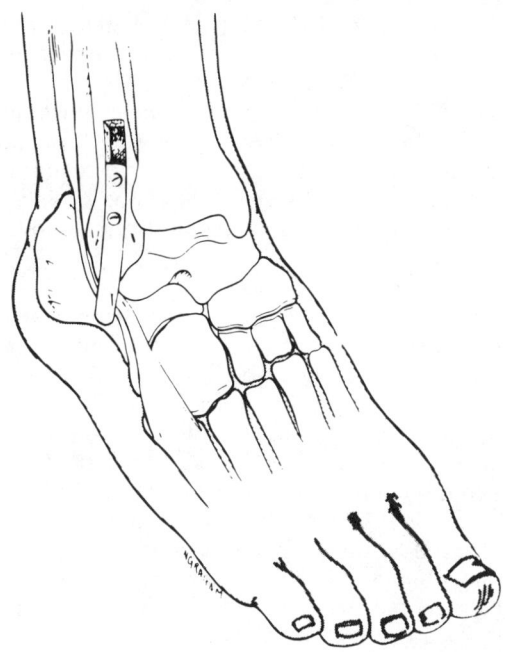

Fig 7–12.—The graft is fixed in its distal position with 3.5-mm cortical AO screws. (Courtesy of Micheli LJ, Waters PM, Sanders DP: *Am J Sports Med* 17:68–71, January–February 1989.)

malleolus is exposed. The distal 7-8 cm of the lateral malleolus is exposed completely by extra periosteal dissection. The osteotomy cuts are marked with margins extending anteroposteriorly from the lateral ridge of the malleolus for 9-10 mm and proximally 6-7 cm from the distal tip of the lateral malleolus. A mini-sagittal saw is used for the proximal, anterior, and posterior cuts. The distal periosteum and soft tissues are left intact. The cortical graft is raised with the distal soft tissue hinge intact. The graft bed is deepened with curettes, and cancellous bone is removed. The cortical graft is slid distally 1-1.5 cm. The graft is first temporarily fixed with a Kirschner wire, then is permanently fixed with two 3.5-mm AO screws (Fig 7-12).

The results of this procedure were excellent in 11 of 12 cases. One patient with bilateral repairs had recurrences of symptoms on 1 side and needed reexploration.

The sliding fibular graft combines the advantages of bone block and groove deepening procedures by recreating a physiologically deeper groove supported by cortical fibular graft and preserving the fibro-osseous groove for tendon gliding. The use of this procedure for patients with this chronic recurrent subluxation of the peroneal tendons can provide consistently excellent results.

▶ Many surgical techniques exist for treatment of subluxing peroneal tendons. These authors present a simple technique with results similar to those of other techniques of repair.— K.A. Johnson, M.D.

Early Postoperative Weight-Bearing and Muscle Activity in Patients Who Have a Fracture of the Ankle
Finsen V, Saetermo R, Kibsgaard L, Farran K, Engebretsen L, Bolz KD, Benum P (Trondheim Univ Hosp, Trondheim, Norway)
J Bone Joint Surg [Am] 71-A:23-27, January 1989   7-19

Postoperative management after internal fixation of a fracture of the ankle still is controversial. In a prospective study, 56 patients with displaced fracture of the ankle necessitating surgical fixation were randomly assigned to 1 of 3 postoperative treatment regimens: no plaster cast or weight bearing, and active exercises of the ankle (no.=18); a non-weight-bearing plaster cast (no.=19); or a plaster walking cast for the first 6 postoperative weeks (no.=19). Duration of follow-up was approximately 2 years.

Any difference in the clinical results between the 3 groups was not consistent, that is, the time lost from work and the proportion of excellent and good clinical results were not influenced by regimen. Radiographs showed no significant differences among groups in the proportion of patients with widening of the ankle mortise. There were no adverse effects from weight bearing with the syndesmosis screw in place.

None of the 3 postoperative regimens proved to be more advantageous than the others in a patient who has a stable osteosynthesis of a fracture of the ankle.

▶ The amount of time that patients remain non-weight-bearing after ankle fractures and after any type of foot and ankle surgery remains largely dependent on the opinion of the surgeon with little supporting objective. This article shows there was no contraindication to early postoperative weight bearing in patients after open-reduction, internal fixation of an ankle fracture and no adverse effects with these patients ambulating before the syndesmosis screw was removed. In addition, they showed no real advantage to early postoperative weight bearing in their group of patients. The postoperative regimen after surgical repair of an ankle fracture remains a clinical decision based on the stability of the fixation, the reliability of the patient, and the experience of the surgeon.—K.A. Johnson, M.D.

Pediatric

Posterior Tibial Tendon Transfer in Spastic Equinovarus
Lagast J, Mylle J, Fabry G (Univ Hosp, Leuven, Belgium)
Arch Orthop Trauma Surg 108:100–103, February 1989   7–20

Most equinovarus deformities of the foot require surgery for correction. To improve the patient's gait and eliminate the need for bracing, a number of different procedures have been advocated. Twenty-eight children (31 feet) had posterior tibial tendon transfers through the interosseous membrane. This operative technique is indicated when no fixed varus deformity is present. Associated lengthening of the Achilles tendon is performed in the event of fixed equinus deformity. After surgery, a cast is applied for 6 weeks and a short walking cast is used for another 3-week period. Most patients require a short leg brace for an average of 9 months.

Twenty-five patients (28 feet) were evaluated at follow-up times ranging from approximately 3 to 8 years. Outcome was subjectively rated very good by 84% of the children or their parents. Correction to neutral position was achieved in 68% of the cases. Five feet (18%) had an overcorrection to valgus, and 4 (14%) showed residual varus deformity. Results were judged poor in 3 cases: 2 children had persistent equinovarus and 1 needed reoperation for excessive valgus deformity.

This operation ideally is performed when a patient is aged between 5 and 10 years. Overcorrection can occur in younger children, and undercorrection is directly correlated with greater age. For this type of transfer to be successful, the tendon must be reinserted near the midline of the foot. The activity of the tibial tendon should be studied during preoperative evaluation; often, in cerebral palsy, there is an increased tension of the posterior tibial muscle.

▶ Deformity of the foot is common in patients with cerebral palsy, and several surgical procedures have been described to correct it. Procedures include anterior transfer of the posterior tibial tendon through the interosseous membrane, posterior tendon tenotomy, transfer of the posterior tibial tendon anterior to the medial malleolus, intermuscular lengthening of the posterior tibial tendon, transfer of the anterior tibial tendon, and split posterior tibial tendon transfer. These authors transferred the posterior tibial tendon through the interosseous membrane, and obtained improvement in gait of all patients, with 82% of them becoming brace free. Dynamic electromyographic studies are useful for this problem in that transfer is most effective when the tendon is active only during the swing phase. In this situation, it acts as a dorsiflexor during swing against the spastic calf muscles. If the tendon is active during both stance and swing phase, a tendon lengthening or split posterior tibial tendon transfer may be preferable (1,2).—K.A. Johnson, M.D.

References

1. Perry J, Hoffer M: *J Bone Joint Surg [Am]* 59-A:531, 1977.
2. Kling T, et al: *J Bone Joint Surg [Am]* 67-A:186, 1985.

Equinovarus Deformity in Arthrogryposis and Myelomeningocele: Evaluation of Primary Talectomy

Segal LS, Mann DC, Feiwell E, Hoffer MM (Southern Illinois Univ, Springfield; Rancho Los Amigos Med Ctr, Downey, Calif)
Foot Ankle 10:12–16, August 1989   7–21

The rigid equinovarus deformities observed in children with arthrogryposis or myelomeningocele are thought to be similar. Both deformities, extremely difficult to treat because of their teratologic nature, are characterized by marked fibrosis and stiffness of the soft tissues and structural tarsal bone deformities that have diminished bone remodeling potential. Nonoperative and soft tissue procedures generally have yielded unsatisfactory results and high recurrence rates. Experience with primary talectomy in children with arthrogryposis and in children with myelomeningocele was evaluated.

Between 1970 and 1987, 16 children with arthrogryposis and 16 children with myelomeningocele underwent operations for equinovarus deformities. Seven children with arthrogryposis involving 14 feet and 2 children with myelomeningocele involving 4 feet underwent primary talectomies, whereas 9 children with arthrogryposis involving 16 feet and 14 children with myelomeningocele involving 22 feet had primary posteromedial releases (PMR). Follow-ups ranged from 13 to 174 months.

Results of primary talectomy in 7 children with arthrogryposis were good in 50% of the 14 operated feet, fair in 43%, and poor in 7%. Results in 9 children with arthrogryposis who had primary PMR were good in 31% of the operated 16 feet, fair in 6%, and poor in 63%. Primary talectomy was clearly more effective than PMR in the treatment of children with arthrogryposis. Four children with arthrogryposis affecting 7 feet needed salvage talectomy after failed index procedures. The results were good in 43% of the 7 operated feet, fair in 29%, and poor in 29%.

Results of primary talectomy in 2 children with myelomeningocele were good in 50% of the 4 treated feet and poor in 50%. Results of PMR in 14 children with myelomeningocele were good in 50% of the 22 treated feet, fair in 23%, and poor in 27%. Salvage talectomies performed in 4 feet of 2 myelodysplastic children had good outcomes in 50% and fair outcomes in 50%.

Primary talectomy clearly was superior to PMR in the treatment of equinovarus deformities in children with arthrogryposis. The role of primary talectomy in myelomeningocele remains controversial. Because of the small number of primary talectomies done in children with myelomeningocele, the role of primary talectomy for this indication cannot be supported or refuted.

▶ This article shows that primary talectomies are effective in the management of severe equinovarus deformities in patients with arthrogryposis and myelomeningocele. Talectomy seems to be an extreme procedure, but arthrogryposis is an unusual disease with severe foot deformities. Posteromedial releases alone were shown to be inadequate in arthrogryposis patients.—K.A. Johnson, M.D.

Long-Term Results of Triple Arthrodesis in Charcot-Marie-Tooth Disease
Wetmore RS, Drennan JC (Newington Children's Hosp, Newington, Conn)
J Bone Joint Surg [Am] 71-A:417–422, March 1989   7–22

The management of foot deformities in patients with Charcot-Marie-Tooth disease is problematic. If the deformity is left untreated, many patients eventually will lose their ability to walk. Triple arthrodesis, which is used to realign and stabilize the hind foot, should be beneficial, but few studies have analyzed the long-term outcome in these patients.

Sixteen patients with Charcot-Marie-Tooth disease had had a total of 30 triple arthrodeses. The patients, whose average age at surgery was 15 years, were followed up for an average of 21 years.

Two patients had excellent results, 5 had good results, 9 had fair results, and 14 had poor results. Four feet with poor results had advanced arthritis and required arthrodesis of the ankle. Five feet had painful residual or recurrent cavovarus deformity, 2 had persistent flail drop-foot deformity necessitating ankle arthrodeses for stability, and 1 patient had an overcorrected valgus deformity of the hind foot with painful degenerative arthritis of the ankle and pseudarthrosis of the talonavicular joint. All 8 patients who did not have arthrodesis required orthoses. In 7 feet that initially had satisfactory alignment, cavovarus deformity recurred as a result of progressive muscle imbalance. Overall, 23 feet had degenerative changes of the ankle and joints of the midfoot.

The large number of poor long-term results among patients with Charcot-Marie-Tooth disease who had undergone triple arthrodesis for deformity of the foot differs from that of patients with poliomyelitis who retained normal sensation and had permanent, stable muscle imbalance. In view of these results, it is recommended that such patients undergo triple arthrodesis only as a salvage procedure. The surgery should be limited to patients who have severe, rigid deformity.

▶ These authors studied a group of patients who had a triple arthrodesis for hindfoot deformity associated with Charcot-Marie-Tooth disease. The long-term results are inferior to those of triple arthrodesis in patients with poliomyelitis. The authors recommend that triple arthrodesis be reserved for those patients who have a severe fixed osseous deformity. For less severe deformities they suggest plantar releases, calcaneal osteotomies, and claw-toe procedures. It is reiterated that Charcot-Marie-Tooth disease is a progressive peripheral neuropathy and that patients need to understand the progressive nature of the disease and the increased risk for deformity and osteoarthritis.—K.A. Johnson, M.D.

Miscellaneous

Operative Ankle Arthroscopy: Long-Term Followup
Martin DF, Baker CL, Curl WW, Andrews JR, Robie DB, Haas AF (Hughston Orthopaedic Clinic, Columbus, Ga)
Am J Sports Med 17:16-23, January-February 1989

Ankle arthroscopy has become commonplace in the treatment of various intra-articular disorders. Data on patients with at least 1 year followup were evaluated to determine the role of arthroscopic surgery in the treatment of ankle disorders.

In 57 patients, 58 ankles met study criteria. In 45% of patients, preoperative diagnosis was synovitis; in 29%, transchondral defects of the talus; in 14%, degenerative joint disease; and in 12%, impinging osteophytes or loose bodies. All patients initially had had conservative treatment. Continued pain, swelling, catching, or radiographic abnormally were indications for surgery. At arthroscopy, preoperative diagnoses were confirmed in 90% of ankles. Charts, radiographs, surgical videotapes, and follow-up results were reviewed. Both subjective and functional ratings were considered at follow-up.

In 64% of all cases, subjective results were good to excellent. Patients with synovitis and those with transchondral defects had the best overall results: 77% and 71%, respectively. Patients with degenerative joint disease had generally poor outcomes, with only 12% having good or excellent results. In addition, 43% of these patients later needed fusion. Overall, the complication rate was 15%, with complications including infections, temporary and permanent paresthesias, and hemarthroses.

Ankle arthroscopic surgery is a useful procedure in selected patients. Good results can be expected in patients with synovitis and transchondral defects of the talus. Results are less predictable in those with loose bodies and osteophytes. Patients with degenerative joint disease are not good candidates for arthroscopy. Because the risk of complications is significant, anatomical knowledge and meticulous technique are mandatory.

▶ Ankle arthroscopy is increasingly popular and has been tried for many indications. These experienced, arthroscopically oriented authors provide information on the long-term follow-up of operative ankle arthroscopy. Their rate of complications is quite high. The authors show that ankle arthroscopy has a morbidity that may be even greater than that of open procedures. Operative ankle arthroscopy may be useful in limited indications. As yet, no one has proved it to be simpler or safer than open arthrotomy procedures.— K.A. Johnson, M.D.

Abnormal Foot Pressures Alone May Not Cause Ulceration
Masson EA, Hay EM, Stockley I, Veves A, Betts RP, Boulton AJM (Manchester Royal Infirmary, Manchester, England; Royal Hallamshire Hosp, Sheffield, England)
Diabetic Med 6:426–428, July 1989   7–24

Increased forefoot pressures have been related to plantar ulceration in diabetic patients, but they also are found in older persons and arthritis patients in the absence of ulceration. To examine further the relationship between high foot pressure, neurologic abnormalities, and ulceration, 37 patients with rheumatoid arthritis who had forefoot deformity and 38 diabetic patients with similar clinical abnormalities, including prominent metatarsal heads and clawing of the toes, were studied. Plantar foot pressures were recorded by optical pedobarography.

One third of the diabetic patients but none of the rheumatoid patients had a history of foot ulceration. Most of the rheumatoid patients had had metatarsal pain. Although several diabetic patients reported neuropathic foot pain, few had symptoms likely to arise from mechanical factors alone. Increased forefoot pressure with reduced toe loading was frequent in both groups of patients. Clinical neurologic deficits were more frequent in the diabetic group. Motor conduction velocity was reduced, and the vibration perception threshold was increased in these patients, but those measures were not related to peak forefoot pressures.

High forefoot pressures are common in patients with deformed feet, regardless of the cause. Diabetic, but not rheumatoid, patients have a loss of protective sensation and plantar ulceration. The findings affirm the critical role of sensory neuropathy in diabetic foot ulceration. An area of mechanical stress usually is present as well.

▶ The pathogenesis of diabetic foot ulcers is multifactorial. Rheumatoid foot patients, like diabetic patients, have increased pressures, but have good sensation and are able to protect their feet. The high pressure, together with the peripheral neuropathy, is responsible for diabetic foot ulcerations. It is unfortunate that no treatment exists for the troubling sensory loss. Efforts to relieve areas of increased pressure will not always be completely effective. Those who commonly treat diabetic foot ulcers have an understanding of this; the article helps substantiate the multifactorial nature of these ulcers.— K.A. Johnson, M.D.

Soft-Tissue Tumors and Tumor-Like Lesions of the Foot: An Analysis of Eighty-Three Cases
Kirby EJ, Shereff MJ, Lewis MM (Hosp for Joint Diseases Orthopaedic Inst; Mount Sinai Med Ctr, New York)
J Bone Joint Surg [Am] 71-A:621–626, April 1989   7–25

The records of 83 patients with soft tissue tumors or tumorlike lesions in their feet were analyzed retrospectively to determine the relative frequency and to identify distinguishing clinical characteristics of these lesions.

Seventy-two (87%) of the lesions were benign, and 11 (13%) were malignant. Ganglion cysts and plantar fibromatoses were the most commonly benign lesions, whereas synovial sarcoma (45%) was the most frequent malignancy. Malignant tumors occurred between the ages of 10 and 40 years, or after the age of 60 years; benign lesions tended to occur in the middle decades. Most of the malignant tumors, especially the synovial sarcomas, tended to aggregate about the ankle (zone 1), heel (zone 2), or dorsum of the foot (zone 3), whereas the sole of the foot (zone 4) rarely was involved. Radiographs were helpful in identifying the nature of lesions in 12% of patients. The sex of the patient, history of trauma, the duration of symptoms, the presence of pain or of neurologic symptoms, and the size of the lesion were not useful in discriminating between malignant and benign lesions.

The relatively increased incidence of synovial sarcoma in this study was verified with Bayes-rule analysis. Synovial sarcoma accounted for 56% of the sarcomas in the foot, a figure comparable to the incidence of 45% found in this study. It appears that synovial sarcoma is the most frequently encountered malignant soft tissue tumor of the foot and ankle.

▶ The authors found an 87% incidence of benign and a 13% incidence of malignant soft tissue tumors of the foot at the Hospital for Joint Diseases. They provide a complete differential diagnosis of the various soft tissue tumors for the orthopedic surgeon treating the foot and ankle.— K.A. Johnson, M.D.

8 Musculoskeletal Neoplasia

Introduction

Metastatic carcinoma to bone continues to represent the most common neoplasia that we as orthopedists have to manage in our practices. With the passing of each year, the management of these patients, both their oncologic management and their orthopedic management, has improved. The fixation equipment at our disposal and our better understanding of the intraoperative and postoperative management of these patients has made surgical management of their fractures significantly better than it was a decade ago.

Despite these advances, some areas of management still are not clear. Orthopedists continue to be faced with patients with metastatic carcinoma from an unknown primary. Nottebaert and associates suggest most of these patients have lung cancer and a poor prognosis. We still do not know when it is best to fix an "impending" fracture of a long bone with internal prophylaxis but Hipp and associates are continuing to study the effects of defects in bone and are helping us make these decisions. Irradiation is the most effective method of treating metastatic deposits, and Poulsen and associates, Latini and associates, and Reinbold and associates have added to our understanding of the role of irradiation in the management of bone metastasis.

Orthopedic oncologists are continuing to search for more accurate predictors of an osteosarcoma's behavior. Treatment has improved during the past decade, but we need better methods to distinguish between patients with osteosarcoma so that their adjuvant treatment can be tailored. We have yet to find biologic markers and still must rely on the traditional indicators: age of patient, size and location of the tumor, level of the serum alkaline phosphatase, histologic grade and subtype of the tumor, and the response of the tumor to preoperative chemotherapy. Taylor and associates, Alvegård and associates, and Bauer and associates have added to our understanding of the risk factors.

Magnetic resonance imaging has increased in its importance to us as a diagnostic tool. Graif and associates and Yuh and associates have added to our understanding of the use of magnetic resonance imaging in the musculoskeletal system. Dollahite and associates have evaluated aspiration biopsy, and Klaase and associates review their treatment of soft tissue tumors by infusional chemotherapy.

The other articles reviewed in this chapter help us better understand a variety of musculoskeletal tumors. Primary bone and soft tissue tumors are uncommon, and our experience with their presentation, natural course, and response to treatment is increased each year. We learn about them from those authors who study these tumors and share their experience with us.

Dempsey S. Springfield, M.D.

Metastatic Carcinoma

Vertebral Compression Fractures: Distinction Between Benign and Malignant Causes With MR Imaging
Yuh WTC, Zachar CK, Barloon TJ, Sato Y, Sickle WJ, Hawes DR (Univ of Iowa Hosps and Clinics, Iowa City)
Radiology 172:215–218, July 1989   8–1

Vertebral compression fractures may result from metastatic disease, trauma, or osteoporosis. In many cases the cause cannot be detected from plain radiographs. Magnetic resonance imaging was performed on 64 patients with 109 vertebral fractures whose cause could not be determined from plain radiographs. The mean age of the 64 patients was 60 years. Both T_1- and T_2-weighted images were obtained. Sagittal T_1-weighted images were classified according to the amount of normal bone marrow signal.

Twenty-five fracture in 21 patients were caused by malignant processes, and 84 fractures in 43 patients were caused by benign processes. Twenty-three benign fractures were known to have resulted from trauma, and 61 fractures were presumed to have been caused by osteoporosis. In 88% of malignant fractures no normal bone marrow was seen in the compressed vertebra. None of the malignant fractures showed increased signal intensity on T_1-weighted images, although this finding occurred in 10% of traumatic benign fractures and in 17% of nontraumatic benign fractures.

Traumatic fractures frequently involved vertebral body fragmentation and disk rupture, but neither was found with malignant fractures. Be-

Secondary Findings

Findings	Type of Fracture		
	Malignant	Nontraumatic	Traumatic
Increased signal intensity on T1-weighted images	0/25	6/61	4/23
Other metastases	22/25	1/61	0/23
Pedicle involvement*	22/25	0/52	5/22
Paraspinal mass*	15/25	0/52	7/22
Fragmentation*	0/25	5/52	14/22
Disk involvement	0/25	1/61	9/23
Other benign fractures	1/25	53/61†	4/23

Note: Numbers indicate number of fractures.
*Axial images were available for only 52 of 61 nontraumatic fractures and 22 of 23 traumatic fractures.
†Twelve of 21 patients.
(Courtesy of Yuh WTC, Zachar CK, Barloon TJ, et al: *Radiology* 172:215–218, July 1989.)

cause a paraspinal mass occurred in both cases (table), this finding does not appear to help in distinguishing benign from malignant fractures.

Magnetic resonance imaging is useful in evaluating vertebral compression fractures. The preservation and configuration of normal-signal-intensity bone marrow is most helpful in determining the cause of fracture. Secondary findings are useful in confirming diagnoses.

▶ We continue to look for a means, short of biopsy, of distinguishing between compression fracture in the spine that is secondary to osteoporosis and one secondary to a malignancy. The magnetic resonance images help and add to our evaluation, but are not always accurate. Combined with other clinical evidence, it is possible in almost all cases to be reasonably certain of the cause of a compression fracture. Patients with histories of malignancy who have compression fractures should be assumed to have metastatic disease until it is proven otherwise, no matter what their other clinical conditions. All patients with compression fractures should have hematocrit, serum calcium, serum phosphate, acid phosphate, alkaline phosphate, immunoelectrophoresis (IEP), erythrocyte sedimentation rate (ESR), blood urea nitrogen (BUN), and creatinine determined as part of their initial screening. A careful physical examination should be done with special attention paid to thyroid glands, lungs, breast, kidneys, and prostate. If these are normal and the patient has no neurologic abnormality, I suggest observation with a presumptive diagnosis of an osteoporotic compression fracture. If a patient's pain is decreased within 1 to 2 weeks, the vertebral body does not collapse further, and other abnormalities are not seen on follow-up x-ray films, I am confident of my diagnosis. If the symptoms do not decrease, if neurologic abnormalities develop, or if further collapse is seen on follow-up x-ray examinations, magnetic resonance imaging (MRI) then can be done and a decision about the possibility of a biopsy entertained. Initial MRI is, in my opinion, not necessary. It does not distinguish accurately a fracture secondary to a malignant process from one secondary to a benign process.—D.S. Springfield, M.D.

Metastatic Bone Disease From Occult Carcinoma: A Profile
Nottebaert M, Exner GU, von Hochstetter AR, Schreiber A (Orthopädische Universitätsklinik Balgrist, Zurich; Universitätsspital, Zurich)
Int Orthop 13:119–123, 1989   8–2

Metastasis from an occult primary tumor occurs in from 3% to 4% of all cancer patients. To delineate skeletal metastases from occult carcinoma, records of 172 patients with skeletal metastases seen in a 20-year period were reviewed.

The primary tumor was not evident at diagnosis of metastasis in 51 patients. The primary carcinoma was finally diagnosed in 33 patients (65%), but in only 15 (29%) was the diagnosis made while the patient was alive. In these 15 it took 3.7 months for the primary cancer to be diagnosed. When the primary tumor was occult, survival was significantly shortened: 55% of patients died within 1 year and 78% died within 2 years.

Patients with skeletal metastasis from an occult source were male in 67% of cases, had spinal metastasis in 75% of cases, had femoral or pelvic metastasis in most other cases, and also had metastasis to other organs in 45% of cases. Back pain was the most common presenting symptom; in 37% the first sign was a pathologic fracture. In contrast to cases with known primary tumor, the site of the occult source was the lung in 52%.

The presence of skeletal metastasis from an occult primary tumor suggests the possibility of lung cancer. Current diagnostic methods often fail to detect the source. An occult primary tumor with skeletal metastasis carries a grave prognosis.

▶ Nottebaert and associates reconfirm that bone metastasis from an unknown primary carcinoma is a relatively common problem but that it is not usually necessary to find the primary unless it arises from the lung (where most metastases from occult carcinoma originate), the breast, the kidney, or the prostate. I recommend that these organ systems be evaluated with physical examination, routine laboratory tests (alkaline phosphatase, acid phosphatase, and urinalysis), mammography, abdominal ultrasound, chest x-ray films, and a chest CT scan if necessary. Any abnormality suggested by a review of systems also should be evaluated. If the primary is not found with these, searching further is not necessary. Chemotherapy for small cell lung cancer is showing promise; as additional carcinomas prove to respond to chemotherapy, finding the primary carcinoma will be increasingly important, but to date there is little reason to know the origin of a metastatic carcinoma. An orthopedist should discuss with the medical oncologist what value an organ-specific diagnosis would be for a patient.—D.S. Springfield, M.D.

Structural Consequences of Endosteal Metastatic Lesions in Long Bones
Hipp JA, McBroom RJ, Cheal EJ, Hayes WC (Charles A Dana Research Inst; Beth Israel Hosp, Boston; Harvard Med School; Toronto)
J Orthop Res 7:828–837, October 1989

Lytic metastatic lesions often develop on the endosteal surface of long bones without penetrating the cortical wall. Current clinical guidelines provide contradictory indications for prophylactic fixation of these defects and do not consider the structural consequences of the lesion. To assess experimentally and analytically the relationships between defect geometry and bone strength for simple endosteal defects and to improve guidelines for prophylactic stabilization of endosteal metastatic lesions in long bones, paired femurs from 52 dogs were studied.

Endosteal defects of various lengths and involving a variable amount of the cortical wall were created with an expanding reamer. Contralateral femurs served as controls. Radiographs and CT were used to determine the geometry of the experimental defects. Finite element models of the canine femurs were used to examine geometric and material parameters during 4-point bending and torsion.

The experimental data showed a significant linear relationship between bone strength and thickness of remaining cortical wall. The length of the defect had little effect on bone strength. Both the experimental and finite element data suggested that minimum wall thickness is the most important geometric parameter governing the structural consequences of an endosteal defect. In addition, a progressive reduction in bone strength was seen as the material properties of a bone along the wall of an endosteal defect were decreased. A need for obtaining accurate geometric data for an endosteal defect was demonstrated, because a critical defect can be missed if the radiographs are not properly oriented or CT scans do not include the thinnest part of the defect.

Minimal wall thickness is the most critical geometric parameter for predicting the structural consequences of endosteal defects. Information on bone porosity around metastatic lesions also should be considered when making estimates of bone strength.

▶ One of the most difficult decisions an orthopedist has to make when managing metastatic carcinoma is when to operate on a lesion in a bone that has not been fractured. The data suggest that those patients who are operated on before their fractures occur live longer and, in general, do better. These are all retrospective studies and may not reflect a real benefit in early stabilization of the fracture, but rather only an unrelated association. In addition, metastatic bone lesions must be irradiated, and if they can be treated with irradiation only, the quality of the patients, remaining lives will be better, but if the bones fracture and must have open reduction and internal fixation, they would have been better off with a prophylactic fixation.

Hipp and associates are trying to determine the effect a metastatic deposit has on the strength of a bone. As they develop their finite element model, they should be able to better predict which bones will fracture and which will not. So far, they have found that the thickness of the thinnest part of the cortex is the determining factor if the defect does not penetrate the entire cortex, and that the properties of the surrounding bone are critical to the strength of that bone when the defect is of full thickness. Prophylactic fixation is most important for a patient with a lesion in the lower extremity when the bone immediately adjacent to the defect is permeated by tumor. Lesions with sharp margins, especially when there is a rim of reactive bone, have little risk of fracture.—D.S. Springfield, M.D.

Palliative Irradiation of Bone Metastases
Poulsen HS, Nielsen OS, Klee M, Rørth M (Finsen Inst, Rigshospitalet, Copenhagen; Univ Hosp, Aarhus, Denmark)
Cancer Treat Rev 16:41–48, March 1989   8–4

Patients with advanced cancer often have painful bone metastases. The appearance of bone metastases generally indicates a poor prognosis, but many of such patients survive for several months or even years and therefore require palliative treatment. Radiation therapy is often used in the treatment of painful bone lesions, but a clear dose-response has not been demonstrated, and the optimal dose and fractionation have not been defined.

Why bone metasteses cause pain is poorly understood. Although it has been suggested that radiation therapy induces pain relief partly by an effect on normal bone cells and partly by killing cancer cells, the mechanism by which radiation therapy induces pain relief is virtually unknown. Even with a wide variety of doses and fractions, only 20% to 59% of the patients with bone pain experience complete relief after irradiation, and 27% of all treated patients have a recurrence of bone pain.

Reportedly, bone metastase originating from prostate and breast cancer respond better to radiation therapy than do metastases from other tumors, but statistically significant evidence has not been provided. Comparative studies that evaluated the feasibility of single treatment schedules at doses from 4 to 18 Gy found no difference in pain relief or relapse rates, either between different single doses or between single doses and fractionated doses. In 1 study in which treatment was delivered to pelvic fields and lumbar spines, single doses of more than 8 Gy caused a higher frequency of nausea and vomiting than did doses of 8 Gy or less. In another study a multifractionated regimen at a dose of 40 Gy was associated with a higher incidence of fractures than was a dose of 20 Gy. Single-fraction treatment at a dose of 5–8 Gy appears to be as effective as fractionated regimens for bone lesions, regardless of the site of the primary tumor or of the bone metastases.

Although wide-field irradiation with the half-body technique has shown some promise in selected patients with multiple bone metastases, it is not known whether this form of treatment is more effective than multiple single-field irradiation. A trial of single upper half-body irradiation showed that pneumonitis often developed in patients so treated, particularly when doses exceeding 6 Gy were applied. The literature has not yet provided answers concerning an optimal use of radiotherapy in the treatment of patients with advanced cancer who have painful bone metastases.

Role of Radiotherapy in Metastatic Spinal Cord Compression: Preliminary Results From a Prospective Trial
Latini P, Maranzano E, Ricci S, Aristei C, Checcaglini F, Panizza BM, Perrucci E (Policlinico, Perugia, Italy)
Radiother Oncol 15:227–233, July 1989   8–5

Metastatic spinal cord compression (MSCC) usually has a negative prognosis, with survival times varying from 2 to 6 months. Therefore, palliative therapy for patients with MSCC should improve the quality of life in a relatively short time without prolonged hospitalization. Recent retrospective studies demonstrated that radiation therapy (RT) alone is as effective as a combination of RT and surgical decompression. In a prospective nonrandomized trial, the effects of surgical decompression combined with postoperative RT were compared with those of RT only in patients with MSCC, with RT alone the preferred treatment.

Fifty-one patients with MSCC were enrolled in the study, but 3 died early. Patients believed to have MSCC were immediately given medium to high doses of parenteral steroids and underwent immediate myelography, with or without CT, to determine craniocaudal extension of the disease. Upon confirmation of MSCC, RT was started within 24 hours. Decompressive laminectomy was done only when stabilization of the spinal cord was essential. Evaluation of response to treatment included assessment of back pain, autonomic function, and motor performance. Pain relief was evaluated by comparing narcotic and minor analgesic use before and after treatment. The median follow-up was 11 months.

Six patients underwent decompressive laminectomy with RT; they were not included in the analysis. Of the 42 patients who had RT only, 54% had complete pain relief, 36% had partial pain relief, and 10% failed to respond. Before RT, 19 patients were ambulatory and 33 had motor dysfunction. After RT, 16 of 33 patients with motor dysfunction had improvement and 17 did not. Six of 17 nonresponders who were able to walk with support before RT did not have deterioration after RT. The walking ability of the other 11 patients worsened after RT. Four nonresponders also had increases in back pain. Four of the 11 nonresponders whose condition deteriorated were paraplegic, and 7 were paraparetic. Twelve of 19 patients who were unable to walk before RT were able to walk after RT, 8 with support and 4 without support. Walking ability did not deteriorate in any of the 23 patients who were ambulatory before RT. Three of 7 patients with autonomic dysfunction had improved. Administration of medium to high doses of steroid probably helped avoid acute radiation damage. Patients in whom MSCC was diagnosed early maintained good motor performance independent of the radiosensitivity of the type of tumor, confirming that the early diagnosis of MSCC remains the most important prognostic factor.

Osteodensitometry of Vertebral Metastases After Radiotherapy Using Quantitative Computed Tomography
Reinbold W-D, Wannenmacher M, Hodapp N, Adler C-P (Univ of Freiburg, West Germany)
Skeletal Radiol 18:517–521, 1989   8–6

The axial skeleton is a frequent site of metastatic tumor, and as much as 40% of all metastatic bone disease diagnosed during life occurs in the spine. Quantitative CT (QCT) was used to measure spinal metastases 3-dimensionally in 19 patients who had osteolytic vertebral metastases. None had received spinal irradiation, chemotherapy, or hormone therapy. Those with metastatic fracture were excluded. Photon radiotherapy totalled 40 Gy in 4 weeks.

Radiotherapy was successful in relieving pain in 13 of the 19 patients. Osteolytic metastases were decreased by 25% in bone density immediately after successful treatment, but were increased by more than 60% after 3 months. Normal bone surrounding the area of osteolysis showed increased density at both times. The relative change in bone density was significant only in successfully treated patients.

Quantitative CT is a reliable means of confirming therapeutic responsiveness in patients with vertebral metastases. A substantial reduction in bone density is associated with successful treatment and is followed by a significant increase in density 3 months later. In patients with osteolytic metastases, reduced nuclide uptake may reflect either regression or progressive disease.

▶ These authors have suggested that fewer patients with metastasis, even to the spine, need surgery than we as orthopedists predict. Although we do not understand how irradiation relieves pain, it does, and most patients have relief sufficient to make surgery unnecessary. Surgery for metastatic carcinoma to bone is to fix pathologic fractures or prophylactically stabilize an impending fracture. Patients who have spine metastasis present difficult problems; the best course is usually not clear. Latini and associates (Abstract 8-5) suggest that few need surgical decompression. It seems clear that those with pain only, who are neurologically normal, and who are walking need only irradiation and that those who come in with complete paralysis may not benefit from decompression, but it probably should be tried.

The difficult case is one in which neurologic findings are just beginning to appear or a neurologic examination is normal but walking is impossible because of "weakness in the legs." I recommend surgical decompression for such patients, especially if they have angular deformity of the spine. Systemic corticosteroids should be used.

Reinbold and associates (Abstract 8-6) have given us x-ray findings that we can use to determine whether irradiation is effective and the bone is healing. Although they noted early decrease in density in the vertebrae shortly after this, the vertebrae's density is increased if the treatment had been effective. When irradiation alone is used it is important to follow up the case until the symptoms are resolved and the bone has regained its density. If these 2 do not happen, operative intervention is advised. If a lesion causes pressure on the anterior portion of the cord, decompression should be anterior. Posterior stabilization is necessary only if the posterior elements are involved.— D.S. Springfield, M.D.

Assessment and Prognosis of Musculoskeletal Tumors

Aspiration Biopsy of Primary Neoplasms of Bone
Dollahite HA, Tatum L, Moinuddin SM, Carnesale PG (Baptist Mem Hosp, Memphis)
J Bone Joint Surg [Am] 71-A:1166–1169, September 1989   8–7

Needle-aspiration biopsy is a simple diagnostic method, but its accuracy in distinguishing malignant and benign bone lesions has been questioned. To assess the value of aspiration biopsy in cases of suspected primary neoplasm of bone, data on all patients who underwent needle-aspiration biopsy during a 10-year period were reviewed, with particular attention paid to patients with primary neoplasm of bone.

From a total of 835 aspiration biopsies performed during these years, 69 (in 57 patients) met criteria for the study. Clinical and roentgenographic evaluation done before the biopsies suggested that 31 lesions were malignant, 26 were benign, and 12 were giant-cell tumors. Tissue samples were obtained by a radiologist and evaluated by a cytopathologist.

Biopsy results included 39 (57%) positive, 23 (33%) negative, and 7 (10%) doubtful. Of the lesions suspected to be malignant, 23 (74%) were positive, 3 (10%) negative, and 3 (10%) were doubtful. Lesions thought to be benign appeared negative in 17 (65%) patients, positive in 6 (23%), and doubtful in 3 (12%). Material in the 17 negative biopsy specimens of suspected benign lesions was insufficient for diagnosis. Ten biopsy specimens (83%) of suspected giant cell tumors were positive; the 2 negative results (17%) were not diagnostic and required subsequent open biopsies.

One of the main problems with needle-aspiration biopsy is the small size of the sample obtained. Accuracy for malignant lesions was 92% for samples with adequate aspiration material, but only 72% for the whole series. Only 23% of suspected benign lesions were correctly identified; in these patients, multiple needle-aspiration samples or open biopsy may be required.

▶ Biopsy is an important part of the evaluation of a patient with a musculoskeletal lesion, but is not always easy and can lead to a wrong diagnosis or complications that make the ultimate management of the lesion more difficult. Open biopsy can be complicated and usually requires an operating room and anesthesia, but provides a pathologist with the best tissue from which to make an accurate diagnosis. Needle biopsy and fine-needle or aspiration biopsy are attractive alternatives to open biopsy because they are easy to do, can be done with a patient in a CT scanner, and do not require anesthesia or hospitalization. If a pathologist can be as accurate from the material provided by needle biopsy and aspiration biopsy as they are from material obtained at an open biopsy, those procedures should be used in place of an open biopsy; if not, their use must be questioned.

Dollahite and associates reviewed their experience with 69 percutaneous biopsies (done by radiologists) in 57 patients with what were clinically primary bone tumors. They conclude that benign lesions are most difficult to diagnosis from needle and aspiration biopsies, but that the overall accuracy of 83% for the malignant lesions, 92% accuracy for the giant-cell tumors, and ease of obtaining biopsy specimens justifies the use of these biopsy techniques.

I am less enthusiastic. Accuracy is dependent not only on the quality and representative nature of the material obtained, but on the experience of the cytologist and, maybe most important, his or her willingness to admit that the material is inadequate. Thirty (43%) of the biopsies in this study were nondiagnostic, and at least 1 major mistake was made when a chordoma was mistaken for a metastatic carcinoma. The authors state that needle biopsies are safer and that "the opportunities for limb salvage are improved," but this is not true if a radiologist puts the needle in the wrong place. Biopsy needle tracts can have local recurrences, and the needle tract (just like other biopsy tracts) should be excised if the lesion requires wide surgical resection. I prefer to use needle and aspiration biopsy to confirm my clinical diagnosis, especially when treatment does not include surgery or if surgery is necessary only after preoperative chemotherapy or irradiation. When a diagnosis is not obvious from the clinical presentation, plain x-ray appearance, or both, and when surgery is the treatment of choice, I use open biopsy.—D.S. Springfield, M.D.

Magnetic Resonance Imaging: Comparison of Four Pulse Sequences in Assessing Primary Bone Tumors
Graif M, Pennock JM, Pringle J, Sweetnam DR, Jelliffe AJ, Bydder GM, Young IR (Chaim Sheba Med Ctr, Tel Hashomer, Israel; Hammersmith Hosp, London; Inst of Orthopaedics, Stanmore; Middlesex Hosp, London; Picker Internatl, Wembley, England)
Skeletal Radiol 18:439–444, 1989

The T_1-weighted spin-echo pulse sequence generally is used to demonstrate tumor within bone, whereas T_2-weighted sequences show the extraosseous component. In 13 patients with primary bone tumors, a comparison was made of a T_1-weighted spin-echo sequence (SE, 544/44); a T_2-weighted spin-echo sequence (SE, 1500/80); a short TI inversion recovery (STIR); and a partial saturation sequence with field echo data collection. Nineteen magnetic resonance (MR) studies were carried out, 13 of them after chemotherapy.

Consensus values of data from the 4 different pulse sequences indicated that the partial saturation sequence most effectively distinguished the soft tissue component of tumor within bone from adjacent red bone marrow. The STIR sequence was best in the presence of yellow marrow. The T_1- and T_2-weighted spin-echo sequences were best for demonstrating bone cortex, periosteal change, and calcification. Plain radiographs were better than MR imaging for studying calcified tissues.

A combination of the partial saturation and STIR sequences will be most sensitive if plain films are available. If it is clear that the lesion will be in yellow marrow, the T_1-weighted spin-echo sequence could be combined with the STIR sequence.

▶ Magnetic resonance imaging (MRI) has introduced a complexity into the interpretation of images that is more than a magnitude greater than the CT scan is from plain x-ray studies. The average orthopedist is not able to keep up with all of the technical aspects of MRI, and we must rely on our radiology colleagues. Graif and associates have compared different "pulse sequences" in evaluation of tumors in bone and suggest that bone tumors be examined with "short TI inversion recovery sequence (STIR)" and with "partial saturation sequence" because of the better definition of the tumor's extent compared with the more usual "T_1" and "T_2" sequences.

I do not understand the mechanisms that explain the differences between these imaging sequences and will not understand them in the near future. Graif and associates have assumed, as well as I can understand, that the criterion for judging the best sequence was the accuracy of image in defining the intraosseous and extraosseous anatomical extent of the tumor. When this is the question to be answered by the examination, I would use the sequences they suggest; but when other questions need to be answered (i.e., diagnosis, effect of preoperative chemotherapy, evidence of local recurrence) other sequences may be better. I ask the radiologist to suggest the best sequence for the specific purpose for which I have requested the MRI.—D.S. Springfield, M.D.

Prognostic Variables in Osteosarcoma: A Multi-Institutional Study
Taylor WF, Ivins JC, Unni KK, Beabout JW, Golenzer HJ, Black LE (Mayo Clinic, Mayo Found, Rochester, Minn)
J Natl Cancer Inst 81:21–30, Jan 4, 1989   8–9

The variability and rarity of osteosarcoma have created problems in studying factors important in survival. The records of 444 patients with verified osteosarcoma admitted to 13 comprehensive cancer centers during a 6.5-year period were analyzed to develop a prognostic scoring sys-

Significant Primary Variables, Their β Weights and P Values

Variables	A. Osteosarcoma death during first 3 yr β	P value	B. Osteosarcoma progression during first 3 yr β	P value
Morphology A (juxtacortical)	—*	—	−1.95	.006
Morphology B (Paget's disease)	3.85	<.0001	1.16	.01
Morphology C (OB, CB, FB, TEL)†	1.15	.008	—	—
Regional spread	0.84	.003	0.62	.0002
High grade	0.60	.06‡	1.34	.0002
Grade not stated	—	—	0.95	.02
Symptoms (<12 mo from onset)	1.93	.0004	0.90	.002
Size (≥20 cm)	1.31	.003	0.86	.01
Site C (head, spine, sternum, rib, pelvis)	0.92	.005	—	—
Site D (humerus, clavicle, scapula, proximal femur)	0.63	.01	—	—
Weight (≥10 lb lost)	0.72	.01	0.72	.002
Swelling at primary site	0.44	.04‡	—	—
Lytic appearance	0.43	.04‡	0.42	.005
Bone expansion	—	—	−0.44	.03

Note: Data derived from step-down regression analyses when end point was death from osteosarcoma during first 3 years and progression of osteosarcoma during first 3 years.
*—, omitted from scores because not significant.
†OB, osteoblastic; CB, chondroblastic; FB, fibroblastic; TEL, telangiectatic.
‡Of borderline significance but retained because of general interest.
(Courtesy of Taylor WF, Ivins JC, Unni KK, et al: J Natl Cancer Inst 81:21–30, Jan 4, 1989.)

tem for this disease. Data follow-up was a maximum of nearly 9 years and a minimum of more than 3 years in more than 90% of cases.

Among the 38 patient and disease characteristics scored for each patient, the following were classified as significant indicators of survival: morphology; spread, grade, and size of tumor; site; weight loss; swelling at the primary site; and lytic appearance (table). Treatment (surgery only or surgery before or after chemotherapy or radiation therapy, or both) had no significant effect on prognosis independent of patient-disease characteristics. The same was true of amputation versus resection. Survival was not related to completeness of surgery, i.e., whether the osteosarcoma was within or extended beyond surgical margins, but completeness was related significantly to progression of disease.

The prognostic scoring system can be used to assess the value of different kinds of treatment, at least among patients treated in a similar period at the same hospital. The scores easily are derived from adequate records. Further testing of this system is encouraged.

Prognostication Including DNA Analysis in Osteosarcoma
Bauer HCF, Kreicbergs A, Silfverswärd C (Karolinska Inst and Hosp, Stockholm)
Acta Orthop Scand 60:353–360, June 1989   8–10

Recent improvements in survival rates for patients with osteosarcoma have been attributed to the use of adjuvant chemotherapy. However, comparisons of treatment have been difficult because of the heterogeneity of tumor features. In a retrospective study of 83 patients with osteosarcoma treated by surgery and adjuvant chemotherapy from 1971 to 1986, clinical course was related to various clinicopathologic features and tumor DNA content. Median age of the 51 male and 32 female patients was 17 years.

Forty-seven tumors required amputation or disarticulation. The median size of the tumors was 9 cm; the most common locations were the distal femur and proximal tibia. In 60 cases DNA analysis was feasible. Four of the tumors were found to be diploid, and 56 were hyperploid. Patients were followed up for a mean of 8 years.

Overall, the 7-year survival rate was 0.44. A poor prognosis was associated with male sex, proximal tumor location, and histologic grade IV. Age, tumor size, and histologic subtype were not predictive of outcome. The DNA variables and nuclear size, according to bivariate Cox regression analysis, offered no prognostic information; extremely high DNA values, however, were associated with a very low rate of survival.

Patients with none of the 3 significant risk factors had a 7-year survival rate of 0.80; the rate for those with 1, 2, or 3 risk factors was 0.59, 0.42, and 0.13, respectively. Ten patients with local recurrence within 1 year had a lower estimated 7-year survival rate (0.48) than the 35 who were disease free at 1 year (0.86). The latter finding emphasizes the importance of obtaining safe surgical margins. Local radiation and adjuvant chemotherapy cannot be relied on for tumor control when margins are inadequate.

Prognosis in High-Grade Soft Tissue Sarcomas: The Scandinavian Sarcoma Group Experience in a Randomized Adjuvant Chemotherapy Trial

Alvegård TA, Berg NO, Ranstam J, Rydholm A, Rööser B (Scandinavian Sarcoma Group; Lund Univ, Lund, Sweden)
Acta Orthop Scand 60:517–521, October 1989   8–11

Except for histologic malignancy grade and tumor size, there is little agreement on which tumor and host factors are predictive in soft tissue sarcoma. The relative prognostic importance of sex, age, tumor depth, localization, extent of tumor necrosis, and intratumoral vascular invasion were analyzed in 138 patients with grades III and IV soft tissue sarcomas of the extremities.

Forty-seven percent of patients had 0 or 1 risk factor and a 5-year metastasis-free survival rate of 73%; 36% of patients had 2 risk factors and a survival rate of 46%; 16% of patients had 3 or 4 factors and a metastasis-free survival rate of only 17% (Fig 8–1). A convariation was noted between increasing malignancy grade and size and between necrosis and increasing size. The importance of tumor size was confirmed, as was the negative influence of male sex and vascular invasion. Based on multivariate analysis, tumor necrosis was not a prognostic factor.

These findings indicate that several clinicopathologic factors should be

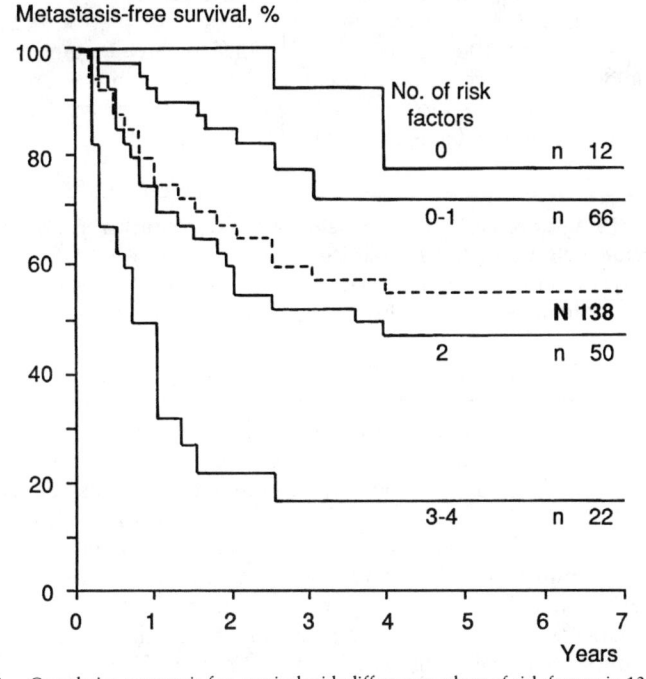

Fig 8–1.—Cumulative metastasis-free survival with different numbers of risk factors in 138 patients with malignancy grades III and IV soft tissue sarcoma, operated with a wide or compartmental margin. *Dashed line*, all 138 patients. (Courtesy of Alvegård TA, Berg NO, Ranstam J, et al: *Acta Orthop Scand* 60:517–521, October 1989.)

considered along with histologic malignancy grade to identify patients with soft tissue sarcoma who have poor prognoses. In this series, the local recurrence rate was low, and the prognostic importance of local recurrence was not analyzed. Further trials might include this factor.

▶ Doctors always have believed that part of their profession is to be able to predict the course of a disease. With increasingly complex methods of treatment, some of which have significant potential complications and side effects, the importance of predicting a patient's course and outcome has become more important and extremely valuable in planning therapy. As we understand sarcomas better, we hope to be able to find specific prognostic markers that will permit more accurate predictions than we have had in the past. These 3 papers are efforts to increase our knowledge for prognostication.

Unfortunately, the prognostic factors that have been identified are of limited value in accurately differentiating patients. Taylor and associates (Abstract 8-9) confirm prior data that histologic grade, size of the tumor, and more central location are prognostic variables for osteosarcoma, but so far, it has not been possible to tailor treatment based on these factors. Alvegård and associates (Abstract 8-11) question even the surgical margin as a prognostic indicator of survival. They reconfirmed that increasing size, histologic grade IV, male sex, and vascular invasion were associated with a work prognosis, but patients with 0-1 risk factor still had 27% incidence of metastases by 5 years. Bauer and associates (Abstract 8-10) did not find DNA ploidy to be predictive, but it is in other tumor systems. There should be a relationship between the DNA pattern and a tumor's metastatic potential; with further research a relationship probably will be found. We need to continue to search for biologic markers that indicate each tumor's metastatic potential.—D.S. Springfield, M.D.

Results of Regional Isolation Perfusion With Cytostatics in Patients With Soft Tissue Tumors of the Extremities
Klaase JM, Kroon BBR, Benckhuijsen C, van Geel AN, Albus-Lutter CE, Wieberdink J (Netherlands Cancer Inst, Amsterdam; Dr Daniël den Hoed Cancer Ctr, Rotterdam, The Netherlands)
Cancer 64:616-621, Aug 1, 1989   8-12

The results of regional isolation perfusion were reviewed for 26 patients with soft tissue tumors of the extremities who underwent 29 perfusions. All but 3 patients had been treated previously. Most patients were perfused because of local inoperable tumor. A cytostatic drug was administered intra-arterially for 1 hour, maintaining physiologic conditions in the isolated limb to the degree that was possible. Doxorubicin was used in 19 perfusions, melphalan in 2, and both agents in 8.

Four patients had a complete remission. Three others with local inoperable tumors had stable disease, but in 10 the disease progressed. Three patients with aggressive fibromatosis and 1 with lymphangiosarcoma had complete remissions. Severe toxicity made amputation necessary in 3 instances. Toxicity remained high even after the doxorubicin dosage was lowered.

Notable results have been achieved with regional isolation perfusion in patients with aggressive fibromatosis. A combination of doxorubicin and melphalan has been necessary to effect remissions. The overall results are not encouraging. At present, only patients with hematogenous metastases and local tumor growth that causes symptoms and is not operable are perfused. More effective and less toxic cytostatic agents are needed.

▶ Direct infusion of chemotherapeutic agents into the vascular supply of malignant tumors is an attractive method of increasing the effect of those agents on the tumor cells and has been tried in a number of tumor systems. It is unfortunate that the advantages of this method are limited and the complications are significant. The risks are greater with perfusion than with infusion methods. In this report, half of the patients had "toxic side effects," and 3 (more than 10%) needed amputations to manage a complication. Among the 17 patients in the inoperable group, 3 of the 4 with complete responses and 1 of the 3 with stable disease had aggressive fibromatosis, a benign tumor. Similar results can be obtained without chemotherapy, and I agree with the authors, who describe their results as "rather negative" and suggest that this method of treatment not be used. The use of systemic adjuvant chemotherapy for soft tissue sarcomas remains controversial.— D.S. Springfield, M.D.

Miscellaneous Bone Lesions

Unicameral Bone Cysts: Natural History and the Risk of Fracture
Kaelin AJ, MacEwen GD (Alfred I duPont Inst, Wilmington, Del)
Int Orthop 13:275–282, 1989
8–13

Unicameral cysts are the most common benign bone lesions in childhood. Standard treatment is curettage of the lining membrane and grafting with homogenous or autogenous bone, but this procedure has been associated with a high rate of recurrence. Treatment of unicameral bone cysts by injection with methylprednisolone acetate first was described in 1974. Because the cysts are benign, the only risk is that of pathologic fracture, but, to date, no reliable means for predicting the risk of this complication or for evaluating the indications for this treatment has been developed.

A new "cysts index" was developed that makes it possible to monitor the progress of a cyst to determine whether the risk of fracture warrants treatment. The cyst may heal spontaneously by bone formation in the cyst's cavity, with the cortex progressively thickening and filling in the cavity. Radiologic findings indicate that the larger the cyst, the more the cortex will be destroyed and the bone will be weakened. The cyst index is expressed as the proportion of the radiographic area of the cyst to the size of the involved bone, measured as the diameter of the diaphysis squared.

The cyst index was measured in 53 pathologic fractures noted on radiograph. The average index in humeral fractures was 6.12, and that in femoral fractures was 4.74. None of these fractures involved the physeal line. If activity was reduced after the first fracture, trauma was likely to

Cyst index	Indications for Treatment or Observation		
	Increasing		Decreasing
High fracture risk Humerus >4 Femur >3.5	Fracture prevention Injection:* If no response, consider operation in the femur		Fracture prevention Injection can accelerate healing
Low/no fracture risk Humerus <4 Femur <3.5	Observation Consider injection.*		No treatment

*Injection of methylprednisolone acetate.
(Courtesy of Kaelin AJ, MacEwen GD: *Int Orthop* 13:275–282, 1989.)

be less severe in subsequent fractures. The index did not show any tendency toward regression of the cyst after a fracture, but all cysts that began healing spontaneously ultimately healed completely. Treatment is successful when the cyst already is healing. A high recurrence rate is related to a rising cyst index, which leads to a higher risk of fracture (table).

Surgical treatment should be reserved for cysts that do not respond to injection and that have a high risk of pathologic fracture and subsequent deformity. Cysts in the femoral neck fall into this category.

Prostaglanding Levels in Unicameral Bone Cysts Treated by Intralesional Steroid Injection
Shindell R, Huurman WW, Lippiello L, Connolly JR (Creighton–Nebraska Health Found; Univ of Nebraska, Omaha)
J Pediatr Orthop 9:516–519, September–October 1989   8–14

The cause of the unicameral bone cyst remains unknown, but elevated levels of prostaglandin have been found in the cyst fluid. A prostaglandin-mediated cycle of osteoclast activities that is interrupted by steroid injection has been proposed. Cyst aspirations were carried out in 7 patients with diagnoses of unicameral bone cyst, and serial measurements of levels of prostaglandins were made in 5. Mean age of the 6 boys and 1 girl was 9 years.

Five of the cysts were in the proximal humerus. Six patients had pathologic fractures. Six lesions were classified radiographically as active. After cyst aspiration 180 to 200 mg of methylprednisolone succinate was instilled.

Levels of prostaglandin E_2 (PGE_2) were elevated in specimens from all the lesions classified radioraphically as active. The latent cyst had a level of 130 pg/mL and was resolved after a single injection. Follow-up levels of PGE_2 were 7% to 53% of initial levels in the 5 patients studied, 4 of whom had definite radiographic signs of resolution. The lesion with a questionable response still had a high level of PGE_2, and it resolved after a second injection of steroids.

If steroids exert an antiprostaglandin effect in this setting, decompression may not be the sole reason why the lesions resolve. Prostaglandins are known to stimulate osteoclast activity and may well have a role in maintaining bone cysts, regardless of the inciting event. The high level of PGE_2 found in active cysts support this hypothesis.

▶ I have not used Kaelin and MacEwen's "cyst index" (Abstract 8–13) but agree that unicameral bone cysts heal spontaneously and their treatment must be reviewed carefully to ensure that treatment is necessary. My indications for treatment are: (1) a lesion in a location that if fractured is likely to cause significant problems (i.e., femoral neck, intratrochanteric area); (2) a lesion that has fractured and the fracture has healed, but the cyst is not healing; and (3) a patient in the teenage years or older who hopes to participate in organized sports and whose lesion is not healing spontaneously. Although we do not understand how an intralesional injection of a corticosteroid stimulates healing of a unicameral cyst, it works and I use the injection of prednisolone as my primary treatment. This injection is done with a patient under anesthesia and contrast is used, but no effort is made to "burst" the cyst. Surgery is reserved for those lesions that do not heal after 3 separate injections, and that fulfills 1 of the 3 criteria above.

We still are trying to understand what causes unicameral bone cyst and to find the best methods for treatment. Prostaglandin E_2 has been found to produce hypercalcemia in some patients with solid tumors by stimulating osteoclast. It is not known whether this action of PGE_2 can produce bone destruction or whether it only increases the release of calcium. It would be interesting to know whether the calcium concentration in the cyst fluid is significantly greater than serum; it should if the increased PGE_2 is a cause of the cyst. If the suggestion by Shindell and associates (Abstract 8-14) that unicameral bone cysts have increased PGE_2 levels can be confirmed, their prediction of a more specific treatment of unicameral bone cyst can be realized.—D.S. Springfield, M.D.

Adamantinoma of Long Bones: A Clinicopathologic Study of 85 Cases
Keeney GL, Unni KK, Beabout JW, Pritchard DJ (Mayo Clinic, Mayo Found, Rochester, Minn)
Cancer 64:730-737, Aug 1, 1989   8-15

Adamantinoma of the long bones is a rare, low-grade primary tumor of uncertain histogenesis. Data on 45 males and 39 females aged 3–72 years with adamantinoma of the long bones were reviewed. One patient's sex had not been recorded. The average age at the time of diagnosis was 26 years (Fig 8–2). Presenting symptoms were nonspecific and included pain and swelling, swelling alone, pain alone, and pathologic fractures; 23 patients had symptoms for more than 5 years.

Seventy lesions were in the tibia, 11 of which also involved the fibula; 6 were in the femur, 3 in the ulna, 2 in the humerus, 2 in the fibula, 1 in the radius, and 1 in the soft tissue anterior to the tibia. About 90% of the tumors were diaphyseal. Most tumors involved both the cortical and medullary portions of the involved bone. Multiple areas of lucency were the most common radiologic finding. Small epithelial islands in a fibrous

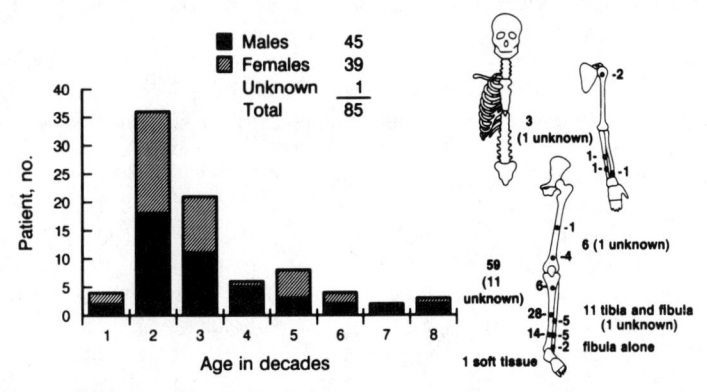

Fig 8–2.—Distribution of long-bone adamantinomas by age and sex of patient and site of lesion. The sex of a 50-year-old patient was unknown; thus the age of this patient is not included in the bar graph. (Courtesy of Keeney GL, Unni KK, Beabout JW, et al: *Cancer* 64:730–737, Aug 1, 1989.)

stroma were the most common histologic finding. Vascular-appearing channels lined by the same type of cells that made up the epithelial islands were observed in 1 tumor.

Twenty patients underwent amputation as the primary treatment, 19 underwent curettage with or without biopsy, and 39 had wide excision or marginal resection. Twenty-six patients had recurrent local disease within an average of 5 years after initial diagnosis, 13 had pulmonary metastasis within an average of 8 years after diagnosis, and 6 had lymph node metastasis within an average of 6 years after initial diagnosis; 1 patient had metastasis to the spine. Rates of recurrence and metastasis for patients treated initially with excision–resection or biopsy–curettage were significantly higher than those for patients treated initially with amputation. Of the 85 patients 41 were still alive without disease 1 month to 47 years after treatment.

Risk factors for recurrence or metastasis included male sex, pain, symptoms of less than 5 years' duration, and histologic lack of squamous differentiation. These data indicate that amputation or wide en bloc resection is associated with the lowest incidence of recurrence and metastasis and is therefore the treatment of choice for patients with diagnoses of adamantinoma of long bones.

▶ Adamantinoma is so unusual that no one surgeon or one institution has sufficient experience to make definitive statements, although these authors from the Mayo Clinic come close. In addition, the histologic criteria for the diagnosis are not accepted universally; cortical lesions in the anterior tibia that have been classified as ossifying fibroma or fibrous dysplasia for years often are changed to adamantinoma when another pathologist is consulted. The clinical presentation of adamantinoma and the osteofibrous dysplasias (ossifying fibroma and fibrous dysplasia of the tibia) are indistinguishable, and the clinical difficulty is in knowing which patient has the malignant tumor (adamantinoma) and which has the benign osteofibrous dysplasia. To compound the problem, adamantinoma and the osteofibrous dysplasias occur together in most cases; a single incisional biopsy negative for adamantinoma is no guarantee that other areas are not malignant. This can be a difficult clinical situation. I agree with the authors that wide surgical resection is the treatment of choice for adamantinoma; this usually can be achieved without an amputation unless a patient has had multiple local resections and recurrences.—D.S. Springfield, M.D.

Pseudomalignant Myositis Ossificans: Clinical, Radiologic, and Cytologic Diagnosis in 5 Cases
Rööser B, Herrlin K, Rydholm A, Åkerman M (Lund Univ, Lund, Sweden)
Acta Orthop Scand 60:457–460, August 1989   8–16

Although myositis ossificans is assumed to be related to injury, one third of the patients have no history of trauma. In these patients the condition is called pseudomalignant myositis ossificans, because the early radiographic appearance and rapid growth of the lesion may suggest a malignant tumor; later, the lesion develops a characteristic radiographic and histologic appearance. The most noticeable feature is the zone phenomenon: the periphery of the lesion contains cancellous bone with radially arranged bony spiculae, and the center contains cellular connective tissue with many proliferating fibroblasts. In 5 patients the lesions were initially thought to be malignant but were confirmed as benign subsequently on biopsy, radiographs, and clinical course.

The rapid growth of pseudomalignant myositis ossificans may indicate a malignant tumor. Radiographs during the early course may suggest an osteosarcoma or chondrosarcoma of soft tissue, and a biopsy specimen obtained from the central proliferating area may also be falsely diagnostic of malignancy at this time. Computed tomography can improve the chances of correct diagnosis of myositis ossificans. The peripheral calcific ring and central low-attenuation area are more clearly demonstrated on CT than on plain radiography.

In 4 of 5 patients reviewed, the mixture of proliferating fibroblasts, osteoblasts, and osteoclast-like multinucleated giant cells suggested either myositis ossificans or proliferative myositis. Symptoms resolved spontaneously, and no patient needed surgery.

Proper and timely diagnosis of pseudomalignant myositis ossificans is important to avoid unwarranted treatments for malignancy. The ability to recognize the characteristic radiographic appearance is important. Computed tomography may be helpful. The rapid disappearance of symptoms in all cases studied suggests that surgery is not indicated in pseudomalignant myositis ossificans.

▶ The myositis called "pseudomalignant" by these authors often is also called "circumscripta." It has the most organized zoning effect, with the periphery composed on mature bone and the center having undifferentiated cells that may be mistaken for malignant cells even by experienced pathologists. This is a lesion that must be biopsied so that the specimen includes both peripheral tissue and central tissue. A surgeon must not allow a pathologist to make a diagnosis until they review the x-ray films and CT scan. Surgery may be necessary if the mass does not resorb, but a limited excision can be done; in my experience, local recurrence, even when excision is done early, does not develop.—D.S. Springfield, M.D.

Chondromyxoid Fibroma of Bone: Thirty-Six Cases With Clinicopathologic Correlation
Zillmer DA, Dorfman HD (Montefiore Med Ctr–Albert Einstein College of Medicine)
Hum Pathol 20:952–964, October 1989   8–17

Chondromyxoid fibroma (CMF) is a relatively rare bone tumor of cartilaginous origins. Misdiagnosis remains a problem. A group of 36 patients with CMF were seen by 1 physician in the past 22 years.

In two thirds of cases the presumptive diagnosis was correct. The peak

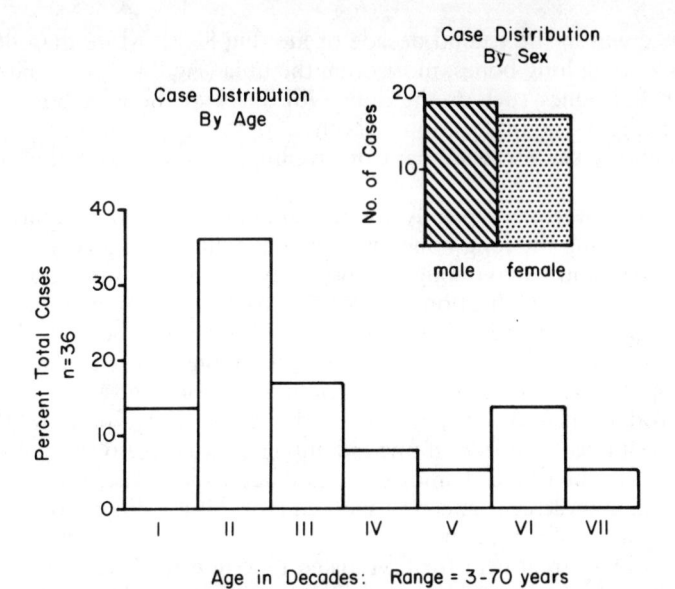

Fig 8–3.—Patient distribution by age and sex. (Courtesy of Zillmer DA, Dorfman HD: *Hum Pathol* 20:952–964, October 1989.)

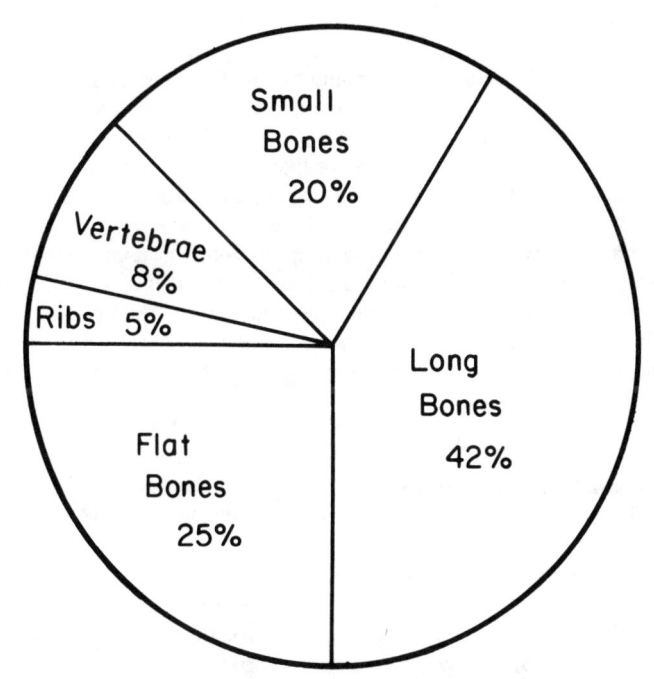

Fig 8–4.—Tumor localization. (Courtesy of Zillmer DA, Dorfman HD: *Hum Pathol* 20:952–964, October 1989.)

incidence was in the second decade of life (Fig 8–3). More than 40% of lesions were in long bones, most often the tibia (Fig 8–4), but one fourth were in flat bones such as the ilium. All but 1 of the long bone lesions were metaphyseal in location. About two thirds of the patients were symptomatic, usually with pain or swelling, or both, over the affected area.

Long bone fibroma typically are benign-appearing oval metaphyseal lesions paralleling the long bone axis. The medullary margins typically are well-defined, but surrounding sclerosis may be absent. Radiographic evidence of matrix calcification is rare. The cortex may or may not be expanded. In small hand and foot bones, CMFs tend to be central and to expand the bone. Flat bone lesions may be large and irregular, or they may appear loculated. Small, eccentric lesions also are seen. Rib lesions may produce fusiform expansion of the bone. The typical CMF is a pseudolobulated tumor with myxoid and chondroid regions separated by zones of fibrous tissue. Tumor cells may be pleomorphic, bizarre, or binucleated. Spindle cells and cells with chondroblastic differentiation stain postively for S-100 protein.

The primary treatment for CMF is en bloc resection. Seven of 8 recurrences were in patients younger than 20 years of age. Unusually aggressive CMFs have occurred; 1 patient died after incomplete excision of a sacral lesion that had produced extensive bone destruction and had spread to the dura.

▶ Chondromyxoid fibroma of bone is an unusual tumor; data about it in the literature are limited. Its occurrence in all decades of life was surprising and reminds us that this benign tumor must not be mistaken for a chondrosarcoma when it is present in a patient aged more than 50 years. I do not agree with the authors that "en bloc resection" is the best primary treatment. En bloc resection often results in significant loss of bone with adverse functional consequences for the patient. None of these underwent malignant transformation, and most were cured with a curettage. I suggest that if an en bloc resection can be done without a functional deficit, it should be the primary treatment, but if it would result in a functional deficit a curettage is better for the primary treatment and a more radical resection can be done for those that recur.—D.S. Springfield, M.D.

Desmoplastic Fibroma of Bone: Radiographic Analysis
Crim JR, Gold RH, Mirra JM, Eckardt JJ, Bassett LW (Univ of California, Los Angeles)
Radiology 172:827–832, September 1989   8–18

Desmoplastic fibroma of bone is a rare, locally aggressive tumor. Previously published and new radiographs of patients with this lesion were analyzed to define the radiographic characteristics that differentiate desmoplastic fibroma from other bone lesions. Findings were reviewed in 107 previous cases and 7 new ones.

Radiographic Features of 3 Cases of
Intraosseous Desmoplastic Fibroma

Features	No. of Cases
Bone destruction	
Geographic	80 (96)
Moth-eaten	3 (4)
Zone of transition	
Narrow	80 (96)
Poorly defined	3 (4)
Marginal sclerosis	
None	78 (94)
<25% of periphery	5 (6)
>25% of periphery	0
Pseudotrabeculation	76 (91)
Bone expansion	74 (89)
Cortical breakthrough	24 (29)
Periosteal new bone	2 (2)
Matrix mineralization	0

Note: Three cases of periosteal desmoplastic fibroma are not included. Numbers in parentheses are percentages.
(Courtesy of Crim JR, Gold RH, Mirra JM, et al: *Radiology* 172:827–832, September 1989.)

Desmoplastic fibroma occurred most often in the mandible, pelvis, and femur. In 96% of the patients with intraosseous desmoplastic fibromas for whom radiographs were available, there was a geographic pattern of bone destruction, with a narrow zone of transition and nonsclerotic margins (table). In 91% internal pseudotrabeculation was noted. Widening of the host bone from gradual apposition of periosteal new bone was common, occurring in 89%, but distinct periosteal new bone was observed in only 2% of the patients with desmoplastic fibromas of intraosseous origin. In 28% the cortex was breached. In 3 patients the lesion arose in the periosteum, which was differentiated radiographically from desmoid tumors of intraosseous or soft tissue origin.

Recognizing desmoplastic fibroma is important, because it is more aggressive than other benign fibrous lesions and requires surgery and long-term follow-up. The criteria defined should aid clinicians in the diagnosis of this rare neoplasm.

▶ This rare bone tumor usually is not included in a prebiopsy differential diagnosis. When encountered, it should be resected completely, if possible, without functional deficit; otherwise, it should be curetted thoroughly. Curettage is recommended, although the recurrence rate is significant, because most resections produce functional deficits. As with chondromyxoid fibroma of bone, local recurrence is not dangerous to the patient and the initial surgery can be less radical in an attempt to control the disease without causing significant functional deficit. More aggressive surgery is reserved for those tumors that recur.—D.S. Springfield, M.D.

Solitary Plasmacytoma of Bone: Mayo Clinic Experience
Frassica DA, Frassica FJ, Schray MF, Sim FH, Kyle RA (Mayo Clinic, Mayo Found, Rochester, Minn)
Int J Radiat Oncol Biol Phys 16:43–48, January 1989

Multiple myeloma, the most common type of myeloma, is a hematologic malignancy composed of plasma cells. Solitary plasmacytoma of bone is much less common, accounting for less than 10% of all plasma cell malignancies. Data on 46 patients treated for solitary plasmacytoma of bone in 1950–1982, were reviewed to clarify the clinical features and prognostic indicators of this malignancy.

The series included 30 males and 16 females aged 16–83 years (median, 56 years), all of whom had solitary plasmacytoma of bone. Presenting symptoms included pain in 80% of the patients, neurologic symptoms in 11%, and pathologic fractures in 9%; 25 patients had spinal involvement. All patients underwent staging studies, including serum and urine protein studies. Follow-up ranged from 30 to 285 months. Forty-three patients underwent radiation therapy; the other 3 patients had successful resection of the lesion.

Of the 46 patients, treatment failed in 31 as manifested by local recurrence, development of multiple myeloma, or new bone lesions without multiple myeloma. The 5 patients with local progression at 7–114 months had received less than 45 Gy of radiation to the primary lesion. The initial results of protein studies were normal in 21 patients and abnormal in 25. Of the latter, 20 had M-protein in serum only, 4 had M-proteins in serum and urine, and 1 had monoclonal light chains in urine only. The median time to progression was 18 months, but 23% of the failures occurred more than 60 months after treatment. Median survival was 96 months, the overall 5-year actuarial survival was 74%, and the overall 10-year actuarial survival, 45% (Fig 8–5). The 5-year disease-free survival was 43%, and the 10-year disease-free survival was 25%. No prognostic indicators could be identified, as neither survival nor dis-

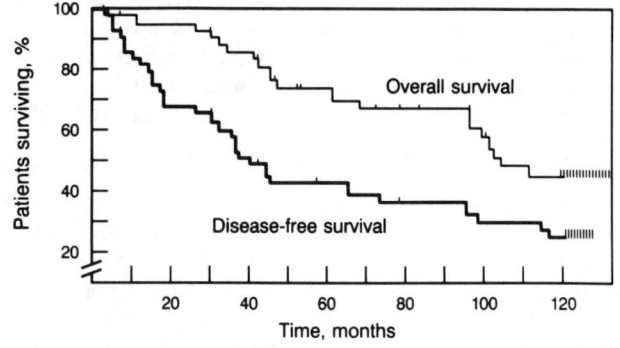

Fig 8–5.—Overall and disease-free survival (Kaplan-Meier method) in patients with solitary plasmacytoma of bone. (Courtesy of Frassica DA, Frassica FJ, Schray MF, et al: *Int J Radiat Oncol Biol Phys* 16:43–48, January 1989.)

ease-free survival appeared to be influenced by the presence of abnormal proteins.

Patients with an apparently solitary lesion at presentation have a much better overall survival than patients with classic multiple myeloma. Therefore, patients with disease progression should be treated aggressively as a substantial proportion of them still will be alive 5 years after treatment failure.

▶ Multiple myeloma is the single most common primary tumor of the bones in adults and always should be considered when an adult first is seen with a radiolucent lesion in a bone. Plasmacytoma is a single foci of multiple myeloma and is usually a prelude to the systemic disease, although there may be a decade between the original plasmacytoma and multiple myeloma. Like an eosinophlic granuloma, a plasmacytoma and the lesions of multiple myeloma may not have increased uptake on a technetium bone scan; when evaluating a patient with a plamacytoma it is important to search for other foci of tumor with a plain x-ray skeletal survey. A patient with a plasmacytoma needs only irradiation and close follow-up, but a patient with multiple myeloma should have chemotherapy in addition to irradiation.—D.S. Springfield, M.D.

Primary Lymphoma of Bone in Children
Furman WL, Fitch S, Hustu HO, Callihan T, Murphy SB (St Jude Children's Research Hosp; Univ of Tennessee, Memphis)
J Clin Oncol 7:1275–1280, September 1989   8–20

Primary lymphoma of bone, formerly called reticulum cell sarcoma or lymphosarcoma, constitutes about 5% of all extranodal lymphomas in adult series. Of 395 children treated for non-Hodgkin's lymphoma in a 7-year period, 11 (2.8%) had a primary site in bone, usually in the femur. The median age at presentation was 13 years. In 7 cases other bones were involved. Most patients had pain that was localized initially to 1 site. Routine laboratory tests were not helpful.

All of the patients had high-grade lymphoma. Large cell immunoblastic lesions were most frequent. Four of 5 patients with localized disease received CHOP chemotherapy and radiotherapy, and 3 of them are in continuous complete remission. Four of 6 patients presenting with multiple bone involvement on both sides of the diaphragm initially received chemotherapy consisting of cyclophosphamide, doxorubicin, vincristine, and prednisone (the CHOP regimen). Two received radiotherapy as well. Three of the latter 4 patients experienced leukemic conversion, and 2 died of progressive disease despite attempted retreatment. One patient died of sepsis during chemotherapy-related granulocytopenia. Of 2 patients who received different multiagent regimens, 1 was in complete remission at last follow-up.

Any child with a small round cell tumor of bone might have lymphoma. The differential diagnosis includes osteomyelitis and eosinophilic granuloma. Scanning with CT can exclude a primary site other than bone. Local resection in the form of amputation is not appropriate for children with primary lymphoma of bone. More aggressive chemotherapy may be necessary if CHOP therapy fails.

▶ Lymphoma, a rare disease in children, easily is overlooked as an explanation for a lesion thought to be osteomyelitis. The treating physician caring for a patient with a lesion of bone that is clinically suggestive of osteomyelitis should include in the differential diagnosis eosinophilic granuloma, Ewing's sarcoma, and lymphoma of bone. This will reduce the chance of 1 of these 3 less common diagnoses being forgotten. Once the diagnosis is made, the patient should be evaluated thoroughly in a search for other foci of tumor. Treatment is controversial, but surgery, except for biopsy, does not play a role. Until proven otherwise, irradiation and systemic chemotherapy are recommended.—D.S. Springfield, M.D.

Subject Index

A

Abductor
  digit quinti perfusion after neurovascular pedicle transfer, 256
Acetabular
  deficiency in adolescence after congenital hip dislocation, 10
  dysplasia, residual, acetabuloplasty in, 11
  fracture (see Fracture, acetabular)
  revision in hip arthroplasty, 164
  wear characteristics against femoral prostheses (in dog), 175
Acetabuloplasty
  in acetabular dysplasia, residual, 11
Achilles tendon
  repair with absorbable polymer carbon fiber composite, 335
  rupture, MR of, 196
Acoustic
  emission in femoral component in hip arthroplasty, 166
Acromioplasty
  clavicular resection and rotator cuff repair in, 120
Adamantinoma
  of long bones, clinicopathology, 362
Adductor
  tenotomy in hallux valgus, 318
Adolescence
  acetabular deficiency during, after congenital hip dislocation, 10
  acetabular fracture during, 42
  femoral lengthening during, 36
  femoral shaft fracture, management, 43
  hallux valgus during, Chevron osteotomy in, 319
  humeral fracture during, triceps-dividing approach in, 47
Aged
  falls in 70 years and older, 232
Air
  inclusion in bone cement, 167
Algodystrophy
  after Colles' fracture, 53
Allergy
  metal, implant in orthopedics in, 160
Allograft (see Graft)
Ambulation
  mechanical performance of, with sping-loaded axillary crutches, 95
Amputation
  below-knee, success of, 89
  level estimation with laser Doppler flowmeter, 91
  after lower extremity trauma, 74
  pain after, fentanyl for, 90
Anesthesia
  epidural, for treatment of knee reflex sympathetic dystrophy, 161
  IV regional, for lower extremity shaft fracture, compartment syndrome complicating, 86
  manipulation under, for frozen shoulder, 122
Angiography
  of gluteal artery in acetabular fracture, 93
  of talipes equinovarus arterial abnormalities, 27
Ankle
  arthroscopy, operative, followup, 341
  fracture (see Fracture, ankle)
  ligament injuries, lateral, reconstruction in, 332
  malleolar fracture, lateral ligament injuries in, 60
  motion, effect of syndesmosis screw on, 325
  syndesmosis injuries, syndesmosis screw for, 326
Ankylosing
  spondylitis, square body pathogenesis in, 291
Ankylosis
  elbow, complete, total elbow arthroplasty in, 136
  of knee with stiffness, arthroplasty in, 231
Anomalies
  extremities, complicated, correction with external fixation, 39
Antibiotic
  prophylaxis in orthopedics, 211
Anulus
  radial tears, MRI and discography in, 289
AO plates
  in osteotomy of metacarpals and phalanges, 262
Arch
  in children, development of, 30
Arteries
  abnormalities in talipes equinovarus, angiography and Doppler of, 27
  gluteal, angiography of, in acetabular fracture, 93
  injuries complicating knee disruption, 202
  trauma to lower extremity, 72
Arteriography
  in extremity trauma, 101

Arthritis
  knee, *Eikenella corrodens* cellulitis in, 214
  osteoarthritis (*see* Osteoarthritis)
  rheumatoid (*see* Rheumatoid arthritis)
  septic, bone imaging in, in children, 41
Arthrodesis
  in Charcot-Marie-Tooth disease, triple, results, 340
  shoulder, by external fixation, 127
  spinal
    cervical, in rheumatoid arthritis, 156
    for spondylisthesis, 22
  in spinal tuberculosis with kyphosis, 310
  subtalar
    in children, 33
    Grice extra-articular, in spastic hindfoot valgus, 35
Arthrography
  of rotator cuff tears, 116
Arthrogryposis
  with myelomeningocele in equinovarus, talectomy in, 339
Arthropathy
  hemophilic, surgery, 154
Arthroplasty
  cemented, lavage during, 158
  elbow
    in elbow ankylosis, 136
    in humeral fracture nonunion salvage, 135
  hip
    cemented, intramedullary plugs in, 169
    femoral component, micromovement and acoustic emission in, 166
    femoral component, subsidence and long-term outcome, 168
    femoral component, torsional stability of, 166
    granulomatous lesions after, 176
    total, aseptic loosening in, in osteolysis, 171
    total, cemented, femur after, 179
    total, femoral head size and acetabular revision in, 164
    total, with infection, C-reactive protein in, 214
    total, with infection, reconstruction of, 213
    total, non-cemented, femoral fracture during, 177
    total, revision, transfusion in, intraoperative autologous, 142
  joint
    total, cardiac isoenzyme values after, 153
    total, postoperative blood salvage with cell saver after, 144
    urinary tract catheterization protocols after, 215
  knee
    angular deformity of, bone graft in, 224
    in ankylosis and stiffness, 231
    cruciate-sparing, gait after, 228
    deformities of, bone graft for tibial defects, 225
    femoral component, failure mechanisms, 229
    pain after, morphine for, 145
    tibial component, failure mechanisms, 229
    total, under 55 years, 230
    total, with infection, spacer block technique in, 218
    total, with infection, treatment results, 217
    total, patellar replacement in, 155
    total, psoriasis and, 216
    in radioscaphoid degeneration, fascial implant, 244
    for rheumatoid wrist with Swanson implant, 246
  shoulder
    in polyarticular rheumatoid arthritis, 124
    total, bone formation in, heterotopic, 126
    total, discussion of, 125
    total, unconstrained, survival in, 125
Arthroscopy
  ankle, operative, followup, 341
  articular cartilage lesion grading at, 191
  of retropatellar pain syndrome, recalcitrant, 189
  in surgery of hip synovial chondromatosis, 183
Arthrotomography
  computed, with MR for shoulder evaluation, 118
Articular
  cartilage (*see* Cartilage, articular)
  chondrocytes, preserved, study of, 162
  intraarticular fracture with elbow dislocation, 131
  surface repair with chondrocyte graft (in rabbit), 195
Aseptic
  loosening in hip arthroplasty in osteolysis, 171
Atlanto
  -axial subluxation, management in children, 21

Subject Index / 373

Atrophy
  spinal muscular, scoliosis in, 17
Avascular
  necrosis (see Necrosis, avascular)
Avulsion
  glenohumeral ligaments, repair approach, 108

B

Back, low (see Low back)
Bacterial
  counts in open fractures, 201
Biceps
  brachii head, tenodesis of, in bicipital tendinitis, 120
  tendon lesions, ultrasound of, 113
Bicipital
  tendinitis, tenodesis of biceps brachii head in, 120
Biodegradable
  internal fixation of ankle fracture, 330
Biomechanical
  analysis of Ilizarov external fixator, 96
  evaluation of rotator cuff fixation methods, 121
Biopsy
  of bone tumors, aspiration, 352
  bone, vs. MR in femoral head ischemic necrosis, 147
  core, in femoral head osteonecrosis, 146
Blood
  preoperative collection of autologous, with erythropoietin therapy, 143
  salvage, postoperative, after total joint arthroplasty, 144
Bone(s)
  biopsy vs. MR in femoral head ischemic necrosis, 147
  cement (see Cement, bone)
  cysts, unicameral
    natural history and fracture risk, 359
    protaglandin levels after steroids, 361
  fibroma
    chondromyxoid, clinicopathology and case review, 364
    desmoplastic, radiography of, 366
  formation
    heterotopic, in shoulder arthroplasty, 126
    new, in femoral head avascular necrosis (in dog), 81
    reduction in non-steroid-treated rheumatoid arthritis, 155
  graft (see Graft, bone)
  imaging, technetium phosphate, in septic arthritis in children, 41
  ingrowth into tibial component of knee prosthesis (in dog), 219
  long
    adamantinoma, clinicopathology, 362
    metastatic lesions, endosteal, 348
  lymphoma in children, 369
  mass
    ethnic and genetic differences in, 236
    reduction in daughters of women with osteoporosis, 235
  metastases (see Metastases, bone)
  plasmacytoma, solitary, Mayo experience, 368
  reaction to silicone metatarsophalangeal joint-1 hemiprosthesis, 315
  resorption after implant, 220
  scintigraphy in reflex dystrophy after trauma, 160
  stiffness of tibial plateau in osteoarthritis, 226
  tumors
    biopsy, aspiration, 352
    MRI of, four pulse sequences, 354
Brace
  functional, in tibial shaft fracture, 60

C

CAD-CAM
  vs. hand made sockets for PTB prostheses, 92
Capitellocondylar
  elbow replacement, total, 133
Carbon
  fiber composite, absorbable polymer, in Achilles tendon repair, 335
Carcinoma
  occult, metastatic bone disease from, 347
Cardiac
  isoenzyme values after joint arthroplasty, 153
Carpal
  kinematics in scaphoid waist osteotomy, 245
  malalignment in Colles' fracture, 54
  scaphoid fracture, thumb-spica cast for, 241
Cartilage
  articular
    fate in osteochondral allograft (in dog), 82
    lesions, grading at arthroscopy, 191
    phenotype maintenance in cryopreserved articular chondrocytes, 162

Cast
  plaster, in unstable Colles' fracture, 55
  thumb-spica, in carpal scaphoid
    fracture, 241
Catheterization
  urinary tract, protocols after joint
    arthroplasty, 215
Cauda
  equina syndrome after lumbar spinal
    stenosis surgery, 300
Cell
  saver for blood salvage after joint
    arthroplasty, 144
Cellulitis
  Eikenella corrodens, in knee arthritis,
    214
Cement
  bone
    air inclusion in, 167
    interface of hip prosthesis,
      radiographic inadequacy for
      evaluation, 181
Cemented arthroplasty
  hip
    femur after, 179
    intramedullary plugs in, 169
    lavage during, 158
Cementing
  of femoral stems, fat embolism in, 158
Cervical
  discectomy with hydroxylapatite fusion,
    268
  myelopathy (*see* Myelopathy, cervical)
Charcot-Marie-Tooth disease
  arthrodesis in, triple, results, 340
Chemonucleolysis
  disc space before and after, 298
Chemotherapy
  adjuvant, in soft tissue sarcoma, 357
Chevron
  osteotomy in hallux valgus during
    adolescence, 319
Chiari pelvic osteotomy
  hip function after, 209
  in hip osteoarthritis, 208
Children
  acetabular fracture, 42
  arch of, development, 30
  arthritis, septic, bone imaging in, 41
  atlanto-axial subluxation, management,
    21
  femoral lengthening, 36
  flatfoot, flexible, corrective shoes with
    inserts in, 31
  hip assessment with radiography, 3
  hip pain in, MR in, 12
  humeral fracture
    condylar, nonunion in, 45
    supracondylar, vascular
      complications, 46
  lymphoma of bone, 369
  spondylolisthesis, spinal arthrodesis for,
    22
  subtalar arthrodesis, 33
  subtalar joint coalition, 32
Chondrocyte(s)
  cryopreserved articular, study of, 162
  effects of salicylate on, in osteoarthritis
    and knee (in dog), 193
  graft for articular surface repair (in
    rabbit), 195
Chondromatosis
  hip synovial, arthroscopic surgery of,
    183
Clamp-on plate
  in forearm fracture, 61
Clavicle
  nonunion and thoracic outlet syndrome,
    102
  resection acromioplasty, 120
Clubfoot, idiopathic
  comparison of surgeries for, 25
  posteromedial release, results with early
    vs. delayed, 24
Collagen
  gel for chondrocyte graft for articular
    surface repair (in rabbit), 195
  types I and III in lumbar disc
    herniation, 290
Colles' fracture (*see* Fracture, Colles')
Compartment syndrome
  chronic exertional, intracompartmental
    pressures in, 204
  complicating anesthesia for lower
    extremity shaft fracture, 86
  MAST-associated, 76
  thigh, acute, 87
Computed arthrotomography
  with MR for shoulder evaluation, 118
Computed tomography
  for osteodensitometry of vertebral
    metastases after radiotherapy, 351
Condyle(s)
  femoral, osteochondritis dissecans of,
    192
  prosthesis, total cemented, 229
Coracoid process
  musculocutaneous nerve and, 104
  or ulna, fracture, 64
Corpectomy
  in cervical kyphosis and myelopathy,
    273
Cotrel-Dubousset
  vs. Harrington rod instrumentations in
    idiopathic scoliosis, 15
Crankshaft phenomenon, 16

Subject Index / 375

C-reactive protein
  in hip arthroplasty with infection, 214
Cruciate ligament
  anterior
    lesions, MR of, 200
    replacement and normal response, 185
    rupture, treatments, 186
    tears, unreconstructed, followup, 187
    transection, effects of salicylate on chondrocytes in (in dog), 193
  in knee replacement, 227
  sparing knee arthroplasty, gait after, 228
Crutches
  spring-loaded axillary, mechanical performance of ambulation with, 95
Cryopreserved
  articular chondrocytes, study of, 162
  osteochondral allograft, articular cartilage fate after (in dog), 82
Cybex
  evaluation of triceps in humeral fracture during adolescence, 47
Cyst
  bone (*see* Bone cyst)
Cytology
  in myositis ossificans, pseudomalignant, 363
Cytostatics
  in perfusion of extremity soft tissue tumors, 358

D

Death
  cause in spinal cord injuries, 281
Deformities
  extremity, complicated, correction with external fixation, 39
Diaphysis
  defect reconstruction after tibial fracture grade IIIB, 73
Disc
  herniation (*see* Herniation, lumbar disc)
  intervertebral, fibrous structure, MRI of, 287
  space before and after chemonucleolysis and nucleotomy, 298
Discectomy
  cervical, with hydroxylapatite fusion, 268
  discoscopy with percutaneous nucleotomy replacing, 299
Discography
  in anulus radial tears, 289

Discoscopy
  with percutaneous nucleotomy replacing discectomy, 299
Dislocation
  elbow
    with fracture, intraarticular, 131
    ligamentous injury study in, 130
  hip, congenital
    acetabular deficiency in adolescence, 10
    failed open reduction, treatment of, 9
    study, 5
  peroneal tendon, fibular graft in, 336
  shoulder
    Putti-Platt procedure in, 107
    recurrent, M. Lange technique results, 106
  sternoclavicular, surgery results, 112
Distraction: rate and frequency, and tissue genesis and growth, 235
DNA
  analysis in osteosarcoma, 356
Doppler
  laser, flowmeter, for amputation level estimation, 91
  of talipes equinovarus arterial abnormalities, 27
Drilling
  in femoral head avascular necrosis (in dog), 81
Dupuytren's disease
  recurrence prediction, 258
Dural
  laceration with burst and laminar fractures, 285
Dysplasia
  acetabular, residual, acetabuloplasty in, 11
  hip, congenital, avascular necrosis in, 7
Dystrophy
  algodystrophy after Colles' fracture, 53
  reflex (*see* Reflex dystrophy)

E

Eikenella corrodens
  cellulitis in knee arthritis, 214
Elbow
  ankylosis, complete, total elbow arthroplasty in, 136
  arthroplasty (*see* Arthroplasty, elbow)
  dislocation (*see* Dislocation, elbow)
  flexorplasty of, 137
  Pritchard Mark II prosthesis, in rheumatoid arthritis, 133
  replacement, capitellocondylar total, 133

in rheumatoid arthritis, synovectomy in, 136
tennis, interosseous nerve decompression in, 131
Wadsworth, failure, rheumatoid arthritis in, 132

Elderly
  falls at 70 years and older, 232
Electromagnetic fields
  pulsed, in osteoporosis prevention, 237
Embolism
  fat, in femoral stem cementing, 158
Ender
  nailing in tibial shaft fracture, 69
Endosteal
  metastases in long bones, 348
Epidural
  anesthesia for treatment of knee reflex sympathetic dystrophy, 161
Epiphysis
  acetabular, absence, and acetabular deficiency in adolescence, 10
Equinovarus
  in arthrogryposis and myelomeningocele, talectomy in, 339
  spastic, tibial tendon transfer in, 338
  talipes, arterial abnormalities in, angiography and Doppler in, 27
Erythropoietin
  therapy with preoperative collection of autologous blood, 143
Ethnic
  differences in bone mass, 236
Extensor
  carpi ulnaris tenodesis in unstable ulna, 259
Extremities
  deformities, complicated, correction with external fixation, 39
  lengthening, modified Wagner method for, 38
  lower
    fracture, reaction time and coordination time in, 66
    fracture, shaft, compartment syndrome complicating anesthesia for, 86
    non-physeal fracture with physeal arrest about knee, 44
    osteomyelitis, MR of, 200
    reconstruction with microvascular free flaps, 70
    trauma, orthopedic and arterial, treatment outcome, 72
    trauma, reconstruction vs. amputation, 74
    trauma, sequelae, long-term, 85

  trauma, soft-tissue reconstruction in, 70
phanton limb pain, fentanyl for, 90
trauma, arteriography of, 101
tumors, soft tissue, perfusion with cytostatics in, 358

F

Falls: in 70 years and older, 232
Fascial
  implant arthroplasty in radioscaphoid degeneration, 244
Fat
  embolism in femoral stem cementing, 158
  graft in lumbar spinal stenosis, 300
Feet (see Foot)
Femur
  anteversion
    hip osteoarthritis and, 13
    hip osteoarthrosis and, 151
  component
    in hip arthroplasty (see Arthroplasty, hip, femoral component)
    in knee arthroplasty, failure mechanisms, 229
  condyles, osteochondritis dissecans of, 192
  decompression in knee avascular necrosis, 148
  dimension changes, radiographic, due to hip rotation, 181
  fracture (see Fracture, femur)
  head
    necrosis, avascular, drilling in (in dog), 81
    necrosis, avascular, intertrochanteric osteotomy in, 210
    necrosis, ischemic, MR vs. bone biopsy in, 147
    osteonecrosis, MR in, 146
    size in hip arthroplasty, 164
    titanium-alloy, causing osteolysis in hip arthroplasty, 171
  after hip arthroplasty, cemented, 179
  lengthening in children and adolescents, 36
  metallic component in hip prostheses, surface changes, 173
  osteonecrosis, capital, MR in, 12
  prostheses, wear characteristics of acetabulum against (in dog), 175
  stem
    cementing, fat embolism in, 158
    in hip prosthesis, cement-bone interface of, 181

Fentanyl
  for pain after amputation, 90
Fibrinolysis
  spinal injury and deep vein thrombosis, 280
Fibroma (see Bone fibroma)
Fibronectin
  in lumbar disc herniation, 290
Fibular
  graft in peroneal tendon dislocation, 336
Fixation stability: and soft tissue preservation, 234
Flap
  gastrocnemius muscle, for jeopardized knee prosthesis, 216
  ligamentous/periosteal, in duplicated thumb, 257
  microvascular free, for lower extremity reconstruction, 70
Flatfoot
  flexible, corrective shoes with inserts for, in children, 31
Flexor
  carpi ulnaris tenodesis in unstable ulna, 259
  tendon repair in zone 2, mobilization after, 254
Flexorplasty
  of elbow, 137
Fluorotic
  cervical myelopathy, 271
Foot
  abnormal pressures not causing ulcer, 342
  arch, development in children, 30
  clubfoot (see Clubfoot)
  crush injuries, skin excision in, 77
  flatfoot, flexible, corrective shoes with inserts in, in children, 31
  hindfoot valgus, spastic, Grice extra-articular subtalar arthrodesis in, 35
  tumors, soft tissue, case review, 343
Forearm
  fracture, clamp-on plate in, 61
Forefoot
  revision, metatarsal osteotomy with compression screw, 320
Fracture
  acetabular
    in children and adolescents, 42
    gluteal artery in, angiography of, 93
  ankle
    biodegradable internal fixation, 330
    immediate internal fixation, 75
    open, immediate vs. delayed treatment, 332
    weight-bearing and muscle activity after treatment, 337
  Colles'
    algodystrophy after, 53
    carpal malalignment in, 54
    triangular ligament repair in, 253
    unstable, 49
    unstable, external fixation of, 56
    unstable intraarticular, plaster cast vs. external fixation, 55
  extremities, lower
    reaction time and coordination time in, 66
    shaft, compartment syndrome complicating anesthesia for, 86
  femur
    early vs. delayed stabilization, 67
    during hip arthroplasty, non-cemented, 177
    shaft, management during adolescence, 43
  forearm, clamp-on plate in, 61
  hip, causes, 233
  humerus
    complex distal, triceps-dividing approach to open reduction during adolescence, 47
    condyle, nonunion in children, 45
    epidemiology, 98
    Hoffmann's external fixation with transcutaneous reduction, 99
    supracondylar nonunion, elbow arthroplasty in, 135
    supracondylar, vascular complications in children, 46
    transcondylar, 128
  intraarticular, with elbow dislocation, 131
  laminar and burst, with dural laceration, 285
  malleolar, of ankle, lateral ligament injuries in, 60
  non-physeal, physeal arrest about knee with, in lower extremity, 44
  occult intraosseous, MR of, 94
  open, bacterial counts in, 201
  quadrangular fragment, radiography and treatment protocol, 266
  radius
    comminuted, ligamentotaxis and bone graft in, 57
    diaphyses, compression plate fixation of, 138
    distal end comminuted, reduction and fixation, 252
  risk in bone cysts, unicameral, 359
  scaphoid
    carpal, thumb-spica cast for, 241

malunion, 242
nonunion, failed bone graft in, 243
spinal, multiple-level noncontiguous, 277
talus dome osteochondral, 327
tarsal navicular, displaced intra-articular, 62
tibia
　grade 1, intramedullary nailing in, delayed vs. immediate, 63
　grade IIIB, reconstruction of diaphyseal defects after, 73
　high energy, early prophylactic bone graft in, 80
　with intramedullary nailing, infection after, 85
　nonunion with infection, Ilizarov technique in, 83
　pleateau, hydroxyapatite as bone graft substitute in, 79
　shaft, Ender nailing vs. external fixation, 69
　shaft, external fixation vs. Ender nailing, 69
　shaft, functional braces in, 60
　shaft, plates vs. external fixation in, 68
　trimalleolar, results after posterior fragment fixation, 59
ulna
　coronoid process, 64
　diaphyses, compression plate fixation, 138
vertebral
　compression, MRI in, 346
　epidemiology in women, 282
Freiberg's disease
　osteotomy in, dorsiflexion, 322

G

Gait
　after cruciate-sparing knee arthroplasty, 228
Gastrocnemius
　muscle flap for jeopardized knee prosthesis, 216
Genetic
　differences in bone mass, 236
Glenohumeral
　instability, 108
　joint subluxation, 110
　ligament avulsion, repair approach, 108
Gluteal artery
　angiography of, in acetabular fracture, 93

Gonarthrosis
　medial, tibial osteotomy in, below age 50, 205
Graft
　bone
　　donor sites, morbidity at, 78
　　failure in scaphoid nonunion, 243
　　in hip replacement, radiography and mobility in, 170
　　in knee arthroplasty angular deformity, 224
　　in radial fracture, comminuted, 57
　　substitute, hydroxyapatite as, in tibial plateau fracture, 79
　　for tibial defects in knee arthroplasty deformity, 225
　　in tibial fracture, high energy, 80
　chondrocyte, for articular surface repair (in rabbit), 195
　fat, in lumbar spinal stenosis, 300
　fibular, in peroneal tendon dislocation, 336
　flap (see Flap)
　neurovascular pedicle, transfer, abductor digiti quinti perfusion after, 256
　osteochondral
　　articular cartilage fate after (in dog), 82
　　for knee resurfacing, 193
　pedicle (see Pedicle)
　strut, in cervical kyphosis and myelopathy, 273
Granulomatous
　lesions after hip arthroplasty, 176
Grice
　extra-articular subtalar arthrodesis in spastic hindfoot valgus, 35
Growth
　plate closure of radius in gymnasts, 261
　of tissues, tension-stress effect on, 234, 235
Gymnasts
　wrist pain and growth plate closure of radius, 261

H

Hallux
　valgus
　　Chevron osteotomy during adolescence, 319
　　Lapidus procedure modification for, 324
　　osteotomy and adductor tenotomy in, 318

Hand
  rheumatoid deformity, metacarpophalangeal reconstruction for, 248
Harrington rods
  in scoliosis, adult idiopathic, with wiring, 307
  vs. Cotrel-Dubousset instrumentations in idiopathic scoliosis, 15
Heart
  isoenzyme values after total joint arthroplasty, 153
Hemiprosthesis
  silicone metatarsophalangeal joint-1, bone reaction to, 315
Hemophilic
  arthropathy, surgery of, 154
Herniation
  lumbar disc
    multifidus muscle changes in, 290
    nucleotomy with discoscopy replacing discectomy in, 299
Heterotopic
  bone formation after shoulder arthroplasty, 126
Hindfoot
  valgus, spastic, Grice extra-articular subtalar arthrodesis in, 35
Hip
  arthroplasty (see Arthroplasty, hip)
  assessment
    with radiography in children, 3
    ultrasound for, in newborn, 1
  chondromatosis, synovial, arthroscopic surgery of, 183
  dislocation (see Dislocation, hip)
  dysplasia, congenital, avascular necrosis in, 7
  fracture, causes, 233
  function after Chiari pelvic osteotomy, 209
  hydroxyapatite titanium, biologic response (in dog), 174
  implant
    hydroxyapatite, experience with, 174
    routine use of custom, argument against, 163
    total, custom-fit cementless, 163
  osteoarthritis (see Osteoarthritis, hip)
  osteoarthrosis, idiopathic, and femoral anteversion, 151
  pain, MR in, in children, 12
  prosthesis (see Prosthesis, hip)
  replacement
    with bone graft, radiography and mobility in, 170
    with knee replacement in rheumatoid arthritis, 231

rotation, femoral dimension radiographic changes due to, 181
Hoffmann's
  external fixation in humeral fracture, 99
Humerus
  fracture (see Fracture, humerus)
  head subluxation after shoulder injury, 103
Hydroxyapatite
  for bone graft substitute in tibial plateau fracture, 79
  fusion in cervical discectomy, 268
  hip implant, experience with, 174
  titanium hips, biologic response (in dog), 174
Hydroxylapatite (see Hydroxyapatite)

I

Ilizarov external fixator
  biomechanical analysis of, 96
Ilizarov technique
  for tibial nonunion infection, 83
  in tibial pseudarthrosis, with infection, 84
Imaging
  bone, technetium phosphate, in septic arthritis in children, 41
  magnetic resonance (see Magnetic resonance imaging)
Implant
  bone resorption after, 220
  fascial, in arthroplasty of radioscaphoid degeneration, 244
  hip (see Hip, implant)
  metal allergy in orthopedics, 160
  metallic, osseointegration of, microscopy of (in rabbit), 221
  Swanson, in rheumatoid wrist arthroplasty, 246
Interosseous
  nerve decompression in tennis elbow, 131
Intertrochanteric
  osteotomy in femoral head avascular necrosis, 210
Intervertebral
  disk, fibrous structure in, MRI in, 287
Intraarticular
  fracture with elbow dislocation, 131
Intramedullary
  nailing (see Nailing, intramedullary)
  plugs in cemented hip arthroplasty, 169
Intramuscular
  pressure recording, injection techniques, 203

Irradiation (see Radiation, Radiography, Radiotherapy)
Ischemic necrosis
  of femoral head, MR vs. bone biopsy in, 147
  of lunate, MRI in, 250
Isoenzyme values
  cardiac, after total joint arthroplasty, 153

J

Joint
  arthroplasty (see Arthroplasty, joint)
  glenohumeral, subluxation, 110
  hip, osteoarthritis, 151
  knee, osteoarthritis, 148
  metatarsophalangeal (see Metatarsophalangeal joint)
  patellofemoral, contact pressures during impact loading, 190
  sacroiliac, movement roentgen study, 295
  sternoclavicular, subluxation, 111
  subtalar, coalition in children, 32
  synovial, continuous passive motion of, 196
  tarsometatarsal, first, biomechanical study, 317

K

Knee
  ankylosis with stiffness, arthroplasty in, 231
  arthritis, *Eikenella corrodens* cellulitis in, 214
  arthroplasty (see Arthroplasty, knee)
  collateral ligament injury, grade III medial, management, 188
  component alignment and tibial load distribution, 222
  disruption, arterial injury complicating, 202
  effects of salicylates on chondrocytes in (in dog), 193
  joint osteoarthritis, 148
  MR of, pitfalls, 199
  necrosis, avascular, femoral decompression in, 148
  osteoarthritis (see Osteoarthritis of knee)
  pain, anterior, approach to, 189
  physeal arrest about, with non-physeal fracture of lower extremity, 44
  prosthesis (see Prosthesis, knee)

reflex sympathetic dystrophy, treatment under epidural anesthesia, 161
replacement
  cemented, total condylar prosthesis in, 229
  cruciate ligament in, 227
  with hip replacement in rheumatoid arthritis, 231
  total, tibial tubercle osteotomy during, 223
  resurfacing with osteochondral graft, 193
  surgery, elective, deep vein thrombosis after, 157
synovitis, pigmented villonodular, radiography of, 152
vascular injury about, 203
Kyphosis
  cervical, corpectomy and strut graft in, 273
  in spinal tuberculosis, arthrodesis in, 310

L

Laminar
  fracture with dural laceration, 285
Lange technique, M.
  results in recurrent shoulder dislocation, 106
Lapidus procedure
  modification for hallux valgus, 324
Laser
  Doppler flowmeter for amputation level estimation, 91
Lavage
  during arthroplasty, cemented, 158
Leg
  cross leg pain and trunk list, 293
Ligament
  ankle, lateral, reconstruction of injuries, 332
  cruciate (see Cruciate ligament)
  glenohumeral, avulsion, repair approach, 108
  injury study, in elbow dislocation, 130
  knee, grade III medial collateral, injury, management, 188
  lateral, injuries in ankle malleolar fracture, 60
  /periosteal flap for duplicated thumb, 257
  triangular, repair in Colles' fracture, 253
Ligamentotaxis
  in radial fracture, comminuted, 57
Limb(s) (see Extremities)

Limbectomy
  in hip dislocation, congenital,
    acetabular deficiency during
    adolescence after, 10
Long bones (see Bones, long)
Low back
  pain, spinal skeletal fixation in, 301
  surgery, outcome assessment, 296
Lumbar
  disc herniation (see Herniation, lumbar disc)
  spine fusions, segmental "floating," 303
  stenosis (see Stenosis, lumbar)
Lumbosacral
  radiculopathy, thermography in, 293
Lunate
  necrosis, ischemic, MRI in, 250
Luque rods
  in scoliosis
    adult idiopathic, with wiring, 307
    neuromuscular, with spinal fusion, 19
Lymphoma
  of bone, in children, 369

M

MACS, 76
Magnetic resonance imaging
  in Achilles tendon rupture, 196
  in anulus radial tears, 289
  in bone tumors, 354
  of cruciate ligament, anterior, 200
  in femoral osteonecrosis
    capital, 12
    head, 146
  of fracture, occult intraosseous, 94
  in hip dislocation detected in early childhood, 198
  of intervertebral disk fibrous structure, 287
  of knee, pitfalls, 199
  in lunate ischemic necrosis, 250
  of meniscal lesions, 200
  of osteomyelitis of lower extremity, 200
  of rotator cuff tears, 115, 116
  in vertebral compression fracture, 346
  vs. bone biopsy in femoral head ischemic necrosis, 147
Malleolar
  fracture of ankle, lateral ligament injuries in, 60
Malunion
  scaphoid, 242
Marrow
  abnormalities in femoral capital osteonecrosis, 12

MAST
  -associated compartment syndrome, 76
Meniscus
  lesions, MR of, 200
  repair, open, technique and results, 184
  tears, non-operative treatment, 185
Metacarpals
  osteotomy of, 262
Metacarpophalangeal
  reconstruction in rheumatoid hand deformity, 248
Metal
  allergy, implant in orthopedics in, 160
Metallic
  femoral component in hip prostheses, surface changes, 173
  implant, osseointegration of, microscopy of (in rabbit), 221
Metastases
  in bone disease from occult carcinoma, 347
  bone, radiotherapy of, palliative, 349
  in long bones, endosteal, 348
  spinal cord compression in, radiotherapy of, 350
  vertebral, after radiotherapy, osteodensitometry of, 351
Metatarsal
  osteotomy with compression screw, 320
  joint
    first, prosthetic replacement, 321
    -1 hemiprosthesis, bone reaction to, 315
Micromovement
  in femoral component of hip arthroplasty, 166
Microscopy
  of osseointegration of metallic implant (in rabbit), 221
Microvascular
  flap, free, for lower extremity reconstruction, 70
Morbidity
  at bone graft donor sites, 78
Morphine
  for pain after knee arthroplasty, 145
Morton
  neuroma, ultrasound of, 321
MR (see Magnetic resonance)
Multifidus
  muscle connective tissue changes in lumbar disc herniation, 290
Muscle
  gastrocnemius, flap for jeopardized knee prosthesis, 216
  intramuscular pressure recording, injection techniques, 203

multifidus, changes in lumbar disc herniation, 290
spinal muscular atrophy, scoliosis in, 17
Musculocutaneous
nerve and coracoid process, 104
Myelomeningocele
with arthrogryposis in equinovarus, talectomy in, 339
Myelopathy
cervical
fluorotic, 271
with kyphosis, corpectomy and strut graft in, 273
Myositis ossificans
pseudomalignant, radiography and cytology in, 363

N

Nailing
intramedullary
in tibial fracture with infection, 85
in tibial grade 1 fracture, 63
Navicular
tarsal, fracture, displaced intra-articular, 62
Necrosis
avascular
of femoral head, drilling in (in dog), 81
of femoral head, intertrochanteric osteotomy in, 210
in hip dysplasia, congenital, 7
knee, femoral decompression in, 148
femoral head, ischemic, MR vs. bone biopsy in, 147
of lunate, ischemic, MRI in, 250
osteonecrosis (see Osteonecrosis)
Neoplasms (see Tumors)
Nerve
interosseous, decompression in tennis elbow, 131
musculocutaneous, and coracoid process, 104
Neuroma
Morton, ultrasound of, 321
Neuromuscular
scoliosis, Luque-Rod instrumentation in, with spinal fusion, 19
Neurovascular
pedicle transfer, abductor digiti quinti perfusion after, 256
Newborn
hip assessment with ultrasound, 1
Nonunion
of clavicle and thoracic outlet syndrome, 102

humeral condyle fracture in children, 45
salvage in humeral fracture by elbow arthroplasty, 135
scaphoid, failed bone graft in, 243
tibia, with infection, Ilizarov technique in, 83
Nucleotomy
disc space before and after, 298
percutaneous, with discoscopy replacing discectomy, 299

O

Operating rooms
ultraviolet radiation in, shortwave, 212
Orthopedics
antibiotic prophylaxis in, 211
implant in, in metal allergy, 160
transfusion in, intraoperative autologous, 142
Osteoarthritis
effects of salicylate on chondrocytes in (in dog), 193
epidemiology, Zoetermeer Survey, 150
of hip
Chiari pelvic osteotomy in, 208
femoral anteversion and, 13
joint, 151
of knee
joint, 148
joint, tibial venous drainage after osteotomy in, 207
tibial osteotomy in, 206
tibial plateau bone stiffness in, 226
Osteoarthrosis
hip, idiopathic, and femoral anteversion, 151
Osteochondral
allograft, articular cartilage fate after (in dog), 82
graft for knee resurfacing, 193
talus fracture, 327
Osteochondritis
dissecans
of femoral condyles, 192
of talus, surgical results, 329
Osteodensitometry
of vertebral metastases after radiotherapy, 351
Osteolysis
in hip arthroplasty causing aseptic loosening, 171
Osteomyelitis
acute, ultrasound in, 40
of lower extremity, MR of, 200
vertebral, pyogenic, 294

Osteonecrosis
  femoral capital, MR in, 12
  femoral head, MR in, 146
Osteoporosis
  bone mass reduction in daughters of women with, 235
  prevention with pulsed electromagnetic fields, 237
Osteosarcoma
  prognosis and DNA analysis, 356
  prognostic variables in, 355
Osteotomy
  Chevron, in hallux valgus during adolescence, 319
  Chiari pelvic (see Chiari pelvic osteotomy)
  in Freiberg's disease, dorsiflexion, 322
  in hallux valgus, proximal closing wedge, 318
  intertrochanteric, in femoral head avascular necrosis, 210
  of metacarpals, 262
  metatarsal, with compression screw, 320
  of phalanges, 262
  scaphoid waist, carpal kinematics in, 245
  tibial
    for gonarthrosis below age 50, 205
    high, tibial venous drainage after, 207
    tubercle during knee replacement, 223
    upper, in knee osteoarthritis, 206

P

Pain
  cross leg, and trunk list, 293
  hip, MR in, in children, 12
  knee, anterior, approach to, 189
  after knee arthroplasty, morphine for, 145
  low back, spinal skeletal fixation in, 301
  retropatellar pain syndrome, recalcitrant, arthroscopy in, 189
  wrist, in gymnasts, 261
Parkinson's disease
  shoulder disturbances and frozen shoulder in, 123
Patella
  replacement in total knee arthroplasty, 155
  retropatellar pain syndrome, recalcitrant, arthroscopy in, 189
Patellofemoral
  joint, contact pressures during impact loading, 190

Pedicle
  neurovascular, transfer, abductor digiti quinti perfusion after, 256
  Wiltse pedicle screw fixation, results, 305
Pelvic
  Chiari osteotomy (see Chiari pelvic osteotomy)
Periosteal
  /ligament flap in duplicated thumb, 257
Peroneal
  tendon dislocation, fibular graft in, 336
Phalanges
  osteotomy of, 262
Phantom limb pain
  fentanyl for, 90
Phenotype
  cartilage, maintenance in cryopreserved articular chondrocytes, 162
Phlebography
  of tibial venous drainage after tibial osteotomy, 207
Pigmented
  synovitis of knee, radiography of, 152
Plasmacytoma
  of bone, Mayo experience, 368
Plaster
  cast in unstable Colles' fracture, 55
Plate(s)
  AO, in osteotomy of metacarpals and phalanges, 262
  clamp-on, in forearm fracture, 61
  compression plate fixation in fracture of diaphyses of radius and ulna, 138
  in tibial shaft fracture, 68
Polymer
  carbon fiber composite in Achilles tendon repair, 335
Pritchard Mark II
  elbow prosthesis in rheumatoid arthritis, 133
Prostaglandin
  levels in unicameral bone cysts after steroids, 361
Prosthesis
  condylar, total cemented, 229
  elbow, Pritchard Mark II, 133
  femoral, wear characteristics of acetabulum against (in dog), 175
  hip
    cement-bone interface, radiographic inadequacy for evaluation, 181
    surface changes in metallic femoral components of, 173
  knee
    bone ingrowth into tibial component of (in dog), 219

salvage of jeopardized with gastrocnemius muscle flap, 216
for metatarsophalangeal joint, first, 321
PTB, CAD-CAM vs. hand made sockets for, 92
silicone metatarsophalangeal joint-1 hemiprosthesis, bone reaction to, 315
Protein
C-reactive, in hip arthroplasty with infection, 214
Pseudarthrosis
tibia, with infection, Ilizarov technique in, 84
Psoriasis
knee arthroplasty and, 216
PTB
prostheses, CAD-CAM vs. hand made sockets for, 92
Putti-Platt procedure
in shoulder dislocation, 107
Pyogenic
vertebral osteomyelitis, 294

Q

Quadrangular
fragment fracture, radiography and treatment protocol, 266

R

Radiation
ultraviolet, shortwave, in operating rooms, 212
Radiculopathy
lumbosacral, thermography in, 293
Radiography
of bone fibroma, desmoplastic, 366
of femoral dimension changes due to hip rotation, 181
of femoral head osteonecrosis, 146
in hip assessment in children, 3
of hip prosthesis, inadequacy for evaluation, 181
in hip replacement with bone graft, 170
of knee synovitis, pigmented villonodular, 152
in myositis ossificans, pseudomalignant, 363
quadrangular fragment fracture, 266
stereophotogrammetric, of sacroiliac joint movement, 295
Radioscaphoid
degeneration, fascial implant arthroplasty in, 244

Radiotherapy
of bone metastases, palliative, 349
in metastatic spinal cord compression, 350
vertebral metastases after, osteodensitometry of, 351
Radius
fracture (see Fracture, radius)
growth plate closure in gymnasts, 261
synostosis after trauma, surgery results, 139
Reconstruction
in ankle lateral ligament injury, 332
in hip arthroplasty with infection, 213
lower extremity with microvascular free flaps, 70
after lower extremity trauma, 74
soft-tissue, 70
metacarpophalangeal, in rheumatoid hand deformity, 248
after tibial fracture, grade IIIB, 73
Reflex
dystrophy
of knee, sympathetic, treatment under epidural anesthesia, 161
after trauma, bone scintigraphy in, 160
Retropatellar
pain syndrome, recalcitrant, arthroscopy in, 189
Revascularization
in femoral head avascular necrosis (in dog), 81
Rheumatoid arthritis
elbow prosthesis in, Pritchard Mark II, 133
elbow synovectomy in, 136
hand deformity in, metacarpophalangeal reconstruction in, 248
hip and knee replacement in, bilateral total, 231
knee arthroplasty in, with patellar replacement, 155
non-steroid-treated, bone formation reduction in, 155
polyarticular, shoulder arthroplasty in, 124
spinal arthrodesis in, cervical, 156
Wadsworth elbow failure and, 132
wrist in (see Wrist, rheumatoid)
Roentgenography (see Radiography)
Rotator cuff
fixation methods, biomechanical evaluation, 121
lesions, ultrasound of, 113
repair in acromioplasty, 120
tear
complete, clinical presentation, 119

MR in, 115
MR, arthrography and ultrasound of, 116
ultrasound of, reassessment, 114
Rupture
Achilles tendon, MR of, 196
cruciate ligament, anterior, treatments, 186

S

Sacroiliac
joint movement, roentgen study, 295
Salicylate
effects on chondrocytes in osteoarthritis and knee (in dog), 193
Sarcoma
osteosarcoma (see Osteosarcoma)
soft tissue, adjuvant chemotherapy of, 357
Scanning (see Imaging)
Scaphoid
fracture (see Fracture, scaphoid)
radioscaphoid degeneration, fascial implant arthroplasty in, 244
waist osteotomy, carpal kinematics in, 245
Scintigraphy
bone, in reflex dystrophy after trauma, 160
Scoliosis
idiopathic
Cotrel-Dubousset vs. Harrington rod instrumentations in, 15
Luque or Harrington rods with sublaminar wiring in, 307
neuromuscular, Luque-Rod instrumentation for, with spinal fusion, 19
in spinal muscular atrophy, 17
Screw(s)
compression, in metatarsal osteotomy, 320
in osteotomy of metacarpals and phalanges, 262
syndesmosis (see Syndesmosis screw)
Wiltse pedicle screw fixation, results, 305
Septic
arthritis, bone imaging in, in children, 41
Shoes
corrective, with inserts for flexible flatfoot in children, 31
Shoulder
arthrodesis by external fixation, 127
arthroplasty (see Arthroplasty, shoulder)
dislocation (see Dislocation, shoulder)
evaluation with computed arthrotomography and MR, 118
frozen
manipulation under anesthesia in, 122
in Parkinson's disease, 123
injury, humeral head subluxation after, 103
in Parkinson's disease, 123
Silicone
metatarsophalangeal joint-1 hemiprosthesis, bone reaction to, 315
Skin
excision in foot crush injuries, 77
Sockets
CAD-CAM vs. hand made, for PTB prostheses, 92
Soft tissue
extremity tumors, perfusion with cytostatics in, 358
metacarpophalangeal reconstruction in rheumatoid hand deformity, 248
preservation and fixation stability, 234
reconstruction in lower extremity trauma, 70
sarcoma, adjuvant chemotherapy of, 357
Somatotype
in spinal canal stenosis, 270
Sonography (see Ultrasound)
Spacer block
technique in knee arthroplasty with infection, 218
Spastic
equinovarus, tibial tendon transfer in, 338
hindfoot valgus, Grice extra-articular subtalar arthrodesis in, 35
Spica cast
for thumb in carpal scaphoid fracture, 241
Spine
arthrodesis
cervical, in rheumatoid arthritis, 156
for spondylolisthesis, 22
atrophy, muscular, scoliosis in, 17
canal stenosis and somatotype, 270
cervical (see Cervical)
cord
injuries, cause of death in, 281
metastatic compression, radiotherapy, 350
deformity in adults, Zielke instrumentation for, 310
fracture, multiple-level noncontiguous, 277

fusion with Luque-Rod instrumentation
  for neuromuscular scoliosis, 19
injury(ies)
  fibrinolysis and deep vein thrombosis,
    280
  multilevel, incidence, distribution and
    neurological patterns, 276
  lumbar, fusions, segmental "floating,"
    303
  plating system, variable, complications,
    306
  skeletal fixation in low back pain
    assessment, 301
  stenosis (see Stenosis, lumbar spinal)
  tuberculosis with kyphosis, arthrodesis
    in, 310
Spondylitis
  ankylosing, square body pathogenesis
    in, 291
Square body
  pathogenesis in ankylosing spondylitis,
    291
Stenosis
  lumbar spinal
    cauda equina syndrome after, 300
    instability in, preoperative and
      postoperative, 302
    spinal canal, and somatotype, 270
Stereophotogrammetric
  study, roentgen, of sacroiliac joint
    movement, 295
Sternoclavicular
  dislocation, surgery results, 112
  joint subluxation, 111
Steroids
  intralesional injection in unicameral
    bone cysts, 361
Stress
  -tension effect on tissue genesis and
    growth, 234, 235
Strut graft
  in cervical kyphosis and myelopathy,
    273
Stump
  pain, postamputation, fentanyl for, 90
Subtalar
  arthrodesis (see Arthrodesis, subtalar)
  joint coalition in children, 32
Swanson implant
  in rheumatoid wrist arthroplasty,
    246
Syndesmosis screw
  for ankle syndesmosis injury
    stabilization, 326
  effect on ankle motion, 325
Synostosis
  radio-ulnar, after trauma, surgery
    results, 139

Synovectomy
  of rheumatoid elbow, 136
  in rheumatoid wrist, results, 247
Synovial
  hip chondromatosis, arthroscopic
    surgery of, 183
  joint, continuous passive motion of,
    196
Synovitis
  knee, pigmented villonodular,
    radiography of, 152

T

Talectomy
  in equinovarus with arthrogryposis and
    myelomeningocele, 339
Talipes
  equinovarus, arterial abnormalities in,
    angiography and Doppler in, 27
Talus
  fracture of dome, osteochondral, 327
  osteochondritis dissecans, surgical
    results, 329
Tarsal
  navicular fracture, displaced
    intra-articular, 62
Tarsometatarsal
  joint, first, biomechanical study, 317
Technetium
  phosphate bone imaging in septic
    arthritis in children, 41
Tendinitis
  bicipital, biceps brachii head tenodesis
    in, 120
Tendon
  Achilles (see Achilles tendon)
  biceps, lesions, ultrasound of, 113
  flexor, repair in zone 2, mobilization
    after, 254
  peroneal, dislocation, fibular graft in,
    336
  tibial, transfer in spastic equinovarus,
    338
Tennis elbow
  interosseous nerve decompression in,
    131
Tenodesis
  of biceps brachii in bicipital tendinitis,
    120
  extensor carpi ulnaris and flexor carpi
    ulnaris, in unstable ulna, 259
Tenotomy
  adductor, in hallux valgus, 318
Tension
  -stress effect on tissue genesis and
    growth, 234, 235

Subject Index / 387

Thermography
 in lumbosacral radiculopathy, 293
Thigh
 compartment syndrome, acute, 87
Thoracic
 outlet syndrome and clavicular nonunion, 102
Thrombosis
 deep vein
  after elective knee surgery, 157
  fibrinolysis and spinal injury, 280
Thumb
 duplicated, ligamentous/periosteal flap in, 257
 -spica cast in carpal scaphoid fracture, 241
Tibia
 component
  in knee arthroplasty, failure mechanisms, 229
  of knee prosthesis, bone ingrowth into (in dog), 219
 defects in knee arthroplasty deformity, bone graft for, 225
 fracture (see Fracture, tibia)
 load distribution and knee component alignment, 222
 osteotomy (see Osteotomy, tibial)
 plateau bone stiffness in osteoarthritis, 226
 pseudarthrosis with infection, Ilizarov technique in, 84
 tubercle osteotomy during knee replacement, 223
 venous drainage after tibial osteotomy, 207
Tibial
 tendon transfer in spastic equinovarus, 338
Tissues
 genesis and growth, tension-stress effect on, 234, 235
 soft (see Soft tissue)
Titanium
 -alloy femoral head, osteolysis due to, in hip arthroplasty, 171
 hydroxyapatite, biologic response (in dog), 174
Transfusion
 intraoperative autologous
  in hip arthroplasty, revision total, 142
  in orthopedics, 142
Transplantation
 osteochondral allograft, articular cartilage fate after (in dog), 82
Trauma
 lower extremity (see Extremities, lower, trauma)

Triceps
 -dividing approach in humeral fracture open reduction during adolescence, 47
Trimalleolar
 fracture, results after posterior fragment fixation, 59
Trunk
 list and cross leg pain, 293
Tuberculosis
 spinal kyphosis in, arthrodesis for, 310
Tumors
 bone (see Bone tumors)
 extremities, soft tissue, perfusion with cytostatics in, 358
 foot, soft tissue, case review, 343

U

Ulcer
 abnormal foot pressures not causing, 342
Ulna
 fracture (see Fracture, ulna)
 synostosis after trauma, surgery results, 139
 unstable, extensor carpi ulnaris and flexor carpi ulnaris tenodesis in, 259
Ultrasonography (see Ultrasound)
Ultrasound
 in hip assessment in newborn, 1
 of Morton neuroma, 321
 in osteomyelitis, acute, 40
 of rotator cuff (see under Rotator cuff)
Ultraviolet
 radiation, shortwave, in operating rooms, 212
Urinary
 tract catheterization protocols after joint arthroplasty, 215

V

Valgus
 hallux (see Hallux valgus)
 hindfoot, spastic, Grice extra-articular subtalar arthrodesis in, 35
Vein
 deep, thrombosis (see Thrombosis, deep vein)
 tibial, drainage after tibial osteotomy, 207
Vertebra
 fracture (see Fracture, vertebra)
 metastases after radiotherapy, osteodensitometry of, 351

osteomyelitis, pyogenic, 294
Vessels
  complications in humeral supracondylar fracture in children, 46
  injuries about knee, 203

W

Wadsworth elbow
  failure, rheumatoid arthritis in, 132
Wagner
  method, modified, for limb lengthening, 38
Weight
  -bearing after ankle fracture repair, 337
Wiltse pedicle screw fixation
  results, 305

Wiring
  sublaminar, with Luque or Harrington rods in adult idiopathic scoliosis, 307
Wrist
  pain in gymnasts, 261
  rheumatoid
    arthroplasty with Swanson implant in, 246
    synovectomy in, results, 247

Z

Zielke
  instrumentation for spinal deformity in adults, 310
Zoetermeer Survey
  in osteoarthritis, 150

Author Index

A

Abels, R., 143
Aboulafia, A., 241
Adelsberg, S., 66
Adler, C.-P., 351
af Ekenstam, F., 253
Aglietti, P., 231
Ahlgren, O., 332
Ahovuo, J., 113
Akelman, E., 245
Åkerman, M., 363
Akeson, W., 193
Alaranta, H., 290
Albanese, S.A., 261
Albrecht, M.E., 193
Albus-Lutter, C.E., 358
Alcheck, D., 224
Alexander, A.H., 189
Alexander, H., 66, 335
Alexander, R.H., 101
Allan, D.B., 296
Allieu, Y., 247
Alsbjørn, B., 91
Alvarez, R., 30
Alvegård, T.A., 357
Amadio, P.C., 139, 242, 252
Aminoff, M.J., 293
An, K.N., 245
Anderson, I.F., 327
Anderson, J.J.B., 236
Andersson, C., 186
Andrews, J.R., 341
Angermann, P., 329
Aprahamian, C., 76
April, E.W., 104
Aristei, C., 350
Arsham, N.Z., 122
Asencio, G., 247
Askew, M.J., 13
Atkins, R.M., 53
Aufdermaur, M., 291
Awaya, G., 183

B

Bach, A.W., 68
Bach, L.A., 235
Bagliani, G.P., 38
Baker, C.L., 341
Ballas, S.K., 143
Bandyk, D.F., 76
Banta, J.V., 19
Bardi, I., 40
Bargar, W.L., 142, 163
Barloon, T.J., 346
Barnes, C.L., 70
Barrack, R., 119
Barrack, R.L., 189
Barrett, W.P., 124
Barron, J., 201
Bartal, E., 12

Bartolozzi, A.R., 116
Bassett, G.S., 9, 32
Bassett, L.W., 366
Bathon, G.H., 87
Bathon, H., 93
Bauer, H.C.F., 356
Beabout, J.W., 355, 362
Becker, D.A., 120
Beim, G.M., 169
Bell, A.L., 181
Bell, M.J., 54
Bell, R.H., 125
Bell, R.S., 158
Benckhuijsen, C., 358
Ben Hamida, H., 40
Benirschke, S.K., 62
Benson, D.R., 142
Benum, P., 337
Berg, M., 212
Berg, N.O., 357
Berg, V., 1
Bergman, B.R., 212
Bergmann, M., 227
Berquist, T.H., 242
Betts, R.P., 342
Bickerstaff, D.R., 54
Biden, E.N., 228
Bigliani, L.U., 104
Bircher, M., 296
Birnbaum, A., 123
Björkenheim, J.-M., 113
Black, K.P., 184
Black, L.E., 355
Blair, R.D.G., 123
Blick, S.S., 80
Bloem, J.L., 198
Blom, H., 145
Boero, S., 38
Bohlman, H.H., 273
Boivin, G., 247
Bollini, G., 11
Bolz, K.D., 337
Bone, L.B., 67
Bonfield, W., 166
Bonfiglioli, S., 17
Booth, R.E., Jr., 218
Boriani, S., 63
Borrie, M.J., 232
Bos, C.F.A., 198
Bosse, M.J., 73, 93
Böstman, O., 330
Botsford, D.J., 301
Botte, M.J., 137
Bottone, E.J., 214
Boulton, A.J.M., 342
Bourne, R.B., 226
Bouyala, J.M., 11
Bowen, M., 110
Bowman, B.E., 15
Bradley, J., 192
Bradley, W.G., Jr., 199
Bradway, J.K., 252
Bragdon, C., 179
Branch, H.M., 321
Brand, R.A., 181

Brandt, K.D., 193
Brandt, T.D., 114
Bray, T.J., 142, 332
Brazier, D., 327
Bredland, T., 1
Breen, T.F., 259
Brennen, M.D., 254
Brenner, B.C., 125
Brodsky, A.E., 303
Brody, M.C., 90
Broom, M.J., 19
Brotzman, T.T., 303
Brougham, D.I., 3
Broughton, N.S., 3
Brumback, R.J., 80, 87, 93
Brunner, R.G., 101
Bruschini, S., 27
Bryan, R.S., 217
Bucholz, R.W., 79
Bulstra, S., 315
Burgess, A.R., 80, 87, 93
Burk, D.L., Jr., 116
Burke, D.W., 179
Butler, D.L., 185
Butler, J.C., 306
Buzzi, R., 231
Bydder, G.M., 354
Byrick, R.J., 158

C

Callaghan, J.J., 153
Callihan, T., 369
Cammisa, F.P., Jr., 285
Campbell, A.J., 232
Candelora, P.D., 306
Capello, W.N., 163
Capra, S.E., 332
Caputo, R.J., 241
Cardone, B.W., 114
Carl, A., 310
Carlsson, Å., 160
Carlsson, Å.S., 214
Carlton, A., 79
Carnesale, P.G., 352
Carpenter, C.W., 261
Carrozzella, J.C., 243
Carter, B.C., 199
Carter, V., 241
Cats, A., 150
Cervellati, S., 17
Chabal, C., 90
Chan, G.P.Y., 57
Chang, J.C.W., 57
Chao, E.Y., 245
Chapman, M.W., 78, 138
Cheal, E.J., 348
Checcaglini, F., 350
Christian, E.P., 73
Christie, M.J., 147
Ciotti, M., 84
Clark, C.R., 156
Clark, R.N., 25

390 / Author Index

Clayton, M.L., 125
Clement, D.A., 46
Cofield, R.H., 120
Cohen, J.L., 306
Coldwell, D.M., 202
Cole, W.G., 3
Collin, J.P., 246
Collins, M.L., 143
Colville, J., 254
Colwell, C.W., Jr., 228
Compston, J.E., 155
Connolly, J.F., 102
Connolly, J.R., 361
Convery, F.R., 169, 193
Cook, A.J., 13
Cook, S.D., 174, 175
Cooney, W.P., 252
Cooney, W.P., III, 242, 245
Cooper, D.E., 161
Cooper, M.E., 235
Cooper, R.A., 327
Crichton, K.J., 327
Crider, R.J., Jr., 27
Crim, J.R., 366
Croucher, P., 155
Crowley, J.P., 143
Crump, J.M., 101
Cummings, S.R., 233
Curl, W.W., 341
Cushnaghan, J., 148

D

Dahners, L.E., 81
Dalinka, M.K., 115, 200
Daluga, D.J., 120
Dandy, D.J., 192
Daniels, J.D., 95
Dannucci, G.A., 82
Darden, B.V., 303
Dargouth, M., 40
Dave, P.K., 207
Davis, L.A., 5
Day, A., 207
DeHaven, K.E., 184, 185
Dehne, R., 102
DeLee, J.C., 161
Del Pizzo, W., 187
Dennis, D.A., 125
Dennis, J.W., 101
DePuy, J., 24
DeSmet, A.A., 196
DeVivo, M.J., 281
DeWaele, M.J., 189
Dieppe, P., 148
DiMartino, P.P., 305
Dines, D.M., 216
Di Paola, M.P., 296
Dobozi, W., 120
Dollahite, H.A., 352
Donati, N.L., 22
Dorfman, H.D., 364
Doyon, F., 211
Drennan, J.C., 24, 340

Drost, T.F., 72
Drouillard, P., 171
Drvaric, D.M., 35
Dubousset, J., 16
Duckworth, T., 53
Dunlap, J., 256

E

Eaton, B.H., 245
Eaton, R.G., 245
Eckardt, J.J., 366
Egund, N., 205, 318
Ehara, S., 294
Einola, S., 290
Eismont, F.J., 285
El Masri, W.S., 276
Emergy, S.F., 321
Endicott, M., 332
Engebretsen, L., 337
Engh, C.A., 177
Eskola, A., 112, 176
Essadam, H., 40
Esses, S.I., 301
Esterhai, J.L., 115, 200
Evrard, J., 211
Ewald, F.D., 222
Exner, G.U., 347

F

Fabry, G., 338
Failla, J.M., 139
Falck, B., 290
Fanø, N., 160
Faris, P.M., 215
Farran, K., 337
Favero, K.J., 266
Feiwell, E., 339
Fenlin, J.M., 116
Fenwick, J.R., 30
Ferlic, D.C., 125
Ferreira, E., 11
Ferron, S., 310
Feuchtgruber, G., 298
Figgie, H.E., III, 135, 136
Figgie, M.P., 135, 136
Find, P.R., 281
Finlay, J.B., 226
Finlayson, D., 296
Finsen, V., 337
Fischer, T.J., 70
Fisher, D.R., 196
Fitch, R.D., 15
Fitch, S., 369
Fitzgerald, R.H., 213
Flandry, F., 152
Flatow, E.L., 104
Fleming, B., 96
Flesher, S.A., 214
Flynn, J.C., 45
Formica, C., 38
Foster, B.K., 41

Fox, J.M., 187
France, E.P., 121
Frassica, D.A., 368
Frassica, F.J., 368
Freeman, B.L., III, 22
Freeman, M.A.R., 166
Frich, L.H., 126
Friedman, M.J., 187
Fritz, W., 298
Froimson, A.I., 122
Fronek, J., 110
Fruensgaard, S., 56
Frye, M.A., 282
Frykberg, E.R., 101
Furman, W.L., 369
Futami, T., 183

G

Galante, J.O., 219
Gallien, R., 33
Garg, A., 222
Garland, D.E., 85
Gebhart, E.M., 124
Gebuhr, P., 91
Geesink, R.G.T., 174
Gellman, H., 241
Gentz, C.F., 131
Gersten, L.M., 60
Gessert, G., 76
Gharbi, H.A., 40
Gibson, C.T., 128
Gilbert, P., 75
Gillquist, J., 167, 185, 186
Glashow, J.L., 200
Goetz, D.D., 156
Gold, R.H., 366
Goldberg, I., 103
Golenzer, H.J., 355
Good, C., 188
Good, L., 186
Goodman, S.B., 144
Goodnough, L.T., 143
Gördes, W., 298
Gordon, J.E., 138
Gorman, P.W., 70
Gorodischer, S., 36
Gould, N., 30
Goulet, J.A., 142
Goutallier, D., 208
Graeber, G.M., 153
Graif, M., 354
Granata, C., 17
Grant, T.H., 114
Grattan-Smith, T., 327
Green, B.A., 285
Green, S.A., 85
Greenberg, B., 216
Griffiths, H.J., 184
Grill, F., 39
Gudmundson, G.H., 133
Gupta, A., 276
Gustilo, R.B., 85

H

Haas, A.F., 341
Habibian, A., 118
Haddad, R.J., Jr., 174
Hagena, F.-W., 227
Hagstedt, B., 205
Haloua, J.P., 246
Hamberg, P., 185
Hammou, A., 40
Hannon, M.A., 89
Hansen, S.T., Jr., 62, 68, 324
Harcke, H.T., 32
Hardaker, W.T., 15
Harner, C.D., 121
Harris, W.H., 179
Hartleben, P.D., 146
Hasegawa, I., 170
Haughton, V.M., 287, 289
Haut, R.C., 190
Hawes, D.R., 346
Hawkins, R.J., 125
Hay, E.M., 342
Hayes, W.C., 348
Hedges, A.R., 157
Heeg, M., 42
Heim, U.F.A., 59
Helmig, P., 130
Hendricks, R.L., 303
Hensinger, R.N., 21
Herndon, W.A., 43
Herring, J.A., 16
Herrlin, K., 363
Hillsgrove, D.C., 81
Hipp, J.A., 348
Hirai, K., 170
Hirooka, A., 195
Hirvensalo, E., 330
Ho, K.-C., 287
Hoborn, J., 212
Hodapp, N., 351
Hoekstra, A.J., 231
Hoekstra, H.J., 231
Hoffer, M.M., 339
Hofmann, G.O., 227
Holbrook, J.L., 69
Holder, L.E., 250
Holm, C., 160
Holmes, R., 79
Homra, L., 147
Hootnick, D.R., 27
Hopper, J.L., 235
Horowitch, A., 305
Hovelius, L., 205
Hoyt, W.A., Jr., 13
Hresko, M.T., 44
Hsu, H.-P., 222
Hughston, J.C., 152
Huiskes, R., 181
Hungerford, D.S., 148, 210, 223
Hurme, M., 290
Hustu, H.O., 369
Huurman, W.W., 361

I

Iannotti, J.P., 115
Ichioka, Y., 170
Ichtertz, D.R., 248
Ikeda, T., 183
Ilizarov, G.A., 234, 235
Ilstrup, D., 164
Ilstrup, D.M., 213, 242
Inglis, A.E., 135, 136, 216
Insall, J.N., 216, 229, 231
Ishii, S., 162
Ivins, J.C., 355

J

Jacobs, M.A., 148, 210, 223
Jacobs, M.E., 181
Jacobsen, F.S., 300
Jacobson, K.E., 119
Jacobson, L., 90
Jacquemier, A., 11
Jakobsson, O.P., 253
Jallay, B., 125
Jalovaara, P., 131
Jarcho, M., 174
Järvinen, M., 290
Jasty, M., 179
Jelliffe, A.J., 354
Jenkins, N.H., 49
Jensen, J., 98
Jensen, P., 329
Jerums, G., 235
Johansen, K.H., 202
Johnell, O., 131
Johnson, K.A., 319
Johnson, K.D., 67
Johnsson, K.-E., 302
Jørgensen, J.P., 91
Josefsson, P.O., 131
Jupiter, J.B., 259

K

Kaelin, A.J., 359
Kaiser, A.D., 166
Kajino, A., 155
Kakkar, V.V., 157
Kalimo, H., 290
Kamisato, S., 183
Kan, S.H., 282
Kanis, J.A., 53
Kanno, T., 170
Karasick, D., 116
Kartus, P.L., 281
Kasper, C.K., 154
Kasser, J.R., 44, 47
Kattapuram, S.V., 294
Katz, R., 200
Kay, J.C., 158
Kay, J.F., 174
Kaye, R.A., 326

Kean, J.R., 25
Kearney, R.E., 72
Keating, E.M., 215
Keene, J.S., 196
Keeney, G.L., 362
Kellerhouse, L., 118
Kelly, M.A., 229
Kelman, G.J., 228
Kemp, W.R., 268
Kerr, D.R., 261
Kester, M.A., 175
Khalil, M.A., 303
Khouri, R.K., 70
Khuffash, B., 293
Khurana, J.S., 294
Kibsgaard, L., 337
Kimura, T., 195
Kinnard, P., 322
Kinnimonth, A.W.G., 57
Kirby, E.J., 343
Kitaoka, H.B., 13
Kjaersgaard-Andersen, P., 126, 130
Klaase, J.M., 358
Klasen, H.J., 42
Klassen, R.A., 319
Klee, M., 349
Kneisl, J.S., 189
Koeweiden, E.M.J., 181
Köhler, P., 92
Kongsholm, J., 55
Konttinen, Y.T., 176
Kooli, M., 40
Kortyna, R., 268
Koržinek, K., 209
Kosmin, M., 143
Kostuik, J.P., 301, 310
Kowalski, M.F., 128
Krackow, K.A., 210, 223
Kraemer, W.J., 226
Kreicbergs, A., 356
Kressel, H.Y., 115, 200
Kristiansen, B., 99
Kristiansen, T., 96
Krödel, A., 106
Kroon, B.B.R., 358
Kruskall, M.S., 143
Kumar, S.J., 32
Kurokawa, T., 127
Kurtz, A.B., 116
Kurtz, D.M., 152
Kyle, R.A., 368

L

Lagast, J., 338
Lakatos, R., 80, 87
Lang, A.E., 123
Lange, R.H., 74
Lanyon, L.E., 237
LaRossa, D., 216
Larsson, S., 332
Lash, E.G., 196

392 / Author Index

Latini, P., 350
Lavernia, C., 169
Lee, J.K., 94
Lee, M.S., 32
Legrain, Y., 258
Lehto, M., 290
Lenes, B.A., 143
Lenkinski, R.E., 115
Leu, H., 299
Leung, K.S., 57
Leung, P.C., 57
Levinsohn, E.M., 27, 261
Levy, D.W., 116
Lewis, M.M., 343
Lidgren, L., 132
Lieber, R.L., 31
Lind, T., 98
Lindén, U., 167
Linder, L., 221
Lindh, L., 92
Lindholm, R.V., 131
Lindholm, T.S., 176
Lindstrand, A., 205
Linscheid, R.L., 242, 245
Lippiello, L., 361
Lirette, R., 322
Lisi, D., 261
Ljung, P., 132
Loback, D., 151
Loeb, P.E., 148
Lombardi, A.V., Jr., 171
Lonstein, J.E., 307
Lotke, P.A., 216, 218
Loudon, J.R., 168
Lucas, G.L., 262
Luck, J.V., Jr., 154
Lund, G., 146
Lundberg, M., 185
Lussiez, HB., 247
Luxhöj, T., 205
Lynch, K.L., 287
Lyon, J.J., 153

M

McAllister, D., 162
McAndrew, M.P., 70
McBroom, R.J., 348
McCann, S.B., 152
McCarthy, J.A., 256
McCluskey, W.P., 9
McDonald, D.J., 213
MacEwen, G.D., 9, 359
McKay, J., 235
McKay, M., 241
McLellan, G.L., 101
McLeod, K.J., 237
Madsen, F., 133
Magone, J.B., 25
Mahnden, R.F., 43
Mäkelä, A., 330
Maletis, G.B., 86
Mallory, T.H., 171
Maloney, W.J., 179
Mann, D.C., 339
Mannarino, F., 204
Manske, P.R., 256, 257
Manz, P., 106
Marandola, M.S., 189
Maranzano, E., 350
Marini, M.L., 17
Markowitz, H.D., 189
Marquis, F., 33
Martin, D.F., 341
Martyak, T., 153
Mason, M.D., 200
Massardo, L., 148
Masson, E.A., 342
Mastragostino, S., 38
Masuda, T., 170
Matsen, F.A., III, 108
Matsuno, S., 170
Matsuno, T., 170
Matsuyama, T., 162
Mattila, M., 290
Mauldin, D., 31
Mauney, C., 201
Maurer, D.J., 85
Mayer, J.G., 177
Mayer, P.J., 300
Mayo, K.A., 62
Mazas, F., 211
Mellish, R.W.E., 155
Melton, L.J., III, 282
Melzer, C., 106
Mendes, D.G., 225
Menelaus, M.B., 3
Menezes, A.H., 156
Menitove, J.E., 143
Mennen, U., 61
Merkle, P.F., 321
Merkow, R.L., 85
Merlini, L., 17
Merritt, P.O., 75
Mestriner, L.A., 27
Meyers, M.H., 193
Micheli, L.J., 336
Miller, C.L., 116
Miller, J., 60
Millis, M., 47
Miranda, F., Jr., 27
Mirra, J.M., 366
Mitchell, D.G., 116
Mittlmeier, T., 227
Moinuddin, S.M., 352
Mok, D.W.H., 188
Möller, H., 160
Moore, J.R., 133
Moore, M.M., 70
Moore, T.J., 85, 201
Mora-Garcia, G., 9
Moran, M.C., 229
Morandi, M., 84
Moreland, M., 30
Morgan, D., 31
Morin, F., 33
Morley, T.R., 157
Moroz, T.K., 226
Morrey, B., 64
Morrey, B.F., 139, 164, 206, 217
Morris, E.W., 296
Mosca, V., 62
Mow, C.S., 135, 136
Muftić, O., 209
Mullen, J.B., 158
Munkacsi, I., 151
Munting, E., 258
Murdock, P.A., 243
Murphy, J.B., 216
Murphy, S.B., 369
Murray, D.W., 220
Myerson, M., 77
Mylle, J., 338
Myllynen, P., 280

N

Nagano, A., 127
Nagao, M., 162
Naidu, M.R.C., 271
Nakamura, S., 151
Nakamura, T., 151
Nakano, J.M., 35
Nawalkar, R.R., 225
Needleman, R.L., 325
Netz, P., 92
Nevitt, M.C., 233
Newman, C., 118
Nielsen, H.K.L., 231
Nielson, P.T., 145
Nielsen, S.-E., 145
Nielsen, S.L., 91
Nielson, O.S., 349
Nienhuis, R.L.F., 231
Nightingale, S., 270
Ninomiya S., 151
Noël, H., 258
Nokelainen, M., 280
Noone, R.B., 216
Norwood, L.A., 119
Nottebaert, M., 347
Noyes, F.R., 191
Nunn, D., 166

O

Obrant, K., 221
Ochiai, N., 127
Ocho, T., 195
O'Connor, D.O., 179
Odenbring, S., 205
Odensten, M., 186
Odor, J.M., 111
O'Fallon, W.M., 282
O'Hara, J.N., 10
Ohashi, Y., 230
Okada, Y., 183
Okinaga, S., 127
Older, M.W.J., 168

Olerud, C., 55
Olney, R.K., 293
Olson, D.W., 76
Ono, K., 195
Origo, C., 38
Osgood, J.C., 189
O'Sullivan, M.M., 155
Owaki, H., 195

P

Paavolainen, P., 113
Packard, D.S., Jr., 27
Padgett, D.E., 230
Paley, D., 96
Paljärvi, L., 290
Palmer, A.K., 261
Panizza, B.M., 350
Parker, R.D., 122
Parkinson, E., 235
Parsons, J.R., 335
Parziale, J.R., 95
Patt, P.G., 250
Pattee, G.A., 187
Paulos, L.E., 121
Pavlisko, F., 335
Pay, N.T., 12
Pazzaglia, U.E., 173
Pearson, R.L., 83
Pedrotti, L., 173
Peek, R.D., 305
Pennock, J.M., 354
Perrucci, E., 350
Perry, C.R., 83, 128
Petäjä, J., 280
Petasnick, J.P., 12
Peters, V.J., 321
Pfeiffer, C.M., 262
Phillips, W.A., 21
Pitman, M., 66
Poka, A., 80, 87, 93
Pollitzer, W.S., 236
Pool, R.R., 82
Pope, M., 96
Porter, R.W., 293
Post, M., 114
Pouliquen, J.C., 36
Poulsen, H.S., 349
Powell, J.N., 277
Pretterklieber, M., 317
Price, T.H., 143
Pringle, J., 354
Pritchard, D.J., 362
Proctor, D., 72
Purry, N.A., 89

R

Rae, T., 220
Rafii, M., 118
Raja Reddy, D., 271
Rajasekaran, S., 310

Ramamurthy, S., 161
Ramella, R., 173
Ranawat, C.S., 230
Rand, J.A., 217
Ranstam, J., 357
Rawlins, B., 224
Redd, R.A., 321
Reddy, P.K., 271
Redlund-Johnell, I., 302
Regan, W., 64
Reicher, M.A., 118
Reid, B., 123
Reilly, S., 296
Reinbold, W.-D., 351
Reinert, C.M., 93
Renshaw, T.S., 19
Resch, S., 318
Resnick, D., 118
Ricci, S., 350
Richard, L., 36
Richards, K., 47
Rifkin, M.D., 116, 321
Riggs, B.L., 282
Riis, J., 56
Riley, D., 123
Ritter, M.A., 215, 228
Robb, G., 73
Roberts, M.C., 115
Robie, D.B., 341
Robinson, H.J., Jr., 7, 146
Rockwood, C.A., Jr., 111
Rokkanen, P., 112, 280, 330
Rombouts, J.-J., 258
Rööser, B., 357, 363
Rorabeck, C.H., 226
Rørth, M., 349
Rosemurgy, A.S., 72
Rosenberg, A.G., 12
Rubin, C.T., 237
Rudnick, S., 143
Rullo, D.J., 189
Rushton, N., 220
Rutt, R.D., 281
Rydholm, A., 357, 363
Rydholm, U., 132

S

Sabetta, E., 63
Saetermo, R., 337
Salter, R.B., 196
Sammarco, G.J., 320
Sanders, D.P., 336
Sanders, R., 69
Sandre, J., 246
Sangeorzan, B.J., 62, 202, 324
Santavirta, S., 176
Sanzén, L., 214
Sarma, U.C., 207
Sarmiento, A., 60, 75
Sartoris, D.J., 118
Sastry Kolluri, V.R., 271
Sato, Y., 346

Savage, J.P., 41
Savini, R., 17
Savory, C.G., 153
Sawka, M.W., 60
Schachar, N., 162
Scheinberg, R., 67
Schenk, R.S., 335
Schernberg, F., 246
Schmitt, E.W., 35
Schneider, M., 200
Schoifet, S., 217
Schray, M.F., 368
Schreiber, A., 299, 347
Schreiman, J., 146
Schurman, D.J., 144
Schwartz, J.S., 115
Schwartz, J.T., Jr., 87, 177
Schwartz, R., 27
Scioli, M.W., 320
Scott, S., 86
Scott, W.N., 200
Scuderi, G.R., 229
Sculco, T.P., 224, 321
Seeman, E., 235
Segal, D., 60
Segal, L.S., 339
Seiler, J.G., III, 147
Sell, L., 76
Selvik, G., 295
Selzer, P.M., 12
Semkiw, L.B., 144
Senter, H.J., 268
Sether, L.A., 287, 289
Sexson, S., 204
Shankwiler, J.A., 60
Shannon, M.A., 7
Sharkey, N.A., 82
Shaw, W.W., 70
Shen, W.Y., 57
Shereff, M.J., 343
Shindell, R., 361
Shoji, H., 155
Shufflebarger, H., 16
Sickle, W.J., 346
Silberstein, L.E., 143
Silfversward, C., 356
Sim, F.H., 368
Singer, W.S., 12
Skipor, A.K., 219
Skrade, D.A., 325
Slätis, P., 112
Sledge, C.B., 124
Slooff, T.J.J.H., 181
Slowman-Kovacs, S.D., 193
Small, J.O., 254
Smith, D.K., 242, 245
Smith, K.J., 143
Sneppen, O., 126, 133
So, Y.T., 293
Sobol, P.A., 60
Sodre, H., 27
Søjbjerg, J.O., 126, 130, 133
Soudry, M., 225
Soundarapandian, S., 310
Sowa, D.T., 250

Spears, G.F., 232
Specchia, L., 63
Speck, G., 31
Spector, M., 222
Spencer, C.W., III, 305
Stabler, C.L., 191
Stauffer, A., 118
Steadman, C.A., 157
Stenström, A., 318
Sterkers, Y., 208
Stern, P.J., 243
Stern, S.H., 216
Stevenson, S., 82
Stiehl, J., 76
Stiehl, J.B., 325
Stockley, I., 342
Stover, S.L., 281
Straight, C.B., 121
Stringer, M.D., 157
Stulberg, B.N., 158
Sturesson, B., 295
Stürz, H., 106
Styf, J., 203
Suezawa, Y., 299
Sugiyama, H., 166
Sullivan, J.A., 43
Sumner, D.R., 219
Sundberg, S.B., 41
Svanström, A., 205
Sweetnam, D.R., 354
Swiontkowski, M.F., 69
Symeonides, P.P., 107

T

Tada, H., 183
Tallet, J.-M., 11
Tallroth, K., 176
Tanner, K.E., 166
Tatum, L., 352
Taylor, W.F., 355
Teitelbaum, G.P., 199
Templeton, A.C., 12
Terjesen, T., 1
Thomas, D.D., 203
Thomas, E.M., 157
Thomas, J.C., Jr., 305
Thomas, K.A., 174, 175
Thomas, S.C., 108
Thomas, W.H., 124
Thornhill, T.S., 124
Tigani, D., 63
Timmerman, L.A., 142
Tjörnstrand, B., 205
Torch, M.A., 25
Törmälä, P., 330
Torsney, B., 296
Transfeldt, E.E., 277
Tredwell, S.J., 5
Trevino, S., 30
Tucker, W.S., 277
Tulp, N.J.A., 136
Turi, M., 15

Turner, D.A., 12
Turner, T.M., 219

U

Udén, A., 295, 302
Unni, K.K., 355, 362
Urban, R.M., 219

V

Vainionpää, S., 112, 330
Valkenburg, H.A., 150
Vandenbroucke, J.P., 150
van Geel, A.N., 358
Vangsness, C.T., 60
van Horn, J.R., 181
Van Peteghem, P.K., 266
van Romunde, L.K.J., 150
van Saase, J.L.C.M., 150
Varnell, R.M., 202
Vastamäki, M., 112
Vaughn, B.K., 171
Vedi, S., 155
Velchik, M.G., 200
Veldhuizen, A.G., 231
Verhaar, J., 315
Vermeulen, A., 315
Verneret, C., 36
Veth, R.P.H., 231
Veves, A., 342
Vihtonen, K., 330
Vince, K.G., 229
Vines, F.S., 101
Visser, J.D., 42, 231
Vollmer-Larsen, B., 91
von Hochstetter, A.R., 347
Von Tress, M., 143

W

Waddell, G., 296
Waddell, J.P., 158, 277
Wadin, K., 253
Wagner, M., 289
Wahner, H.W., 282
Wakitani, S., 195
Walenkamp, G., 315
Walker, P.S., 222
Wallas, C.H., 143
Wanivenhaus, A., 317
Wannenmacher, M., 351
Warren, R.F., 110
Wasmer, G., 227
Watanabe, A.T., 199
Waters, P.M., 336
Watson, J.T., 158
Watson, R.C., 86
Watt, I., 148
Wedge, J.H., 151

Weigelt, J., 67
Weiland, A.J., 133, 250
Weiner, D.S., 13
Weinstein, J., 305
Weiss, A.B., 335
Weiss, A.-P.C., 133
Weiss, C.A., 114
Weiss, C.B., 185
Wendeberg, B., 131
Wenger, D.R., 31
Westholm, F., 217
Wetmore, R.S., 340
Wetzler, M., 60
Whitecloud, T.S., III, 306
Whitelaw, G.P., 60
Whitelaw, G.P., Jr., 189
Whiteside, L.A., 166
Widell, E.H., Jr., 305
Wieberdink, J., 358
Wiencek, R.G., 203
Willner, S., 302
Wills, R.P., 133
Wilson, R.F., 203
Wilson, W.J., 142
Wiltse, L.L., 305
Windsor, R.E., 216, 229, 231
Winia, W.P.C.A., 136
Winsberg, D.D., 122
Winter, R.B., 307
Wiss, D.A., 75
Wolff, A.M., 223
Wood, M.B., 137
Wood, V.E., 248
Woolson, S.T., 144
Wukich, D.K., 153
Wyatt, M.P., 228

Y

Yahiku, H., 248
Yao, L., 94
Yasui, N., 195
Yngve, D.A., 43
Yoneda, M., 195
Yoshino, S., 155
Yosipovitch, Z., 103
Young, I.R., 354
Younger, E.M., 78
Yu, S., 287, 289
Yuh, W.T.C., 346

Z

Zachar, C.K., 346
Zalenski, E.B., 179
Zatti, G., 173
Zdeblick, R.A., 273
Zembo, M.M., 84
Zillmer, D.A., 364
Zimmer, T.J., 319
Zissimos, A.G., 138
Zlatkin, M.B., 115, 118, 200